Rejuvenating Medical Education

Rejuvenating Medical Education:

Seeking Help from Homer

By

Robert Marshall and Alan Bleakley

Cambridge
Scholars
Publishing

Rejuvenating Medical Education: Seeking Help from Homer

By Robert Marshall and Alan Bleakley

This book first published 2017

Cambridge Scholars Publishing

Lady Stephenson Library, Newcastle upon Tyne, NE6 2PA, UK

British Library Cataloguing in Publication Data
A catalogue record for this book is available from the British Library

ISBN (10): 1-4438-9564-4
ISBN (13): 978-1-4438-9564-4

BY WAY OF AN APOLOGY

This book is tough on medicine and medical education, but for good reasons – our aim is to encourage constant quality improvement to provide best patient care and safety. We do not set out to engage in "doctor bashing" – we recognise that most doctors are doing an exceptional job under extreme pressures, the foremost being organisational pressure due to lack of resources. We applaud English NHS junior doctors for their widespread resistance in the face of this political situation.

Our concern in this book is another set of pressures on performance that can remain unconscious for many doctors but that need to be unearthed and addressed. These include lingering subscription to the historical and cultural legacy of metaphors and practices of "heroic medicine", no longer fit for a contemporary team-based, patient-centred approach. There are also persistent problems in medical education such as failing to address patient safety issues grounded in poor clinical teamwork. Finally, poor self-care persists amongst some doctors, and this is not good for them, their patients or their colleagues. Such doctors should be offered understanding and support. We hope that our audience, many of whom will be doctors, see our book as encouragement for improvement and not as finger-wagging from a moral high ground!

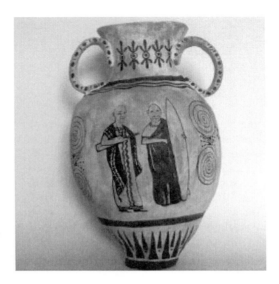

Figure a-1: The authors as Greek warriors and adventurers, Marshall of the cricket bat and Bleakley of the surfboard.

TABLE OF CONTENTS

Acknowledgements xi

Foreword xiii
Trish Greenhalgh

Introduction 1
"Thinking Otherwise" with Homer
    How we got into this epic mess
    Where does medical education fit in?
    The Homeric imagination
    Why Homer?
    Using Homer in new ways to refresh medical education

Chapter One 15
Heroes
    The mortality gene
    From two types of hero to the hero with a thousand faces
    Emergence of the anti-hero
    A new wave of heroes and heroines

Chapter Two 27
Heroes (Are Yesterday's Men)
    Heroes satisfy a need in those who are not heroes
    The heroic tradition celebrates masculinity
    Heroes are individuals
    Heroes must embrace mortality
    Heroes have a stand-in, or ritual substitute
    Heroes have a cult after death
    Heroes are flawed psychologically and morally
    Heroes are transgressive
    Heroes are charismatic as well as skilled
    The behaviour of heroes is excessive
    Today's heroes are not as good as yesterday's men
    Homeric heroes are generally of two types: force or craft
    Heroes are a bloody mess
    Conclusion

Chapter Three 48
Putting it Bluntly
    Can "thinking otherwise" with Homer really help doctors to improve
        communication?
    The Embassy
    Embassy scenarios in the clinic and on the ward

Chapter Four.. 63
Lost in Translation
    Receiving a history
    Translation matters
    Issues of translation in healthcare contexts
    Translating Homer
    Faithfulness to the original
    Identity
    Power
    Contingency
    Conclusion

Chapter Five 83
Sing, Muse
    Medical history as oral tradition
    Songs in hospital
    The medical history and genre
    The aesthetic worth of the case presentation
    The effect of oral traditions
    The creation of identity
    Telling the same story to different audiences
    The next crisis

Chapter Six 104
Compassion
    Communication: skill or style for life?
    Pity in Homer
    Communication, virtue, virtuosity
    A return to pity
    Conclusions: empathy ancient and modern

Chapter Seven... 122
Lyricism
    Waxing lyrical
    Medical genres
    The erosion of care
    The lyrical body in Homer
    Finding a place for the lyrical
    Coda

Chapter Eight... 135
Anger
Written in collaboration with Dr David Levine
    Medicine as epic
    Medicine as war
    Alternatives to medicine as war
    The return of the repressed
    Rageaholics and civility
    Transformations of anger
    Conclusion

Chapter Nine.. 155
Error
Written in collaboration with Jacob King, Elin Barham and Kirsten Leslie
    Homer and error
    Medicine and error: from individuals to systems
    Errancy and reparation
    Doctors too are wounded by their errors
    Conclusion

Chapter Ten 177
Whistleblowing
Written from an original idea by, and in collaboration with,
Victoria Rodulson
    Dilemmas of "speaking out"
    Whistleblowing and virtue ethics
    Whistleblowing in the flesh
    Speaking out against social injustice
    Anonymity or open confrontation?
    Speaking truth to power
    Conclusion

Chapter Eleven 193
Abuse
    Encounter with a surgeon
    Ritual humiliation in medicine
    Can Homer help?
    Abuse in Homer
    "Honour-shame" and "Guilt" cultures
    Aidos
    Conclusions and solutions

Chapter Twelve 211
Bone Tired
    Bone tired and ready for sleep
    Durational misperformance
    Embracing Hypnos through a new medicine

Chapter Thirteen 224
Resilience
    Medicine's "Achilles' Heel"
    Definitions
    What quality do we need?
    Grit
    "Thinking otherwise" about resilience and grit through Homer
    Bouncing up, not bouncing back
    Moving forward

Appendix: Synopses 245
    The *Iliad*
    The *Odyssey*

Bibliography 267

Index 300

ACKNOWLEDGEMENTS

Robert Marshall dedicates this book to his wife Annie, with love and thanks.

Alan Bleakley would like to acknowledge the loving support of his wife Sue and his family, who recognise that writing can turn you by turns into recluse, grump, and unsavoury beast, according to current theme and topic. This is amplified in the case of Homeric epic, where every twist and turn is lived out psychologically and metaphorically, if not literally. Homer has made me bone tired in the best possible way.

The authors have benefitted enormously from conversations with Professor Helen King (Open University), Dr Elton Barker (Open University), and Dr Katherine Harloe (University of Reading).

We are grateful to the following journals, in which earlier versions of some of these chapters appeared: *Medical Humanities* (*BMJ* group), *Performance Research*, and *The Review of Communication*.

Our students at Peninsula Medical School (latterly Peninsula College of Medicine and Dentistry), Universities of Exeter and Plymouth, and then the University of Exeter Medical School and Plymouth University School of Medicine and Dentistry, have afforded inspiration and hope for the future of medicine, medical education and the medical humanities. We are particularly grateful to those medical students who made up our first two cohorts for the 4th year Special Study Unit "Homer and Communication in Medicine".

Special thanks go out to Dr David Levine, Victoria Rodulson, Jacob King, Elin Barham and Kirsten Leslie, who helped with some of the research and writing in three chapters.

Trish Greenhalgh, Professor of Primary Care Health Sciences at the Nuffield Department of Primary Care Health Sciences, University of Oxford, has been very generous in her support of our Homer and medicine project, and kindly agreed to write a Foreword to this book.

Alice Oswald, who read Classics at Oxford and has subsequently become one of the UK's leading poets, generously gave feedback on parts of this book.

Finally, we encourage all readers to keep copies of the *Iliad* and the *Odyssey* at the bedside. You never know when you might need them. They are our desert island books.

Authors' Notes

Translations of the *Iliad* and *Odyssey* are by Robert Marshall, except where stated otherwise. Line numbers for the epics refer to the Oxford University Press editions in the bibliography.

The names of Homer's characters and places, when rendered into English, can be a contentious issue. We have used names that will be familiar to most readers or that are currently widely accepted.

Synopses of the *Iliad* and *Odyssey* are given as an appendix, and readers unfamiliar with Homer may like to start there. We usually repeat those events in the epics that are the subject of each chapter, for the convenience of readers not intimate with them.

FOREWORD

PROFESSOR TRISHA GREENHALGH

In a book chapter called *The Silent Crisis*, philosopher Martha Nussbaum (2010) announces that "We are in the midst of a crisis of massive proportions and grave global significance".[1] Across the Western world – and indeed, much of the non-Western world too – we have abandoned the teaching of the humanities ("useless frills") in favour of a narrow focus on what are commonly known as the STEMM subjects (science, technology, engineering, mathematics and medicine).

The result of this shift, suggests Nussbaum, is not merely that generations of citizens are emerging who are unable to engage at a sophisticated level with literature and the arts. The problem is much more sinister: such citizens (to a greater or lesser extent) lack moral imagination and are unable to make judgements about what is right and reasonable:

> Thirsty for national profit, nations, and their systems of education, are heedlessly discarding skills that are needed to keep democracies alive. If this trend continues, nations all over the world will soon be producing generations of useful machines, rather than complete citizens who can think for themselves, criticize tradition, and understand the significance of another person's sufferings and achievements. The future of the world's democracies hangs in the balance (Nussbaum 2010, p.2).

The humanities, she argues, teach us to reflect, to consider different framings of an issue, to deliberate and to place ourselves imaginatively in the position of others. We gain these skills and qualities most especially through the study of stories as we are drawn into different real or imaginary settings and follow characters who encounter, and try to resolve, different kinds of trouble. We learn that despite the open-ended nature of story, literature – and indeed life itself – follows a small number of basic plots (quest, comedy, tragedy and so on) because humans interact in ways that are both totally unique and highly patterned. Through stories, we learn that the world is not fair; that situations are ambiguous; that no text is self-interpreting; that men and women are not born equal in terms of either their material circumstances or the character traits they can bring to bear on those circumstances; that hopes and dreams and traditions are important; and that all choices have moral significance and unintended consequences.

In this book, Robert Marshall and Alan Bleakley offer a detailed worked example of how one classic contribution to the humanities – perhaps the greatest adventure-and-homecoming epic in the whole of literature – could inform and enrich the teaching of a subject which, perhaps more than any other in recent years, has fallen prey to the inexorable march of scientific reductionism, abstraction and standardisation with a concomitant devaluing of perspectives that are viewed as subjective, unquantified and relativistic.

The assumption underpinning this shift is that *through* reductionism (pursuing scientific "truth" through bounded rationality and ever-smaller units of analysis), abstraction (distilling a generalisable and analytically neat "essence" from our untidy, idiosyncratic and emotionally-charged real-world experiences, and then exploring and manipulating these essences as if they were reality) and standardisation (establishing a single "correct" and parsimonious way of doing everything, monitoring performance closely against that standard and driving "quality improvement" with reference to it), we will achieve with ever-greater efficiency the time-honoured goals of the medical profession: to heal the sick, to alleviate suffering, to comfort and console, and to support the patient in living well with illness.

This flawed line of reasoning runs increasingly through every medical specialty and also, troublingly, through the generalist fields of family medicine and geriatric medicine. Take heart failure, for example. Randomised controlled trials, accumulated over three decades, have informed a weighty collection of "evidence-based" clinical practice guidelines. According to these, patients should be prescribed the maximum tolerated dose of three different classes of drug (a practice known as "up-titration"), be monitored using an agreed set of biomarkers (such as body weight, blood pressure, blood oxygen level, atrial naturietic peptide and – using novel implantable technologies – variables like pulmonary artery pressure) and given structured education with a view to them learning to adjust the day-to-day dose of their own medication without the need for clinical intervention ("self-management"). All this is directed at a set of predefined outcome measures: improved left ventricular ejection fraction, longer survival, fewer hospital admissions and increased self-efficacy scores (allegedly, a measure of "empowerment").

Any practitioner's (or clinical team's) management of heart failure can be assessed in terms of performance against quantified targets derived from evidence-based guidelines. What proportion of the denominator population is on the maximum recommended dose of ACE inhibitors, beta-blockers etc (high is good)? What proportion of this denominator population has had a hospital admission in the last year (low is good)? What proportion is self-managing in response to changes in their biomarkers (high is good)? Thus, the rationalist pursuit of defined targets becomes the dominant logic in heart failure management at both an individual and a system level.

Where in this model of heart failure management is the uniqueness of the individual patient? Where are surprise, ambiguity, paradox and uncertainty? Where are suffering, despair, compassion and sensibility? Where are deference, trust, confidence and commitment? Where is the unfolding story of a person-in-context – and where is the witness to this story? Where are the symbolic meanings and moral implications of technologies and practices? Above all, where in the evidence-based algorithm are the unique, case-based judgements that engage with these human, interpersonal and societal dimensions of illness?

Of course, evidence-based guidelines are not inherently inhumane, and their judicious use can be, and often is, a key component of humanistic care rather than its antithesis. But this best-of-both-worlds scenario will happen only if (and to the extent that) both these dimensions of professional practice (and with them, professionals as flawed heroes with characters and virtues) are valued and nurtured. As Martha Feldman (2000) has pointed out, "Routines are performed by people who think and feel and care. Their reactions are situated in institutional, organizational and personal contexts. Their actions are motivated by will and intention."[2] A protocol cannot be meaningfully studied in isolation from the person who follows it (or who chooses not to follow it, or finds themselves unable to follow it) in a particular setting.

The focus of this book is what happens when rational science and the managerial efficiency of healthcare systems is pursued *at the expense* of attention to what it means to be human. It is an attempt, through close analysis of a story (and what a story!) to reclaim such things as "community, the human spirit, manners, character, ethical conduct and learning" (see introduction) in the medical curriculum. It uses the adventure-and-homecoming literary genre to press home the point that travel – both literal and metaphorical – broadens the mind, develops professional virtues and nurtures the moral imagination.

Like many doctors, I have read the detailed and systematic public inquiries that were conducted into "system failures" such as Alder Hey, Bristol and Mid-Staffordshire, hoping to glean transferable lessons on how to prevent such failures ever occurring again. Marshall and Bleakley offer us a different lens on such tragedies: there are no fixes – but by studying the emplotted fortunes of heroes, villains and victims in such systems, we will enrich our understanding of healthcare systems in general and how to improve them.

For example, on page 159, they say, "The mid-Staffordshire Hospital scandal provided a case study for widespread error and neglect due to poor management, lack of resources, and habitual negligence amongst care staff where ethical concerns were sidelined by subscription to crude managerialism". Notwithstanding these fundamental system flaws, a "Homeric" analysis of the events at Mid-Staffs highlights the heroic efforts of individual staff members and illustrates how honesty, courage, kindness, humility and diligence shone through even in a culture that did *not* value or nurture these virtues, while also illustrating how vices like pride, vengeance and cruelty were allowed to flourish.

Virtues cannot be protocolised, nor can vices be over-ridden by leaving them out of the algorithm. As Martha Nussbaum (2010) so eloquently explained in *Not for Profit*, we hone our understanding of virtue ethics through close reading of stories as well as through a more general engagement with the arts.

I enjoyed revisiting the *Iliad* and the *Odyssey* (two books forgotten since school), though I did not find this book an easy read. Those who would take the advice of Marshall and Bleakley and use Homer (or indeed, other classic narrative texts) to enrich a flagging medical education system will have their work cut out to convert his central message into the kinds of learning objectives and assessable competences that pervade the contemporary curriculum. But if Nussbaum is right, undertaking precisely that task is not merely desirable but essential and urgent.

Notes

1. Nussbaum, M. "The Silent Crisis". Chapter 1 in: *Not for Profit: Why Democracy Needs the Humanities*. Princeton University Press, 2010.
http://press.princeton.edu/chapters/s9112.pdf
2. Feldman, M.S. "Organizational routines as a source of continuous change." *Organization Sci* 11 (2000): 611-29.

Trisha Greenhalgh is Professor of Primary Care Health Sciences at the Nuffield Department of Primary Care Health Sciences, Medical Sciences Division, University of Oxford. She is an internationally recognised academic in primary health care and a practicing GP.

INTRODUCTION

"THINKING OTHERWISE" WITH HOMER

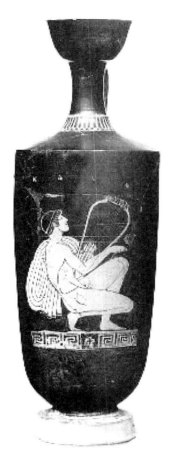

Figure b-1: "Sing, Muse"

How we got into this epic mess

Over a decade ago one of us (AB) suggested to the other (RM) that he should revisit his undergraduate classical studies and think what might inform the teaching and learning of medicine. This was also in the context of the exciting development of a new and innovative medical school – Peninsula – in which both of us were involved. Those classical studies began as a four years' undergraduate course at Oxford, studying *Literae Humaniores* – "More Humane Letters", as this course is known there. More humane than what is unstated, but presumably than any other possible course of study. Humanity, at any rate, seemed a good place to look for a connection between classics and medicine.

The return visit to the classics was primarily to Homer's *Iliad*. Progress was initially very slow, with frequent recourse to a Greek lexicon kept from Oxford for over 30 years (Liddell and Scott's lexicon; Liddell the father of the Alice who fell down the rabbit hole). Gradually, I (RM) could read the Greek more fluently, and it became one of the day's highlights to get home and immerse myself in the rhythm of Homeric epic poetry. It was a profoundly moving experience.

My (AB's) route into classics was quite different and profoundly unscholarly, but nevertheless passionate and had been on the boil for around 25 years. After studying zoology and psychology, and prior to a career in medical education, I had trained as a psychotherapist within a post-Jungian, Archetypal Psychology tradition primarily based on the work of James Hillman. My DPhil from the University of Sussex too was in the same field. Central to the architecture of this approach to psychology is the use of classical myth and poetic structures. I had soaked myself in reading such myth in translation, constantly returning to Homer.

Our reading of and around Homer, brought alive through subsequent conversation, made it natural and inevitable that we would bring the content of his work,[1] and his style or poetic sensibility, to bear on the study, research and practice of medical education. We found immediately that "thinking with Homer" bore fruit – a "thinking otherwise" about largely habitual approaches to medicine and medical education. Within the context of a nascent but developing medical humanities culture, we took a leap and started to write collaboratively about key topics in medicine and medical education that could be re-visioned through the lens of key Homeric characters and scenes.

In analysing such scenes and characters from the *Iliad* and *Odyssey* we asked readers in a series of articles to re-think, for example, what is a "communication skill" and what we mean by "empathy"; in what sense medical practice is formulaic, like a Homeric "song"; what is lyrical about medical practice; how doctors function as translators of the patient's story; and how uninvited anger, bullying and violence appear all too frequently in hospitals and clinics while, paradoxically, medicine still clings to its guiding martial metaphor ("medicine as war"). We used "thinking with Homer" as medium and metaphor for questioning the habitual in contemporary healthcare practice. Homer provided the grit, and we hopefully made some pearls in terms of both insights into, and practice change suggestions for, certain habits – rusted and rutted - crying out for attention, and leading to potential improvements in patient care and safety.

Often, those who reviewed our work asked "Why Homer?" Our answer is the text of this book, but the question has also been answered over and over by others writing about Homer, especially in the modern age.

Paul Cartledge (2002, pp.1-7), for example, starts his account of *The Greeks* with an address by President George Bush to the United Nations in 1991 concerning the violent ethnic division of Yugoslavia and the collapse of the Soviet Union. Caroline Alexander (2009, p.xi) says early in her book that: "Today, headlines from across the world keep Homer close by". One of those headlines was of the bodies of U.S. Rangers dragged behind their killers' jeeps, just as Achilles dragged the dead Hector behind his chariot. Barker and Christensen (2013, pp.1-2) begin their book by showing how Homer is not highbrow, permeating popular culture in its language, product branding, literature and film. Jonathan Shay (1994, 2002) enriches modern understanding by going directly to Homer to shed light on the trauma inflicted on those who fought in the Vietnam War, for example, showing how difficult it is for combat veterans to simply slip back into the skins of civilian identities. Adam Nicolson (2015, pp.1-7) perhaps gives the best personal answer to the question "Why Homer?", describing the effect of his first adult reading after surviving a storm at sea: "Here was a form of consciousness that understood fallibility and self-indulgence and vanity, and despite that knowledge didn't surrender hope of nobility and integrity and doing the right thing."

Medical education is generally interpreted, inside and outside medicine, as the teaching of medicine to undergraduates. It is much more. Graduation creates one of the unnatural and unhelpful barriers in medical education - between undergraduate and postgraduate education; the other is between postgraduate training and education for "junior" doctors, and their appointment to consultant status within hospital medicine or as qualified general practitioners, conferring the status of "expert". We believe that doctors learn, and want to learn, from the first day of medical school until they stop practising medicine and probably beyond. This book is then

written with that large group of learners and teachers in mind. It is not
intended purely as an academic study, although we provide the necessary
academic apparatus, but to change medical practice. We write this book
for the benefit of doctors in particular, who would never dream of turning
to Homer faced with an abusive colleague, a dysfunctional health system,
or ongoing disaffection and fear of burnout. A classical education used to
be regarded as essential for the study of medicine. Perhaps it still is, but, in
a postmodern, now "post-truth", age, perhaps it needs to be presented in a
way that intrigues as well as informs.

We hope that this book is of interest beyond that group, however.
Classicists have always been interested in modern and innovative, even
unusual, reception of their areas of study. We have had helpful discussions
with some of them and outcomes are woven in to our book. For others, our
level of classical expertise has been suspect and we have been asked: "who
is this book for? If it is for classics scholars, are we not a little
presumptuous, and if it is for doctors and healthcare professionals
interested in education, isn't the Homer bit simply ostentatious?" One can
only hope that a little learning has seeped in over several decades of study
through our collective interest, and besides, much of what we write about
is actually pedagogy, common to all disciplines.

There is a fourth potential cohort of readers beyond the medical,
classics and education communities. The issues we discuss are, most of
them, relevant to everyone – how we speak to each other, and how we
speak to the powerful; issues of empathy and compassion; whistleblowing;
abuse; exhaustion in the workplace; developing the resilience to cope with
work and the world outside. We completed this book at the beginning of
2017, with the new President of the United States issuing a raft of
executive orders that will have a profound effect throughout the world, and
which disgust many. Homer's *Iliad* starts with a prophet scared to resist an
oafish king – or speak truth to power - the latter's petulant anger when the
truth is told, and his unreasonable reaction and subsequent demands,
leading to a large toll of deaths for his people. We see parallels in all
autocracies (including the traditional autocracies of medicine), where
potential democracy is masked or distorted.

But for any non-specialist reader we would hope that this book serves
as an introduction to the pleasures of reading Homer for the first time, and
moving on to read the many generalist books about these two great epics.
We hope that, like Adam Nicolson (2015, p.6), they may ask: "Why has
no one told me about this before?"[2]

Where does medical education fit in?

Junior doctors are now entering a far different world from their predecessors – there is greater emphasis upon prevention rather than cure; doctors work in collaborative, interprofessional teams; patients' hospital stays have been radically shortened, compromising continuity; patient encounters occur more in the community than in hospitals, yet most medical education for students and juniors occurs on the wards; women will soon constitute the majority of the medical workforce; and junior doctors in England have become overtly politicised, recently striking over conditions of work (unthinkable in previous generations); the patterns of presenting symptoms are changing as mental illness becomes more dominant; and finally, there is a realisation that iatrogenic illness, caused by medical intervention itself, is a major problem, resulting in greater patient safety awareness and action.

As passionate medical educators, we actively resist medical education's habitual forms, established for over a century since the major overhaul resulting from Abraham Flexner's famous 1910 Carnegie Report (on medical education in North America) (Flexner 1910) and 1923 Report on Medical Education in Europe (Flexner and Pritchett 1923). We will continue to agitate for necessary and radical reform, drawing from sources that have been ignored in the past. Despite innovative responses to the established Flexnerian orthodoxy from a new Carnegie Report (Cooke et al 2011) demanding overhaul of North American medical education, and a parallel response from UK medical educators (Bleakley et al 2011), necessary innovation is frustratingly slow. We believe that medicine's historical legacies must be challenged, transforming hierarchy into democracy (to include patient participation), with male domination and "heroic" medicine morphing into a more feminine, collaborative care.

As we look forward to such radical change, we argue in this book that transformation in medical education can be informed by looking back, a long way back – to ancient Greece. In Homer's *Iliad* and *Odyssey* we find a wealth of learning and inspiration to inform and shape current medical education. This connection, perhaps surprising at first sight, has shaped this book.

The Homeric imagination

Surprised at how difficult it still is to introduce the arts and humanities into the medicine curriculum (even to explore the intrinsic beauty of science), we have worked hard over the years to show how the medical humanities can benefit medical education. An important part of that process for us has been a return to Homer to illuminate and "think otherwise" about communication and professionalism in 21st century medical practice. If "Homer" (recognising the issue of authorship) were here today, he would perhaps say "only over my dead body should people ignore the legacy of my texts" - the epics of the *Iliad* and the *Odyssey*. Helene Foley (2001) describes "the Homeric imagination" as "an evolving historical reality". In other words, Homer never dates, but is a constant source of inspiration.

At the beginning of Homer's *Odyssey*, we are introduced to the "song" of Odysseus who "wandered off far and wide ... he saw the cities of many peoples and knew their mind". What a liberal idea from a book written down in the eighth century BCE from a much older oral tradition – that a person should experience "otherness" so that he or she can think differently, or in our term, "think otherwise". Odysseus may already have been open-minded, but exposure to otherness through travel confirms his identity, or complex multiple identities, as "versatile": "the man of many twists and turns", and "the one who could change in many different ways who he was".

Odysseus' epithets include *polymetis* (of many counsels), *polymechanos* (resourceful, inventive), and *polytropos* (turned every way). Nicolson (2015) refers to him as the "poly" man. Where Odysseus gets to know different ways of thinking through exposure to otherness, so he gets to know how to think differently in himself, or acquire what we now call "critical reflexivity" (Bleakley 1999). In short, he is ultimately adaptive, sensitive to what he can learn from new, often challenging, encounters and new frameworks for thinking and responding. Such education into cultural relativism and psychological reflexivity seems a modern notion, but Homer prefigures this outlook. We suggest that education into tolerance of ambiguity, grounded in learning from the "other", is central to a successful medical education that properly addresses communication, professionalism, ethics, and the expression of considerate, humane values.

Carol Dougherty (2001) suggests that travel educated Odysseus into "mind leaps": "As when the mind leaps, the mind of a man who has travelled across/ much territory and thinks with shrewd intelligence, 'If only I were/ there or there' and wishes many things ..." (*Iliad* Book 15). The earliest use of the term *theoria*, says Dougherty (2001, p.4), "designates the process of traveling". Theory is then a direct result of seeking active exposure to the "other" or "travelling" to seek encounters with the other. We can read "travel" both literally and as a metaphor for scanning possibilities rather than dogmatically jumping to conclusions.

For medical students and doctors, travel is common: between ideas and competing theories; in traversing differential diagnoses; between clinical sites and hospital-based placements as an apprentice, and finally across specialties to arrive at a career focus. The object of such "travel" is to encounter the widest variety of views, patients and clinical contexts early in a career to build a flexible yet subtle medical imagination. This project deserves the best and most refined support from medical educators.

In a key talk from 2005, Professor Lee Shulman, then President of the Carnegie Foundation for the Advancement of Teaching, describes the orthodoxy of the "signature pedagogy" for medical education (Shulman 2005). Strip away the pre-clinical years of classroom-based anatomy and science learning, and the main focus for a medical education is hospital-based bedside teaching, as a traditional apprenticeship. Despite, as noted above, the fact that many more patient presentations (largely chronic care) occur in General Practice than in hospitals, and that patients now spend far fewer days in hospital than they used to - making continuity of study difficult for medical students and junior doctors - nevertheless, the rituals concerned with acute care bedside teaching remain high profile, and not much has changed in this respect since Shulman's account a decade ago.

Shulman describes the signature pedagogy of medical education as a "formation of character". He goes on to say that when, in 2005, he attended a team at a major medical school hospital to observe clinical rounds, this was something he had not done since "about 1972" when he was intimately involved in medical education. In the intervening 33 years, he noted that not much had changed about the signature pedagogy except that patients - the curriculum content - did not stay in hospital as long and so continuity was disrupted. Shulman notes an extraordinary continuity elsewhere: "what was fascinating is the routinisation, almost to the point of ritual, of clinical rounds". What he did not say was that routinisation might be a symptom of stale practice, or lack of innovation in response to the rapidly changing context of healthcare.

"Ritual", from the Latin *ritualis*, means not only "custom", but also "correct performance". This is a scripted performance, an habitual and strongly socialised way of behaving, that is the primary focus of Homer's epics, based around two main principles: the glorification/ honouring of heroes, and the primacy of hospitality. The latter is, in turn, based upon two sub-principles – the solidarity of family and the conditional welcoming of strangers into a household. We say 'conditional' because ancient Greek hospitality is a formalised "gift exchange" process. While I am taken into your home as a stranger, bathed, fed and entertained, the expectation is that I will do the same for you.

These two principles – the honouring of heroes and hospitality - their sub-principles, and the rituals associated with them, have also historically defined modern medicine. Doctors are potentially heroes and the hospital is the site of hospitality. Until recently, junior doctors were called "house officers" or "housemen" and slept on site at the hospital. Doctors are the head of the family of healthcare teams and patients are offered conditional welcome and respite under care. The "condition" contemporary societies place on the availability of healthcare is that it can be resourced, somehow, either through taxes (such as a national health system "free" at point of service), or through health insurance.

In Homeric epic, ritual is tied with reciprocity (to which hospitality is central (Reece 1993)), where, as long as the rules of hospitality are followed, tragedy is avoided. In the tragic genre, however, the order of reciprocity is disrupted as family members feud and outsiders are treated with suspicion and judged (Seaford 1995). Where the curve of the epic narrative includes the hero's homecoming or a celebration of the death of the hero doomed by fate (Allums 1992), the tragic narrative concludes in a painful mess, leaving scars and stains (Hall 2010).

These archetypal frameworks are important for understanding medicine because it is the only profession in which tragedy (illness, suffering and death) provides its *raison d'être,* but the profession itself must not be engulfed by that tragedy. Rather, it must maintain its epic structure of ritual and reciprocity/ hospitality to not allow itself, as a social institution, to be engulfed by the very tragedy that it treats. As doctors and medical managers alike will tell you, medicine cannot afford to suffer. Yet it does, and it is this suffering of medicine that is the subject of this book and upon which a return to Homer can offer some illumination. We need to stress that we celebrate the achievements of medicine and the daily hard work of doctors and healthcare staff, but it is medical culture's symptoms that intrigue us and that we address in this book from an unusual angle.

Again, medicine is, historically, grounded in the epic genre with the making and honouring of heroes at its core (see chapters one and two), in order to "fight" (medicine is replete with martial metaphors) disease, where disease and suffering advertise the genre of tragedy. The paradox of this position is that the harder medicine fights off the tragic, the more this genre comes to inhabit medical culture and the lives of doctors as a return of the repressed. The tragic returns in distorted or unexpected forms, the most obvious being iatrogenesis – where medicine itself unintentionally harms patients, for example through hospital-based infections, or medical error such as misdiagnosis, dysfunctional teamwork or prescribing error (see chapter nine). As medicine treats symptoms, so it displays its own symptoms. And these must be treated.

This historically formed state of medicine is changing rapidly and this book responds directly to such flux. We are now recognising the limits of epic medicine and learning how to accept elements of tragedy within medical practice that might be suitably addressed, such as compassion fatigue (see chapter six), anger and abuse (see chapters eight and eleven), and burnout (see chapters twelve and thirteen). Homer, again, provides a suitable guide to "thinking otherwise" about these encompassing issues in medicine and how we might address them through reformulating medical education.

Medicine too is formed by comic and lyrical genres (see chapter seven), although we recognise that humour in medical circles is often "black" and at patients' expense (Piemonte 2015), and a lyrical medicine has found it difficult to gain a foothold in the last five hundred years of martial, heroic medicine in the Metropolitan West.

It is in ritual as routinisation that medical students learn how to position themselves within the medical hierarchy, to make diagnoses and check these with superiors, to arrange treatments, and to record information. This all seems very mechanical. Indeed, the habitual or routinisation part is mechanical and previously scripted (as historical legacy, made so clear by Shulman's remarks above). We find its parallel in the structure of Homer's poems as sets of songs originally learned by heart and performed for an audience (see chapter 5). The performance of medicine in part mirrors this routinisation. However, within this inflexible structure - a means of memorising facts - is a field full of opportunity for interpretation. Medical work is never as routine as Shulman's signature pedagogy suggests. It is full of surprise, ambiguity and the unexpected. Learners must be able to think on their feet, adapt and be creative according to new context – in particular communicating with such a wide variety of patients, whose symptom presentations and narratives are necessarily unique.

While the structure of Homer's poems as we read them from the page in modern translations is largely formalised, what the characters and stories do to us as audience is open-ended and an invitation to invention. Reception of Homer invites thinking imaginatively, and Homer's tales, while again patterned or formulaic, invite open and inventive reception. As Carol Dougherty (2001) argues, we must read Homer ethnographically, as travellers meeting "otherness" that serves to re-formulate our values and practices. In this ethnographic work, we merely repeat what Homer has taught us through the figure of Odysseus – that we learn by comparing and contrasting our values and actions with those of others.

Why Homer?

This book is then an invitation to think otherwise about medicine, medical education and the identities of doctors using Homer's *Iliad* and *Odyssey* as the media. While doctors undertake a well-documented socialisation into a uniform character, the reality of their work is that they are constantly adapting to a liquid clinical context through meeting a variety of patients. Hence, we ask the reader to think otherwise particularly about the identities of doctors exposed simultaneously to a conformist medical culture and a range of otherness in the procession of patients throughout their careers.

In spite of its grounding in Bronze Age events, filtered through an Iron Age song and oral poetry tradition, Homer's work offers a foundational text for understanding and re-imagining such multiplicity in the human condition. Homer's work is not just a convenient medium. Rather, it is an Ur-text about community, the human spirit, manners, character, ethical conduct and learning. From reading Homer, we have learned that medical culture and medical education can be re-visioned thoroughly, providing radical insights. Of course this might be achieved drawing on the Bible, the Vedas, Virgil, Dante, Chaucer, Milton, Shakespeare, Cervantes, Chekhov, Tolstoy, or Proust for example, but Homer resonates with medicine for two particular reasons.

First, from the doctor's point of view, for at least 500 years, the central metaphor for medical intervention has been "medicine as war". However much this continues to stigmatise patients, doctors continue to "wage war" on cancers and "mobilise forces" against invading armies of bugs. The *Iliad* is the West's primary war text, focused on forty or so days in a decade long conflict between the Greeks and Trojans, grounded in an illicit love affair between the Trojan Paris and the Greek Helen, and crystallised in deeply personal and brutal warring encounters of body and feelings between Achilles and his king Agamemnon, and then Achilles and his foe Hector.

Second, from the patient's point of view, illness has been framed as a "journey" and errancy. Through the figure of Odysseus, the *Odyssey* describes human wandering, the wandering mind, and the mindset and values needed to deal with the unexpected. Whatever the current standing of these two metaphors - and their usefulness for contemporary medicine has been deeply questioned - we are bound to understand them if we are to stand under medical culture and practice to gaze at its normally hidden belly. We must gain new perspectives on how medical students are educated and socialised, or acquire identity as a doctor. Our current understanding is limited, divisive, and even hampers medical education where it reproduces unproductive hierarchy and fails to deal with young doctors' emotional needs.

It was once assumed that students entering medicine would have received an education in Classics, beginning in Homer. This could be seen as preparation for what we now call "professionalism" - the ability to carry out one's job ethically and humanely. Where communication with patients, healthcare colleagues and junior doctors was once framed as benevolent paternalism, doctors were male and viewed as heroes, reproducing the Homeric themes of "honour and glory" (*kleos*) in "war" (clinical practice), and strong leadership in captaining the ship in "homecoming" (*nostos*) (successful outcomes to clinical interventions).

But we see potential in reading Homer with a sideways glance to think otherwise with the texts of the *Iliad* and *Odyssey* for better understanding of contemporary themes in medicine: in particular the roles of women and the feminising of the culture, and the rise of patient-centredness and inter-professional teamwork – all aspects of a democratised medicine concerned with social justice that may be summarised as the democratic dispersal of the medical gaze. This is a medicine in which medical students are politicised and actively challenge social injustices. Allied with this is the steep rise in interest in narratives in medicine and the importance of metaphor within medical discourse (Bleakley 2017). Our project then, in mobilising Homer, is more radical than "thinking medicine with Homer" – it is, again, "thinking medicine *otherwise* with Homer". Thinking otherwise is to think imaginatively, radically, aesthetically, ethically and with humanity.

"Communication" and "professionalism" in medicine for us go beyond face-to-face consultations with patients and teamwork with colleagues. The historical, cultural and social contexts for medical practice demand investigation to ask "why do we do things this way, now?", "are our practices appropriate?" and "if not, then how can we change them?" As noted above, we must understand, for example, why junior doctors are suddenly, and radically, politicised (at the time of writing, we have just seen the first wave of doctors' strikes as a protest against work conditions in the NHS in England); how medical institutions such as hospitals can be understood as complex, adaptive systems; and why many medical students see their future as a job rather than a vocation. To address issues such as these, we need to mobilise background contexts, the first of which is history. Western literary history begins with Homer.

Again, why return to Homer rather than, say, Shakespeare or Milton? And why, for example, does Ulysses keep getting re-invented? - the latter question answered by W.B. Stanford's *The Ulysses Theme* (1968) invoking an archetypal perspective. These books - first written down in the 8th century BCE from oral storytelling set in the Late Bronze Age Aegean - have provided a primary inspiration not only for the Western literary imagination but also for practical and ethical co-existence in society.

The *Iliad* is a book of war and the *Odyssey* a book of adventure and homecoming; both have themes of forgiveness and hospitality (see the appendix for summaries of both books). While the kind of heroism portrayed by Achilles and Odysseus, the main protagonists of the *Iliad* and *Odyssey* respectively, may seem brutal to us – their brand of heroism depends upon creating victims who suffer a loss of esteem in their presence – they are complex and paradoxical, rather than flawed, heroes. It is by entering these worlds of complexity and paradox that we can shed new light on social issues in medicine such as the emotional lives of doctors.

G.K. Chesterton (1999/1908, p.63) remarked that: "Tradition means giving votes to the most obscure of all classes, our ancestors. It is the democracy of the dead. Tradition refuses to submit to the small and arrogant oligarchy of those who merely happen to be walking about". Invoking Chesterton's "democracy of the dead", we might treat any contemporary issue through calling on the voices of tradition; and for medicine, why not call on Homer? We follow Hernandez's (2007) "Reading Homer in the 21st Century" in allowing the voices of the oral poets who sang Homer to resonate in our own times, as a "reproduction of knowledge kept by the Muses". We have merely joined the legion of singers or *rhapsodes*, as part of a procession or parade.

Just as we stick strictly to Homer (for example, "thinking medicine otherwise" with Hesiod's pastoralism and lyricism would be a separate book), so we stick to medicine and do not stray into wider healthcare, although there is no reason why that should not happen. Our agreed agenda is medical culture. Within medicine, we have strenuously avoided repeating the outcomes of work already done on Homer, the body and medicine. For example, Homer's graphic depictions in the *Iliad* of bodies rent in war offers a mini anatomy lesson - a distinction is made between wounds that are fatal and those that are not; and bandaging and herbal treatments for various battlefield wounds are also described (Friedrich 2003). Further, there are idiosyncratic observations, such as Hector's breathlessness on the battlefield suggesting asthma (Jackson 2010). These anatomical and physiological concerns are not something we pursue. Our focus is elsewhere and we have nothing to add to what has already been thoroughly researched concerning Homer and war wounds or medical conditions on the battlefield.

Using Homer in new ways to refresh medical education

What then, is different about our approach in contrast to this body of literature? Our focus is, again, illustrating how we can use Homer to think differently and creatively about issues associated with the human side of medicine, in particular the construction and management of identity through styles and modes of communication (for example, the "hero" identity discussed in chapters 1 and 2). This includes ethics and professionalism, within which are nestled the thorny issues of communication lapses, collapses, inability to jump synapses, and other mis-takes. Doctors and patients might speak differing languages that call for cross-translations, where much may still be lost in translation (chapter 3), where frustrations can readily spill over into anger and abuse (chapter 11), and errors accumulate (chapter 8); there is a range of styles of communication with both patients and colleagues, some wholly inappropriate, unreflective, and unskilled (chapter 5); and there are pitfalls of contemporary medical education in reducing communication to blunt-edged "skills" and "competences", where refinement, aesthetics and creative communication are abandoned for common "core" practices (chapter 5).

Just as we might be straining out the art of communication as an unintended consequence of simulation-based clinical skills training, so we miss, through the blunting or an-aesthetising processes of socialisation and identity construction of a doctor - overworked, over-tired, and over in another ward when needed urgently - the opportunity to appreciate the rituals and habits of clinical work as "song" (chapter 4), and as lyrical (chapter 7), where medicine again deals with the tragic (suffering, facing death), and works according to the epic (heroism and homecoming).

Some doctors and surgeons are "unteachable", habitually abusive, difficult, or "serial errorists" disguised as charming villains (chapter 8). Colleagues and students alike are encouraged to whistleblow where they see clear ethical transgression, but how do you manage this in an ingrained culture of opacity and protective inward focus, even as a culture of public transparency and reparation for mistakes is emerging (chapter 9)? Can doctors, already "bone tired" through work exhaustion and expectations of perfect performance (chapter 12), show weakness and fragility, even shame (chapter 8) in the face of error?

These, amongst others, are our key questions. In some cases, we suggest provisional answers – tactics, strategies and scaffolding of learning. But in other cases, the best we can do is to raise issues of consequence that are historically determined, and second-guess the future from current trends. In these areas, we ask readers to join us in tolerating the ambiguity of knowing that we don't know. But, as we hope you will agree, we are not short of ideas. Our hope is that we stir up a passion to revisit Homer and re-discover the riches of the *Iliad* and the *Odyssey*. We are sure that you will agree with us that the connections between Homer's work and medicine's work are far from tentative. Our wider project is to advertise the value of application of classical literature and philosophy to contemporary medical practice and education. Classical literature, in particular, except that about ancient medicine, has been very little examined for its potential to affect the care of patients and shape the practices of medical education.

Notes

1. Probably "his" rather than "hers", although Andrew Dalby (2006) would disagree.
2. We agree with Furbank (1992, pp.33-46) that enthusiasts can go too far and irritate the non-classicist: Chapman's "Of all books extant in all kinds, Homer is the first and best", for example. We hope to make our case and ask our readers to bear with us.

CHAPTER ONE

HEROES

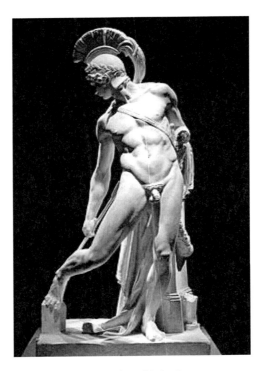

Figure 1-1: Achilles pulling the arrow from his heel

The mortality gene

As Homer, in the *Iliad,* begins with songs of heroes, so we will consider the heroic in medicine as an opening frame. Later, we will contest the value of the heroic in 21st century medicine. But to understand such contestation, we must first look at the parallels between Greek heroes and senior doctors. This is written primarily from our knowledge of doctors in the UK, Canada, and North America, but we believe will resonate with many nationalities. The ancient Greek hero (we include the heroine), unlike ordinary men and women, can be close to the gods as the offspring of a god and a mortal (such as Achilles). In modern secular terms, this means that the hero has a special, elevated talent or ability that affords status. The hero has a gift or ability beyond the norm, but may also carry a wound or vulnerability.

This extraordinary gift may be special knowledge and skill (Odysseus), exceptional courage linked to depth of feeling (Achilles), guile (Odysseus), humanity and faithfulness (Hector), brute strength (Ajax), or extreme patience and tolerance (Penelope). In each case, there is a species of ethical wisdom – models for living. We know that the ancient Greek hero, while dreaming of immortality, is usually destined to die young and in combat, or, as Gregory Nagy (2013) puts it, what distinguishes heroes from gods is that heroes have the "mortality gene". The hero of song, myth and story is then a paradox who bears a burden: his life is short, an intense flame that burns fiercely, burns out, and then lives on after death, as this flame both illuminates and warms the lives of others, a burning memory rekindled in differing ways across generations.

A pathological fascination with mortality is a distinguishing mark of the hero, who accepts fate or destiny as sacrificial victim. Since the times of Palaeolithic hunter-gatherers, shamans or priests have offered animal sacrifices to the gods as a way of ensuring that the hunted animal flourishes and appears next season (Campbell 1984). In farming societies, the sacrifice is the death and re-birth of the harvest (Campbell 1988). As societies grow more complex, so heroes are marked as "sacrifices" through their destinies to die fighting for a cause. The Homeric epics detail how extraordinary humans sacrifice longevity - in recognition of their destinies - usually in combat and in order to be re-membered forever through epic song, and then literature. The hero then gains eternal life through repetitive appearance in cultural lore – or, the hero is regularly re-embodied in the body politic of a community. This counts for much in human culture as our ancestors are usually forgotten after only three generations. What do you, reader, know of your great-grandparents?

There are upper case and lower case heroes in Homer: descriptions of the deaths of soldiers appearing as minor characters constitute about one eighth of the book, which the poet Alice Oswald (2012), in *Memorial,* foregrounds as "the *Iliad's* atmosphere, not its story". Strip away the *Iliad's* narrative and an ecology emerges, despite the epic's concern with just a few days in a decade-long battle that the poet Christopher Logue

(2003) captures as "All Day Permanent Red", referring of course to the brutal hand-to-hand, blood-spilling combat between Trojans and Greeks. Oswald does include the big hitters - or upper case heroes - Patroclus (Achilles' "foster-brother" and perhaps lover), and Hector, whose wife was Andromache: "One day he looked at her quietly/ He said I know what will happen/ And an image stared at him of himself dead" (Oswald 2012, p.69).

But *Memorial*, in stripping away the main narrative and allowing the sub-text of a parade of deaths or sacrifices to express itself, raises these footnotes to the status of text, or affords heroism for every one of the soldiers mentioned in the *Iliad*. Today's "foot soldier" doctors might fruitfully be compared to this group of minor heroes, constituting the atmospheres of medicine in health services across the world as they generate the weather under which patients receive care.

The death of the upper-case hero constitutes a sacrifice for the greater good of the future body politic. Great figures, now dead, are recycled for their key qualities as ethical models. As the hero is re-membered (just like a sacrificial animal was once dis-membered), or put back together in memorial, the people come together to celebrate, reconstitute, and further the body politic where memories act as compost for new growth. This is why the desecration of the hero's body is such a taboo, because the body must be intact for it to be buried so that it can be subsequently re-membered whole. The errors committed by both Hector, in desecrating Patroclus' body, and Achilles, in later desecrating Hector's body in revenge for the death of Patroclus, are deep moral transgressions. The dead, as it were, feed the living organ by organ. The courage and depth of feeling of Achilles must drip-feed the procession of culture organ by organ: for example, Achilles' *phrenes* or "spirited anger" infects the heart and lungs of the body politic and inspires the community to take courage and breathe deeply.

This cultural trope is repeated particularly in medicine where there is a tradition of reverence for great historical figures treated as heroes: Hippocrates, Galen, Vesalius, Harvey, Edward Jenner, Elizabeth Blackwell, Joseph Lister, Ignaz Semmelweis, William Osler, Christiaan Barnard, and so forth. They too, according to specialism, feed the organs of the living. Christiaan Barnard will forever be remembered in our hearts, even *as* the hearts of transplant recipients. Even the lower case heroes inspire where their portraits line the wood-panelled walls of medical schools' lecture theatres, and these ex-Deans and Great Surgeons of the attached hospital are kept alive in generational procession as their achievements are lionised amongst faculty and students.

The ancient Greek hero is in our blood, lodged in our minds, a cultural archetype given with the mortality gene. Our lives are by turns epic and tragic as they are touched by illness; and medicine, in response, shapes the identities of doctors as responses to the epic and tragic – the expression of the mortality gene. Homer's epics, sadly, remain unread by most of us; but worse, science manuals replace them that offer literal accounts stripped of poetry, metaphor and quality. If you Google "telomere" you will find out how we age and die in the 21st century:

> Telomerase counteracts telomere shortening. An enzyme named telomerase adds bases to the ends of telomeres. In young cells, telomerase keeps telomeres from wearing down too much. But as cells divide repeatedly, there is not enough telomerase, so the telomeres grow shorter and the cells age. (http://studylib.net/doc/10242809/are-telomeres-the-key-to-aging-and-cancer%3F-inside-the-nuc...).

In stark contrast, here again is the poet Alice Oswald (2012, p.15), re-membering Homer's characters from the *Iliad*. Pherecles, a boat-builder, "Died on his knees screaming/ Meriones speared him in the buttock/ And the point pierced him in the bladder". Here is a sharp anatomy lesson for medical students and an early handshake from death, a figure or presence they will subsequently meet daily. Of course medical students need their science, and science can be inspiring and of great beauty. But medical students too need their humanity, a moral imagination and a conscience.

From two types of hero to the hero with a thousand faces

Homeric characterisations of the hero come from song cycles composed and transmitted orally over two and a half thousand years ago in the Iron Age, about events that occurred in the much earlier Bronze Age from around four thousand years ago. These song cycles, that we call epic poems, celebrate the cult of the hero, such as Achilles, an extraordinary human situated between mortals and immortal gods (the offspring of the nymph Thetis' liaison with the mortal King Peleus). Doctors, too, particularly surgeons, have been stereotyped as close to the gods. A popular medical joke runs:

> Q. What's the difference between God and an orthopaedic surgeon?
> A. God doesn't think that he's an orthopaedic surgeon.

The work of heroes consists of grappling with conflict close to death, modelling in particular two human virtues – courage, or going straight for the jugular (Achilles); and cunning, or outwitting the enemy (Odysseus). These become styles of life. Courageous heroes like Achilles die at an early age, but, as already described, are immortalised through collective memory and celebrations (song, drama, visual representation, and poetry) through successive generations.

Homer's *Iliad* is the story of the single-minded Achilles, whose rage and stubbornness brought calamity to the Greeks until he was spurred into a frenzy of mindless battlefield brutality and a final act of reconciliation with the enemy. The *Odyssey's* hero is different - the many-sided Odysseus, whose twists and turns characterise the adaptive hero who is also a trickster, staying alive through guile on a long and tortuous journey home; but once at home, Odysseus too enacts a brutal mass slaying to purge that house of the many suitors who had courted his wife Penelope during his long absence, sure that he had died. Unlike doctors, Homer's heroes slay for principles rather than save lives on principle.

"Quick-burn" Homeric heroes, of whom Achilles is the supreme model, are characterised by choosing glory (*kleos*) over life, inviting death in a blaze of glory on the battlefield (Nagy 2013). While Achilles' death is not recorded in the *Iliad*, it is foretold, and the audience of the epic would know of other tales that tell of the death of the great hero. For example, in the *Odyssey*, Odysseus visits Achilles in the underworld. The focus of Achilles provides the model for specialists.

"Slow-burn" heroes, of whom Odysseus is the supreme model, are characterised by adventure and homecoming (*nostos*) (Nagy 2013). After fighting in the Trojan War for ten years, Odysseus' journey home takes another ten. The *Odyssey* invokes the Muse to sing of a versatile man who veered from his path and learned many different things from different people. The adaptability of Odysseus provides the model for generalists.

Homeric heroes suffer fleshly wounds and die gloriously in war to gain a posthumous life in cult; or undertake a series of adventures and trials to emerge wiser and to rule over a kingdom. Doctors as heroes of the first type are confrontational, impulsive risk-takers, stereotypical old-school surgeons. Medical students gain places because they are high achievers academically, but this is often accompanied by a personality profile of perfectionism and impulsivity; put this into the pressure cooker of early, stressful work as a junior doctor, and some fallout is inevitable, such as alcohol and substance abuse and mental health issues (Carpenter 2014, Peterkin and Bleakley 2017). Heroes of the first type can fly too close to the sun.

Heroes of the second type are career doctors, polymaths and talented, even astounding, clinicians, such as William Osler (1894-1919). In "Healing and Heroism" in the *New England Journal of Medicine*, Wheeler (1990, p.1540) describes Osler as a "hero to the public as well as to the medical profession". But heroes of the second type can be wily, passive aggressive, and schemers. They may lose their clinical colleagues' respect as they climb the greasy pole of management to become Clinical Directors, Deans and CEOs, seemingly losing their humanity along the way. Scandals may beckon the higher they climb, where heroism equates with "leadership".

The birth of the hero moves us from mythology to history, from tales of the gods to those of special mortals. But hero cults too are grounded in myth and legend. Indeed, as Joseph Campbell (1949) insists in *The Hero With a Thousand Faces*, the life of the hero is shaped by a foundational myth with a universal plot. The hero (1) responds to a call or vocation; (2) sacrifices himself to a bigger purpose putting his life at risk; (3) undergoes an arduous set of initiations and a journey, involving trials (such as dragonslaying); (4) resists temptations; and (5) achieves a goal that benefits others (releasing a captive princess, returning stolen treasure, bringing back stolen fire). The perils of the journey include encounters with death or visits to the underworld. Wheeler (1990, p.1540) says:

> ... if you practice medicine conscientiously, you are indeed a hero, in Campbell's sense of having surrendered your personal desires to a greater goal — the welfare of your patient. Hero myths assure us that in serving others, we also fulfill our own destiny.

Doctors traditionally tick every box of the hero cycle: (1) responding to a call or vocation; (2) sacrificing their lives to a bigger purpose; (3) undergoing an arduous initiation or socialisation; (4) resisting temptations to stray from the path; and (5) achieving a goal that benefits others (cheating death, healing against the odds). The military and fire service may also tick these boxes, but they do not require the high levels of technical knowledge and skill, acquired through a long apprenticeship, that medicine demands.

The hero myth requires that doctors are shaped by a guiding martial metaphor – disease is to be conquered and medicine requires both warriors to fight the disease and cunning to outwit it, the latter fed in to innovative research strategies. For heroism to flourish in medicine, it must be practiced in a metaphorical climate of war and violence ("the battle against cancer"). Should this metaphorical frame be displaced, classic heroism may fail as an appropriate strategy for medicine. In an age of collaborative healthcare - patient-centred and team-based - the guiding martial metaphors for medicine are challenged. Perhaps doctors of the future will be anti-heroic, washing feet rather than going to war (Miller 2014).

We began this chapter by saying that hero includes heroine, and this remains the case. Heroines in Homer are not attracted to the orbit of *kleos* or glory. Helen's heroic power is unabashed eroticism, while Penelope's is faithfulness and patience shaped by guile. However, the classical heroic mould is unashamedly masculine, as is medicine's primary metaphorical framework of violence and war. It is unusual to find portraits of women deans and high-flying surgeons hanging in the corridors and boardrooms of the more traditional medical schools (there are exceptions, such as the Royal Free in London). Women are still hugely under-represented at the highest levels in academic medicine (although in 2014, the UK Royal College of Surgeons elected their first woman President, Miss Clare Marx, an orthopaedic surgeon).

In the wider culture, of course, the notion of what constitutes a hero now readily embraces heroines and finds alternatives to martial contest. The black gymnast Simone Biles was the poster girl of the Rio 2016 Olympics and is a self-confessed flawed heroine who suffers from Attention Deficit Hyperactivity Disorder (ADHD).

Great heroes in sport, such as Lance Armstrong, quickly fall from grace if found to be flawed - for example caught cheating through illegal doping. Traditionally, to be real heroes doctors too must remain squeaky clean, somebody to be looked up to in the local community. Recent studies suggest that 10-15% of North American doctors suffer from substance abuse, a rate slightly greater than the general population (Reese 2015). Shelly Reese notes:

> Physicians' perfectionistic tendencies enable them to perform well in the workplace even as their marriages fail, their personal lives crumble, and their abuse becomes deeply entrenched. "The big issue is the hiding," says Christopher Welsh, MD, an associate professor of psychiatry at the University of Maryland School of Medicine in Baltimore. "Physicians are very good at hiding their problem."
> (http://www.medscape.com/viewarticle/843758).

Emergence of the anti-hero

We are in the midst of a sea change in medicine – a transition from a paternalistic and heroic era of self-willed senior male doctors, hierarchical teams, and passive patients to a democratic world of flattened hierarchies and informed patients, where women doctors constitute the majority. Heroic metaphors have shaped Western medicine for 400 years, but this will change (Bleakley 2017). Only 25 years ago, the distinguished vascular surgeon and educator H. Brownell Wheeler (1990, p.1548) could write of medicine that:

> Our patients need us to be heroic. They face suffering and death. They desperately need the emotional support of a competent and dedicated physician who cares for them and will try to help. If we can meet their needs, we will have succeeded not only as physicians, but also as human beings. In a quiet and unassuming way, we will be their heroes.

While Wheeler's heroic doctor is lower case, in a minor key, unassuming rather than brash, he nevertheless remains rooted in the paternalistic tradition. Nietzsche described the modern superman as a moral relativist unafraid to say that he or she does not know in the face of others' blind faith, and can live with that uncertainty. We doubt that Wheeler's post-WWII heroic doctor or surgeon is from the same stamp. We think that he would be intolerant of ambiguity, sure of his diagnosis and treatment regime; and that the patient's voice would remain secondary to that of the doctor or surgeon as expert (meritocracy), but also as higher on the social ladder (paternalism). Such doctors assert that medical expertise should not be worn lightly – seniority affords a right to inhabit not just the knowledge high ground, but also the moral high ground.

Today's medical students and young doctors prize differing values to those shaping previous generations - by not being afraid to say "I don't know" and that I can live with ambiguity; and by treating medicine as a job rather than a vocation. This does not mean that they do not take the job seriously and act professionally; but they generally eschew the tradition of heroism. In an era of standardisation (all must satisfy common, assessable competences), in which collaboration is preferred to competition and patients have become experts in their own illnesses thanks to the ready availability of information (the internet, patient support groups, television medi-soaps and helplines), have we moved beyond Wheeler's assertion that doctors are heroes because patients need them to be? Indeed, "hero" can also offer an embarrassing tag where clinical teams look after patients collectively, so all must have prizes, and autonomy generally works against the grain of collective activity. Medical educators now vigorously promote this new landscape of democratic medicine and healthcare.

The new heroes in medicine are perhaps anti-heroes. They are the collective picket line demonstrating against unfair work conditions and cuts to health services. It is not that the hero (and heroine) is going away – it is an archetype – rather, the hero is presenting in new and radical forms. Our aim in this chapter and the following one is to use Homer as a background against which we can think differently, and imaginatively, about the hero. We articulate an understanding of this post-modern transformation of heroism as it applies to medical culture.

Some would claim that old-style heroism is as strong in medicine and surgery today as it was for Wheeler's and previous generations. Indeed, it can be argued that a self-promoting "hero factory" has recently emerged through a new genre of medical autoethnography and doctors' pathographies, as a form of identity construction. The genre was established in the early 1970s by the American surgeon Richard Selzer (1996), and is continued in recent publications such as the British neurosurgeon Henry Marsh's (2014) *Do No Harm*, and the late American neurosurgeon Paul Kalanithi's (2016) *When Breath Becomes Air*.

Reading these accounts, it is difficult to not see them as heroic. No matter how hard the authors try to be self-effacing, the epic natures of their work and life struggles offer self-publicity as hero. Kalanithi (2016, p.98) summarises responsibility in medicine as: "In taking up another's cross one can get crushed by the weight". Not "doctor washing feet" but doctor as sacrificial victim and medicine as a Herculean task. In the late Kalanithi's case, his autoethnography mirrors Homer's figures dying in combat as he struggles to work in the face of "battling" stage IV metastatic lung cancer, demonstrating that doctors and surgeons are particularly poor at accepting the inevitability of the mortality gene expressed in those ever-shortening, pesky telomeres.

While quick to praise heroes in their blaze of glory, we are just as quick to condemn them for their flaws. This shows that we idealise, and have forgotten that Homer's heroes are complex and flawed for a reason. It is in entering these psychological cracks that ordinary mortals can identify with heroes. Heroes must have vulnerabilities.

We do not withhold Odysseus' status of heroism from him because he had years of what seemed like satisfying (but unfaithful) sex with Calypso (although he was "entranced" – but isn't being in love to be entranced?); and that, under his leadership, he allowed the narcotics and easy life of the Lotus Eaters to tempt some members of his crew. Neither do we judge Helen for running off with Paris and causing the Trojan War, for Aphrodite entranced her, or she could not help but flaunt her eroticism. So, we might turn heroising into empathising when we hear of doctors who have fallen from pedestals as a result of undue stress for example. Sometimes, the hero needs to be understood and helped.

A new wave of heroes and heroines

Everyone can be a hero(ine) these days it seems: the first black South African cricketer to score a century for his country (McKenzie 2016), or a striking junior doctor who leaves the picket line to help a man collapsing in the street (Wheatstone 2016). No longer warriors, but sports stars and media celebrities too are heroes. George Clooney gained cult status as an actor playing a doctor in the medi-soap *ER*. It wasn't playing a doctor that made him a hero, but rather his classic chiselled looks. This reinforced the stereotype set by the early TV series Dr Kildare, that the truly heroic doctors are also handsome. David Bowie's 1977 pop song "Heroes" – telling the story of two lovers divided by the Berlin wall - says that you can be a hero for a day, while Andy Warhol suggested that everybody should have fame for 15 minutes, finally aligning heroism with populism. In the wake of David Bowie's recent death, the German government thanked him for "helping to bring down the Wall", adding the final compliment: "you are now among Heroes" (Hall 2016).

So, "hero" has perhaps become so devalued that we lose all notion of what is truly heroic. While dictionary definitions may include divine ancestry, endowment with great courage and strength, renown for bold exploits (often in battle), being favoured by the gods, and being reverenced and idealised, this is the archetypal hero as declared by Joseph Campbell (1949) (including the trickster hero of the kind modelled by Odysseus, who relishes the disruption of the status quo). Beyond this, the dictionary definition is tepid – both heroes and heroines are persons "admired for their courage, outstanding achievements, or noble qualities" (Shorter *OED*).

This can include persons who have overcome disabilities to achieve remarkable things (such as Stephen Hawking, or para-Olympians); or the sister next door who saved her sibling from drowning. We cannot just dismiss this as vanilla heroism – rather the qualities of a hero have become elastic. Mother Theresa and Malala Yousafzai (who won the 2014 Nobel Peace Prize for championing women's rights to education) are shoo-in heroes, but Lionel Messi (multiple winner of the *Ballon d'Or* as Footballer of the Year) too has achieved hero status (actually, flawed status as he was found guilty of massive tax evasion by a Spanish court).

While the hero must still have achieved something that is extraordinary, what is different about modern day heroes is that they are idealised and cleansed of complexities. Heroes who are too complex pall in the public imagination, and heroes who fall from grace through moral flaws or transgressions may be stripped of their knighthoods, even posthumously, such as Jimmy Savile – once a national treasure and now a notorious sex fiend. (Again, scrutiny through contemporary mores of the sex lives of Achilles and Oedipus would leave their reputations in tatters!) Or, some heroes smudge and fade as time progresses, such as Elvis Presley, so daring in his youth and then a caricature with an eating disorder in his sunset years.

In the modern era, we generally think of heroes as those who strive against adversity and make an effort that is almost beyond human - such as doctors working in Aleppo under the most terrible combat conditions with meagre resources and often treating young, defenceless children with horrific injuries. But of course the people of Aleppo who suffer from a war they did not create are heroes too, simply because of their strength of spirit. The Ebola epidemic in 2014-15 in West Africa called for behaviour from local and foreign healthcare staff that most would regard as truly heroic (Green 2014, Saidu et al 2016).

We have seen that the poet Alice Oswald, in *Memorial*, foregrounds the deaths of the ordinary foot soldiers in the Trojan War in a re-configuration of Homer's *Iliad*, and we are touched in a way that the audience who first heard the so-called "*Iliad*" as a performed song would probably not have been. The death of these soldiers is everyday and incidental to the main protagonists who are pinnacle warriors, such as Achilles, Hector and Patroclus. Yet Oswald brings the badge of heroism for the foot soldiers too, as a gesture of poetic democracy.

Jessica Zetteler (2005, p.644), a psychologist who researches health, mulls on "what is a hero?" in the *British Journal of General Practice.* She suggests that "It's probably best not to take the subject of heroes too seriously" although we might use them as lighthouses to guide our way. We disagree with Zetteler on this point – it is extremely important to take heroism seriously, particularly in medicine, for the very reasons that we have already set out. Heroism was once part and parcel of the fabric, the very being of a doctor, an identity "must". Yet now we are confused about what heroism means and unsure of its historical trajectory within medical culture. We must work out where medicine stands in relationship to classical heroism if we are to treat medicine's symptoms, so that medicine can better treat patients.

Zetteler (ibid.) suggests that heroism is "more than just bravery, compassion or wisdom alone" and reminds us of several definitions. In the psychological literature, North and colleagues (North et al 2005) do not conflate heroes and celebrities, as we have done above, but distinguish them on the basis that heroes produce ideas or objects that persist through time, where celebrities are characterised as transient - phenomena of the moment. Celebrity status is then not heroic status. Well, people are still talking about Mae West, Charlie Chaplin, Fred Astaire and Ginger Rogers for example. But perhaps these were innovators, and not just "15 minutes" celebrities that Andy Warhol promoted. The psychological literature also suggests that a characteristic of heroes is their prosociality, where heroes often endanger their bodies or lives for others.

The issue here is that this excludes people such as Bill and Melinda Gates who are not only the richest couple on earth, but also the most generous in terms of philanthropy. If you can afford to be generous, does this make you a hero? The "putting your body on the line" argument also rather mocks the heroic status of people such as Stephen Hawking, whose disability means that his body is permanently on the line. How often do we think of disabled medical students automatically as heroes? Yet the courage they show in making this commitment already marks them out as exceptional.

Zetteler's own heroine is Camila Batmanghelidjh, founder of Kids Company, a day centre for young people in South London. Zetteler (2005, p.645) said that: "Not many people that I speak to have heard of her, so she is a very personal hero". Yet Batmanghelidjh has since become a well-known public figure, and just as dramatically has fallen from grace as a charity boss who transgressed certain rules of the game. Today's heroes are transient.

Zetteler conducted an informal survey of 48 staff members from the Department of Community Based Medicine at the University of Bristol, who generated a wide-ranging list of 71 heroes, including firemen, mountaineers, naval commanders and people who have overcome disability or other adverse situations, as well as doctors. Four respondents said that they did not have a hero, and two were cynical about the concept of heroism in today's world. Included in the list of heroes were the cyclist Lance Armstrong, since vilified for doping. How fragile our heroes may be! The list also puts the Dalai Lama and Nelson Mandela alongside Eddie the Eagle and the fictional Han Solo from *Star Wars* (described as a "smuggler" and "scoundrel" as well as a "hero" on his internet profile), demonstrating again how wide-ranging definitions of hero can be and how they might say more about their audiences than themselves.

CHAPTER TWO

HEROES (ARE YESTERDAY'S MEN)

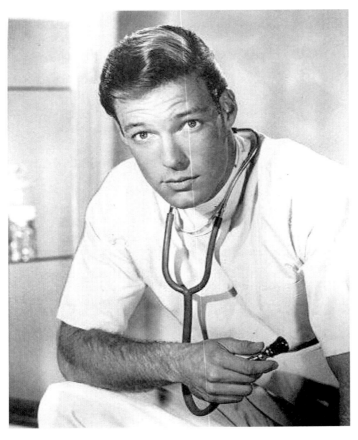

Figure 2-1: Richard Chamberlain as Dr Kildare

In *Catcher in the Rye*, J.D. Salinger (1951, p.169) says: "The mark of the immature man is that he wants to die nobly for a cause, while the mark of a mature man is that he wants to live humbly for one". This casts the Achillean heroic mould as problematic, even symptomatic of a juvenile personality. Salinger prefers to reverse heroism, or perhaps even erase heroism entirely, seeing the traditionally anti-heroic characteristic of humility as something to be embraced. Two years after his success with *Catcher in the Rye* Salinger turned his back on the public gaze. America's (arguably) greatest post-war novelist Thomas Pynchon has also become a recluse, although he continues to be a prolific writer. Are these acts of walking away from the limelight in their own way heroic?

Below are 12 things we know about heroes and their relationship to medicine. From this, we can see how the heroic can be re-visioned for 21st century medicine and medical education.

Heroes satisfy a need in those who are not heroes

Where Joseph Campbell's (1949) *The Hero with a Thousand Faces* concentrates on the appearance of the hero across cultures as the expression of an archetype fulfilled in myth, Lucy Hughes-Hallett's (2006) *Heroes: Saviours, Traitors and Supermen* looks at the hero's emergence not so much as an expression of myth but as satisfying a popular need. Campbell says the hero is made in the image of the archetype or eternal form, a transcendental mould; Hughes-Hallett says the hero is a product of everyman's need for a hero. Campbell's model is paternalistic, where Hughes-Hallett's perspective echoes the Hegelian view that there is no Master without the Slave (therefore the slave has power); or, there is no doctor without patients (the view of humanistic, patient-centred medicine). There is a dark side to the view that crowds source the heroes they need. We forgive our heroes their corruption and transgressions, dictatorship and immorality; and their plain stupidities. In heroising this way, we can normalise bad behaviour that usually insults.

To those without the expertise, doctors and surgeons can appear to do miraculous things in diagnosis and intervention, because they inhabit the same turf as heroes – the fringe between life and death. The initiations – learning anatomy through dissection, exposure to death, overcoming disgust, engaging in intimate examinations professionally; and inhabiting territories that become entirely familiar, such as consulting rooms, morgues, operating theatres, and wards of hospitals – remain largely alien and mysterious to the public.

The heroic tradition celebrates masculinity

Mother Theresa, the black gymnast Simone Biles who won four golds at the Rio 2016 Olympics, the singers Madonna and Taylor Swift, the sculptor Louise Bourgeois: the modern-day hero is just as likely to be a heroine. As more women than men enter medicine and are now practicing in medicine (although a larger proportion of women than men are working part-time), let us briefly consider how the archetype of the heroine may impact upon medicine. Bleakley (2014, chap. 9) asks whether or not the future numerical dominance of women in medicine will produce important quality consequences: (1) for feminising the culture of medicine; (2) for shifting the centres of power away from men towards women in terms of senior clinical, management, and academic positions, where men still dominate; (3) whether this will touch surgery, that remains a staunchly masculine concern in terms of numbers, power and values; and (4) most importantly, how will this gender shift affect patient care? Research clearly shows that women doctors are generally better at the human side of medicine than their male counterparts.

There remains a largely unwritten critical-historical story of women's place in medicine and the emergence of heroines in the field (Greene 2001, McIntyre 2014). For example, The London School of Medicine for Women, established in 1874, was set up as a protest to medical schools in the UK not accepting women applicants. Any one of the pioneering women doctors could be seen as heroines – especially Sophia Jex-Blake, who had attempted to gain admission to the then men-only medical schools. Isabel Thorne and Jex-Blake later founded the Edinburgh School of Medicine for Women, in 1886. In 1876, a UK Medical Act allowed authorities to licence qualified women as well as male applicants, but women found it difficult to gain places at medical schools and thus to qualify. Famously, when Abraham Flexner set out a blueprint for the radical reform of North American medical schools in 1917 he recommended closure of many schools that were under-resourced. These were precisely the schools that served women and minority entrants. It has taken medical education a century to recover from this error of judgement (Hodges 2005).

While we are discussing gender as a key issue in the changing status of heroism in modern life and medicine in particular, celebrity status is now afforded to gay, lesbian, bi-sexual, transgender and questioning individuals on the basis of their championing of sexual orientations especially within climates of repression or outright prejudice. Medicine, however, makes lukewarm statements about the gender choices of doctors on the basis that such choices sit outside codes of professional and ethical

practice (Peterkin and Bleakley 2017). But this misses the point in an era
in which young doctors are increasingly politically aware and active.

Proactive support of sexual identity choices within medicine sends out
a positive message to patients with minority sexual orientations or who are
questioning and confused. Many of these patients may suffer from mental
health issues. Our model here is the importance of the relationship
between Achilles and Patroclus to the unfolding narrative of the *Iliad*. It
seems that they are lovers, not just friends; and it is because of the death of
Patroclus (disguised in Achilles' armour) at the hands of the Trojans that
Achilles decides to rejoin the Trojan War, redoubling his effort.

Medical education cries out for feminist revision, reading and
reconceptualisation, and could learn much from feminist approaches within
Homeric scholarship (Doherty 2009). This should include radical readings
and revisions, such as Andrew Dalby (2006) making a case for the
"Homer" of both the *Iliad* and *Odyssey* as a woman, or more likely,
women. He elaborates on traditions of women oral poets to suggest that
prior to writing out the epics, women may well have performed them.

Heroes are individuals

Heroes, by definition, do not work well in teams. They are an odd fit and
far too unpredictable. Heroes then are surely on the way out in medicine as
we establish an era of authentic, collaborative teamwork. Some, however,
may claim that heroes simply transform, to become the leaders of those
teams as an emergent property of the team system's adaptive complexity.
Or, heroism is now distributed across team members, as social capital
turned into common property. Mennin and colleagues (Mennin et al 2016,
blurb) make "the assumption that every health professional/teacher is a
leader, and that every leader is a teacher". This democratises leadership
(and pedagogy), spreading heroism like butter on toast, to be shared by all.
One might think that this open access leadership is a million miles from
the styles of Achilles and Odysseus, but in fact there are many instances of
collective decision-making in the *Iliad* that David Elmer calls a "poetics of
consent" (Elmer 2012). This is where doctors need to be "re-skilled" rather
than "de-skilled" in gaining "tools for conviviality" (Illich 2006).

Heroes must embrace mortality

The hero was born in death and "is touched by it", says Carl Kérenyi
(1974), returning us to Nagy's "mortality gene". Kerenyi (1974, p.15)
further notes that: "the healing god Asklepios was taken from his mother

Koronis on her funeral pyre by Apollo", so the patron god of medicine was born in the midst of death; and medicine as a vocation obviously repeats this motif, as death is ever present. Doctors are tempered in this funeral pyre – introduced to death early in their careers through dissection of corpses as a key initiation, and thereafter committing themselves to working within the web of suffering and death, with the threat of burnout a constant companion. (It should be noted that some medical schools have abandoned learning anatomy through dissection for learning surface and living anatomy through study of live, virtual and plastic models, where initiations into medicine then take differing forms such as early clinical experience).

Studies over more than 25 years (Thorson and Powell 1991, Asadpour et al 2016) show that medical educators still do not devise appropriate support and other curriculum interventions to help medical students to cope with the patient deaths they encounter, and no body of work addresses their responses to deaths of senior colleagues or peers (for example through suicide).

Hull (1991) found that some medical students' encounters with death were traumatic, with no counselling or support available. Ratanawongsa and colleagues, in a North American setting, found that students on placement in End of Life Care settings coped well with death because of such a developed culture of care and compassion in their rotation settings (Ratanawongsa et al 2005). Kelly and Nisker (2010), in a Canadian setting, showed that final year medical students responded differently to deaths of patients according to the circumstances of death and the quality of support and debriefing that they encountered from clinical teachers around patients' deaths.

Smith-Han and colleagues (Smith-Han et al 2016, p.108), in a UK setting, followed a group of medical students longitudinally through their clinical years and investigated their responses to patient deaths. This recent study is important because, although the sample was small and the results cannot be generalised, the study may well have taken the temperature of a new generation of contemporary "anti-heroic" medical students, where there was "a change in students' perceptions from an heroic curing view of the doctor's role to a role of caring". The study found that as students experienced more deaths, instead of becoming hardened and more capable, they felt "emotionally diminished" and were concerned about this dampening of emotions. They put this in context through appreciating the "ordinariness" of death in a hospital environment. Yet, despite the formalising of their roles in responding professionally to patients' deaths, they rationalised this professional distance in terms of formal responsibility for patients. This is where classical heroism transformed into contemporary care.

The difference between Homer and medicine is that heroes in Homer know that their fate is plotted out – in Achilles' case, again, an early death in a blaze of glory (*kleos*). In the *Iliad*, despite the fact that both he and the audience listening to the epic know Achilles' fate, Achilles is (strangely) told that his fate is in his own hands. He can apparently choose between a long life of anonymity at home surrounded by wife and children, or a glorious death at Troy, to become the subject of songs for ever. Actually, once Patroclus, his lover, is killed on the battlefield, mistaken for Achilles because he is wearing Achilles' armour, Achilles' fate is sealed.

He sets out on what the Norse heroes called "berserker" behaviour, completely driven to slay every Trojan who comes his way, until the final and fateful meeting with Hector, the best of the Trojan warriors. Achilles is the greatest of heroes partly because he died young: "In this he is typical of all doomed heroes whose short careers reflect in their crowded eventfulness the bursting ardours of the heroic soul" (Bowra 1978, p.131). Achilles then differs from the new wave of doctors we discuss above - who have absorbed the traditional nursing role of care into their traditional work of cure – as his care is highly selective and not given unconditionally.

Can doctors really be said to – traditionally - embrace mortality as heroes? Certainly, generalisations from surveys suggest that, historically, doctors are notoriously uninterested in their own health, carrying delusions of invincibility (Wiskar 2012); while a recent survey showed that 80% of doctors report concerns with mental health such as depression and anxiety arising from stress (Oxtoby 2016).

For lesser mortals at Troy, their fate is less clear. The fragile nature of their existence is described twice in a memorable simile, once by the Trojan Glaucus, when he comes up against Diomedes on the battlefield:

As the leaves on the trees, so are the generations of men. Some leaves the wind blows to the ground, while others the tree puts forth in bloom at the next spring season (*Iliad* 6. 146-8).

And the second time, more cynically, by the god Apollo when he refuses to fight another god, Poseidon, because it would be stupid to fight for wretched mortals

who are like the leaves, blossoming forth brightly at one moment, eating the fruits of the earth, the next wasting away lifeless (*Iliad* 21. 462-6).

Doctors are, traditionally, notoriously pragmatic and not prone to philosophising. Their proximity to death is what they signed up for – a central part of the job. The standard approach is to "get real" about illness and death and get on with the job at hand. And so begins the very tricky balance between maintaining empathy for others in suffering and grief and allowing cynicism to creep in, followed closely by cults of medical slang and black humour. It is in this ground between empathy and cynicism that medical education, including ethics and humanities, is seeded and hopefully flourishes.

Outside the *Iliad*, great heroes can have some sort of existence as a demi-god or cult figure; in it, there is only death (Schein 1984). In the *Odyssey*, Odysseus descends to the underworld and meets the ghost of Tiresias, the great seer, who tells him that Odysseus' own death will come painlessly, as an old man:

> For you a very gentle death shall come, away from the sea, and take you worn out by a gentle old age (*Odyssey* 11. 134-6).

So, the fate of a hero can be the option of homecoming and gentle demise, supposedly rejected by Achilles but actually already scripted out for him in his unfolding fate. This suggests his fate is to make it home. But when Odysseus meets the shade of Achilles, the latter is miserable. Achilles asks Odysseus not to humour him over being a great Lord in the Underworld:

> Do not make light of death, bright Odysseus. I'd rather be a serf serving a landless man who has nothing, than rule over all the dead and perished (*Iliad* 11. 488-91).

The choice of heroic glory is then a major sacrifice.

The relationship of the modern doctor with death is complex. We have already noted that going to work in medicine is metaphorically framed as going to war. The difference, again, is that the medics are there to save lives not destroy them. James Hillman (2004) tries to understand our "terrible love of war", citing one soldier's memory of battle: "I felt like a god … I was untouchable", where heroism is overtaken by inflation. Surgeons too can talk in this way when everything in the battlefield of the operating theatre seems to be going their way (Selzer 1974).

Hillman reminds us that Ares (Mars) the god of war is best removed from the battlefield through his passionate relationship with Aphrodite (Venus) (see also Burkert 2009). Only the passion of seduction and sex can take Mars' mind away from the brutality of the battlefield – a mythological emblem that has spawned the most common plotline for medical soap operas – relationships and sex between clinical colleagues.

While medical soap operas make much of the link between the fast-paced and demanding work of intensive medicine, surgery and emergency medicine and post-work drinking and sex, there is little research on the subject. Grandinetti (2000), in a North American survey study, found that – true to stereotype - orthopaedic surgeons claim to be the most sexually active amongst the specialties, with 20% of respondents claiming that they have sex more than 10 times a month and 18% admitting to affairs outside marriage. However, they are near the bottom of the league table of specialties in terms of reporting satisfaction from sex – perhaps a result of their perfectionism? Recall that every hero is vulnerable.

In a war scenario, the bravery of medics (and this would include a variety of personnel) often excites comment. This bravery is unlikely to be above that of other servicemen, but differs perhaps in its necessary *sang froid*. It must be hard to assess injuries and carry out delicate first aid and operations when one's own life is at risk. Admiration is easily found in reports from the First and Second World Wars:

> A scrutiny of the casualty lists reveals the fact that the number of RAMC officers who have fallen or been wounded is, proportionately, very great. And those who have been in the firing line know with what courage the doctors have gone about their work, how again and again, they have penetrated to the trenches under fire, and how small a weight considerations of personal safety have been given in the direction of their actions.
> (http://1914-1918.invisionzone.com/forums/index.php?/topic/82799-captain-harry-sherwood-ranken-ramc/).

It could be said that doctors in these situations chose the risk when joining the armed forces and are then following military rules. More evidently heroic are those who put their lives in danger by volunteering to work in dangerous situations, often related to conflict. So, for example, the British vascular surgeon David Nott, who worked in Syria, was told that the hospital in which he was poised to carry out an operation on a severely injured young girl was about to be bombed; the hospital was evacuated, but he stayed with his anaesthetist colleague to complete the operation (http://www.bbc.co.uk/programmes/b07djzyq#play).

Another type of bravery was shown during the outbreak of Ebola virus infection in West Africa in 2014-15. Ebola is highly infectious and has a high mortality rate of around 50% (http://www.who.int/mediacentre/fact sheets/fs103/en/). Those in contact with the sick, family and carers, are at great risk. In one area, 66 of 145 local and volunteer healthcare staff became infected, and about 70% died (Green 2014, Senga et al 2016).

A different, subtler awareness of mortality also pervades the medical profession. All doctors are aware (and are constantly being told) that they rank highly in suicide ideation and suicide ratings across professions (Brooks et al 2011), although this is contested (Hawton et al 2001). This is related to the stress of their work and the driven, perfectionist nature that they bring to it. Doctors therefore examine the pressures of their work as never before and, now, are more assertive in limiting their workload. Nevertheless, external pressures are applied.

The authors have seen the natural deaths of at least three colleagues, where excessive work was generally agreed to have been a contributory cause to an early death. They cannot be unique. None of the three was obliged to work as hard as he did (all were male), but were clearly driven personalities. Driven by what? All were widely respected, even loved, across a wide range of staff, patients and medical education colleagues, yet they did not obviously seek the "the praise of men" (*klea andron*). That is the main driver of the Greek hero: "For the suffering that he must bear in life and for the ineffable horror of annihilation in death, Homeric man knows only one compensation – glory" (Frankel 1975, p.84), where "Fame ... is a kind of surrogate immortality" (Clarke 2004, pp.77-78). The praise of men lives on only a short time after a medical death, and does not render the doctor "imperishable" (*aphthitos*), as it did Achilles.

The great Greek heroes assumed totemic status long after Homer and it remains to this day. Again, great doctors have their portraits hung in the boardrooms of their hospitals or Royal Colleges in the UK, but few of the living know anything about them. William Osler is often mentioned, but seldom read or discussed critically; rather he is lionised as hero (Wheeler 1990). Some medics live on as eponyms for diseases but few doctors today know much about Cushing, Addison or Graves. For most, an eponymous disease is their best hope of heroic immortality. Most medics would feel that the respect, at least, of their colleagues is an important driver of performance; working hard, sometimes to excess, can be part of that performance.

For Achilles, again, "the creed of heroism is that the fame of great deeds defeats death" (Hainsworth 2000) – but look at how miserable Achilles is in death as Odysseus visits him in Hades. That the ancient Greeks could cast the dead in the image of the living is not such an existential challenge – as psychoanalysts and psychologists since Freud have shown, the Greek underworld can be paralleled with our vividly experienced world of dreams (Hillman 1979). Psychiatrists are experts in this field, but few turn their expert gazes on the health of their colleagues or their profession as it transitions between traditional heroism and contemporary anti-heroism. There is much work to do on the meaning of this transition.

Heroes have a stand-in, or ritual substitute

Heroes have stand-ins who are also their sidekicks, apprentices and maybe lovers - Batboy to Batman in comic book heroes. Achilles has his closest friend, or lover, Patroclus as ritual substitute (*therapon*). Indeed, Achilles and Patroclus are said to share the same *psyche* or soul. Patroclus famously wears Achilles' armour to battle the Trojans, as if he is taking on the persona of Achilles. In turn, Achilles, as boss, warns Patroclus not to get into trouble by straying too close to the walls of Troy. Impersonation can only go so far, but it can be said that they share a common imagination. Similarly, registrars (fellows, residents) act as stand-in for consultants (attending physicians) as an important part of their apprenticeship ritual in medicine, sharing a common medical imagination.

Heroes have a cult after death

As we have seen, heroes gain a kind of immortality as their tales are passed down across generations. In ancient Greece, the heroes' tales are told by *rhapsodes* – both actors and singers. In medicine too, some hero figures have gained immortality, such as William Osler, for their clinical acumen and wisdom – in Osler's case enshrined in many memorable aphorisms or maxims; Anton Chekhov too, who called medicine his "lawful wife" and literature his "mistress". Medicine has its *rhapsodes* – medical students and junior doctors who sing the praises of the best clinical teachers; and "medicine watchers" such as medical educators who are not physicians, but sing of the best way to teach physicians.

The latter is illuminated by Plato's *Ion* – a dialogue in which Socrates demonstrates through artful argument that the *rhapsode* Ion cannot claim to have a learned profession like a doctor, but is in fact directly inspired by the Muses. The "medicine watcher", in turn, has no original skill or even a particular identity, but has a knack of being able to see into the workings of the profession of medicine and to explore how doctors gain an exclusive cognitive identity. Medicine watchers are tolerated by the medics they watch only because they bring interesting insights to practice that are difficult to gain from the position of being fully embedded in the practice. Homer of course is our medicine watcher here.

Heroes flower after their deaths, or stimulate a cult. The ancient Greeks described the hero put into the earth at death and providing a particularly fertile ground, a source of prosperity (Antonaccio 1995). The memory of the hero is turned and turned, to offer new revelations. Inevitably, heroic status is re-assessed. Abraham Flexner has been seen as the founder of modern medical education through his influence on introducing structures and standards to North American medical schools. His reputation peaked at the centenary of his work, and then began to dip as critiques appeared (Bonner 2002). As mentioned above, Brian Hodges (2005) notes that Flexner's reforms closed down the less well-resourced medical schools as the most vulnerable, but these were also the schools that took in women and minority applicants. It can be said that Flexner created the blueprint for a century of male-dominated medicine.

This was reinforced by adopting the German model of cold, detached and rational laboratory science as the primary initiation into medicine, prior to clinical exposure. This reinforces the masculine frame for medical education where *logos* supplants *eros*. Doctors must first learn cold detachment before they meet the warm living flesh of patients. We wonder how medical education, and then medical practice, would have been shaped over the past century if Flexner had preferred the French to the German system. The former includes a longer initial education with a broad humanistic base, to include languages, ethics, and psychology.

Heroes are flawed psychologically and morally

Our modern views of heroes may suffer from idealisation. Comic book heroes provide the stereotype: selflessly at the service of others, conscientious, and supremely adept. It is others who trick or stain them. Heroes are slotted in to a bigger archetypal polarity of Good versus Evil. Doctor Kildare, the American TV and comic book hero from the early 1960s, fits this bill, with not a bad moral fibre in his being (figure 2.1). Homeric heroes, however, are fatally flawed both psychologically and morally, so that, as discussed earlier, mere mortals can identify with them. Achilles is trussed by a fierce pride and independence, and is finally brought to a frenzy of violence in the grip of revenge. Odysseus too, at the close of the *Odyssey* is gripped by the deepest need for revenge. Both heroes lose the ability to discriminate as the red mist of revenge descends upon them.

The contemporary turn in the medical imagination, away from heroism and idealisation, is relatively recent. Compare the portrayal of doctors in early television soap operas such as Dr Kildare (NBC 1961-66) and Dr

Finlay's Casebook (BBC 1962-1971) with contemporary TV medical soap operas. In the former, doctors are squeaky clean, in the latter they are portrayed as complex and flawed. For example, in the most successful of all medi-soaps, Hugh Laurie's character Dr Gregory House in "House MD" is cast as heroic (he has an uncanny ability for diagnostic acumen or sleuthing), charismatic (a likeable rogue), but flawed (addicted to painkillers, acerbic and almost pathologically anti-social), and transgressive (he constantly ignores protocols).

Heroes are transgressive

Achilles' anger can be put to good effect on the battlefield, although even here his actions are excessive. He goes berserk, slaughtering without mercy and prepared to fight a river god with impunity. His anger also causes him to act against the interests of his comrades, to put himself above the common interest. He moves beyond the pale and becomes impossible to work with. It is possible to give this a positive interpretation by emphasising the uniqueness of the hero: "(Achilles) is the champion of individualism against the compromising demands of the community, the defender of the loner's purity against the complex imperfections of the group" says Hughes-Hallett (2004). Try telling that to champions of democratic clinical teamwork who have worked tirelessly to educate for authentic inter-professionalism.

However, following his quarrel with Agamemnon, Achilles retires to his encampment, refusing to fight. This leads to disastrous reverses for the Greeks. The Greek commanders, as the battle turns against them, send three senior figures to urge him to change his mind. We discuss this embassy scene at length in the following chapter. Here, it will remind any older doctor in the UK NHS of attempts to bring a colleague whose behaviour was giving concern back into line. Before the major management reorganisations starting in the 1980s, difficult and intransigent senior doctors in hospital medicine could be truly unmanageable. One way of trying to deal with them was through a system, strikingly similar to that used by the Greek generals, known as the "three wise men". This involved three senior doctors talking to the difficult colleague to persuade him or her to modify his or her behaviour. Few threats or penalties were available to them and they had to rely on appeals to custom and ethos much as Homer's ambassadors. In one case in which one of the authors (RM) was closely involved, an approach was made by the "three wise men" and was wholly unsuccessful. The situation they were attempting to resolve unwound over a long period of time with much hurt to almost everyone involved.

Heroes are charismatic as well as skilled

A feature of medical transgressors is that, like Greek heroes, they can be charming and seductive characters. As a manifestation of that, they often have a loyal band of followers and supporters. Achilles comes to Troy with a force of his own countrymen, the Myrmidons. Homer says little of their devotion to their commander, but they support his withdrawal from action, and mourn with him the death of Patroclus. When the Greeks are beaten back to their ships and losses are great, Patroclus come in tears to Achilles to beg to be allowed to lead their men into battle. Achilles replies with one of the epic's memorable similes: "Why are you crying, Patroclus, like a little girl begging her mother to pick her up, clutching her skirt, dragging her back as she hurries along, gazing at her until she is picked up?" (*Iliad* 16. 7-10).

Scenes such as this perhaps demonstrate a softer – at least more lyrical - side to Achilles (although the remark can be seen to be sarcastic and scornful), and enlist the sympathy of the audience. Those who are transgressive, outrageous and difficult, if they are to stay in the limelight, must have a base of support. This tends to be a particular group on whom they exert their charm. Their bad behaviour, excessive anger and flagrant bullying are, equally, often directed at particular groups, usually those who find it difficult to fight back – students, junior doctors, nursing staff or particular patients.

The behaviour of heroes is excessive

Greek heroes are unrestrained in their behaviour. They embody one particular quality to excess, and because of it are often flawed characters. Achilles is the finest warrior of the Greeks. His comrades acknowledge it and he knows it. But his sulk is excessive and his rage is beyond comprehension. When he goes on the rampage after Patroclus' death, he kills Trojans at will, in the most bloodthirsty way. For example, he wounds Deucalion in the forearm, so that it hangs limply by the Trojan's side and in this moment Achilles slices off Deucalion's head with a single blow, along with the helmet. Homer describes the marrow oozing from Deucalion's spine as he lies dead on the ground.

While this is excessive and is berserk battlefield behaviour, our point is that it is on the spectrum of anger and impulse. Take the behaviour down several gears and you find the outbursts typical of some doctors and surgeons that we describe in chapter eight (on anger). Anger or rage (*menis*) is the first word of the *Iliad*, and shapes the whole epic.

"Impulsiveness" has come to describe the stereotypical surgeon who will cry out "don't just stand there, do something", and who lampoons non-surgeons with the reversal: "don't just do something, stand there!"

Achilles' impulsiveness is brought to the attention of the audience early on in the *Iliad* where, angered by Agamemnon's bullying, Achilles is on the point of drawing his sword to kill the leader of the Greeks, and is only restrained when the goddess Athene pulls him back by his hair (figure 2.2), turning impulse into reflection.

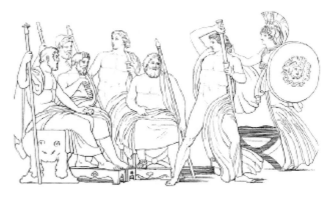

Figure 2-2: Achilles, about to kill Agamemnon, is restrained by Athene

Other warriors, as might be expected, express anger at other times in the *Iliad*, but other words are used, such as *cholos* (from which we have choleric). Such anger is not the absolutely cold, brutal rage that runs through Achilles, and where *menis* is used elsewhere in the *Iliad* it describes a state beyond human anger, generally the wrath of the gods. So, for example, Athene restrains Ares from joining battle in support of the Trojans: "Let us withdraw and so avoid the wrath of Zeus" (*Iliad* 5. 34).

The use of *menis* at the beginning of the *Iliad* is to emphasise that Achilles' response to Agamemnon is beyond what is reasonable, even what is human. Not his immediate response, which is that of a young man without self-control, but its sequel, which is an implacable refusal to rejoin the battle even when his comrades are being slaughtered and driven back to their last defences. It is not the rage that sustains him in battle but "the principled fury that kept him off it" (Hughes-Hallett 2004, p.20). His response to the three ambassadors in book 9 (see chapter three) makes clear that he has gone beyond reason when he rejects the very different arguments and pleas of three senior, respected colleagues. His anger is beyond reasonable limits, at the spectrum's end.

Fieldwork observation of some doctors and surgeons at work confirms that such unreasonable anger has parallels in medical practice, as we note above (see chapter eight). From our own experience we have several anecdotal accounts. An example is a gynaecologist who was the last of his team to arrive for a theatre list. He found in the changing room that his boots had been inadvertently taken and worn by another, so he refused to operate ("vowed he would take no further part in the action") until they were returned. The culprit could not be found, and the consultant was true to his word so that the half-day of operations had to be cancelled.

From direct experience in the field, Wen Shen (2014, online), a surgeon himself, reports: "On more than a few occasions, I witnessed senior surgeons throw instruments in anger, leaving the staff cowering". And from the research literature, a 2011 American College of Physician Executives survey of 840 doctors found that 14% had witnessed colleagues throwing objects (https://www.advisory.com/daily-briefing/2011/05/26/bad-behavior-26-percent-of-physicians-admit-to-being-disruptive).

The point in myth is that the hero is constantly reminded of his humanity through a kind of frailty - of character or actions – to deter from *hubris* (excessive pride or self-confidence). Among the heroes of today – in the UK often decorated in the honours lists, although they account for only a small proportion of that list – are those successful in business, the big CEOs. These are also the grossly high earners. A recent Australian study showed that one in five CEOs (of 261 surveyed) were clinically psychopathic – devoid of empathy, cold-hearted, superficial, insincere and manipulative (Agerholm 2016).

Many-talented, but slippery, Odysseus is perhaps a more complex character than Achilles, certainly as regards extreme and inappropriate behaviour. In many ways, he is the opposite of Achilles - older, wiser, more experienced and careful to weigh up a situation before he acts. Still, he is capable of perplexing actions. After ten years fighting at Troy and a further ten wandering the Aegean, he reaches his home on Ithaca. There, a gang of badly behaved suitors has harassed his wife Penelope, keen to marry such a rich widow, and depleting the resources of the house. With the help of his son, Telemachus, Odysseus kills them all, savagely.

The behaviour of the suitors has been gross – breaking all the rules of hospitality - and they had threatened to kill Telemachus, so Odysseus' reaction may seem reasonable in the context of his time. But he then goes on to order the deaths of those of his women servants who had sided with, and slept with, the suitors. It is odd, savage behaviour by a wise and battered hero, not the result of the anger that typifies Achilles, but a much colder, calculating impulse. Later, the relatives of the suitors approach the palace to exact revenge and Odysseus and his son are poised to continue the slaughter, but the goddess Athene, on Zeus' counsel, arrives to restrain them, thus preventing bloodshed at the end of the *Odyssey* as she had, tugging at Achilles' hair, at the beginning of the *Iliad*.

Today's heroes are not as good as yesterday's men

The generation before yours was always the one with the true heroes. This is especially so in medicine. In the action of the *Iliad*, fighters lift stones that Homer tells us "two of today's men could not lift": Diomedes "took a rock in his hand which two men of today's generation could not lift, a great feat. But he brandished it easily on his own" (*Iliad* 5. 302-4). The words are repeated almost verbatim when Aeneas fights Achilles later (*Iliad* 20. 285-7).

Yet these mighty heroes were themselves preceded by a finer race of men. After the quarrel between Achilles and Agamemnon, Nestor, a venerable Greek councillor, tries to make peace between the protagonists. His credentials to do this, he says, are that he has given council in the past to much better men and was heeded:

> How delighted the Trojans would be if they heard you … . But listen to me. I have been the companion of men better even than you and they did not despise me. I never saw nor shall see such men as Peirithous and Dryas. They were the strongest men that earth has nourished. They were the mightiest and fought with the mightiest …. . No man alive on the earth today could fight with them. (*Iliad* 1. 255-72).

Later, Agamemnon is exhorting Diomedes to enter the battle. He does this by comparing him unfavourably with his father Tydeus, giving a long description of the latter's athletic and military excellence and ending with an insult: "Such was … Tydeus. But his son is a lesser man in battle, though he may be better at talking" (*Iliad* 4. 370-400). This is part of a decline, described in Hesiod's *Works and Days*, in the generations of men from the godlike Golden Race to a fifth generation of Iron, in which the poet lives. The heroes of the *Iliad* belong to a fourth generation and are often performing feats beyond the power of Homer's (and our) generation.

Recall that Homeric heroes are lodged between gods and mortals. Christopher Jones (2010) traces how the qualifications for the status of "hero" were relaxed after Homer. Indeed, the *Odyssey* already embraces a wider notion of hero than the *Iliad*, where some women, such as Epicaste (both the wife and mother of Oedipus), while not called "heroines" are referred to as "the wives and daughters of heroes" (Jones 2010, p.5). See our panorama of the heroic landscape, ancient and modern, in the previous chapter. Modern heroes and heroines, it seems, can be soap opera stars and fictional characters, even "post-truth" public figures.

Ordinary mortals cannot imagine the powers of superheroes, although Nietzsche recalled the Superman (or Overman) from the summit and brought him within the grasp of ordinary mortals. Nietzsche's formula was elegant – humans are constrained by their arrogance in thinking that they can set out a value system that suits all other humans. The superman engages with the "transvaluation of all values" by first admitting that values are relative historically and culturally; and second, by engaging with the notion that one can critically examine one's own value system for its limits and foster tolerance of the values of others. For Nietzsche (2013), this was a mark of grand moral courage.

Such moral relativism was easily lampooned as an "anything goes" perspective, but Nietzsche did not condone this. Relativism included arguing cogently for the value of your own views and against the views of those who you thought peddled destructive values. The anti-heroism of Nietzsche now powers contemporary medical education with its central principles of "reflective practice" and "critical reflexivity" (Bleakley 1999).

One of us (RM) was of the generation that regularly worked over 100 hours a week, on rotas that could be one in two, and often one in three nights and weekends on call for 24 hours, and could work continuously from Friday morning to Monday evening with only a few hours' sleep (see chapter twelve). Currently, with the working time regulations under which the UK NHS works, doctors in training should not be working more than 48 hours per week, though the rules are flexible. Trainee doctors become irritated by the reflections of their seniors on how much harder life was for them. But those seniors had no sympathy from their consultants who, in the 1940s and 50s, had no rotas because they lived for a year, after qualifying, in hospital and were always available, only allowed out with special permission. And their consultants were doing the same but without pay. And so it went on, maintaining another pillar of medicine's mythology (Sinclair 1997).

When *The British Medical Journal* recently (White 2016) considered changes in the working conditions of doctors since the 1950s, the title of the piece – "Was there ever a golden age for junior doctors?" – echoed Hesiod's description of succeeding generations showing decline, from gold to iron.

Homeric heroes are generally of two types: force or craft

The *Iliad* and the *Odyssey* offer two styles of hero: Achilles models courage and force while Odysseus models craft or guile. Achilles' death and Odysseus' plan for the Wooden Horse are not recorded in the *Iliad*, but in the *Odyssey*. Of course it is an oversimplification to think of just two types of hero, but what Homer provides is a host of examples of how a variety of figures respond to these two complex hero archetypes, and under what circumstances their respective styles are successful and unsuccessful.

Heroes are a bloody mess

Achilles cuts and slashes the enemies' bodies amongst a stench of blood and gore. Surgery has often been seen as a microcosm of this, with the patient's body as the battlefield and the surgeon as the warrior flown in to save the day. As medicine is now cast as a business, so senior management take on the heroic roles of cutting and slashing, but now with budgets, and even senior surgeons must kowtow to these managers, who in turn are wrestling with senior politicians. Like Achilles wrestling the river, personified as the river-god Scamander, so CEOs wrestle with the flow of money and resources through their organisations.

But the flipside of this heroism is the collective daily acts of tenderness that doctors and healthcare practitioners show to their patients in distress. Medical students and junior doctors who come into medicine with heroic intentions need to remind themselves that wrestling the current is already a tired, nearly exhausted, metaphor that must change for a more caring medicine to emerge. They should go to the bed of the river they are wrestling, to discover that a patient is trying to rest. But the patient attempts to rest in vain, as pain kicks in. The young doctor might then test his or her approach to the bedside and linger a while, resisting being pulled away by the bigger current of frantic hospital routine and demands.

Importantly, can the young doctor allow himself catharsis in the face of such suffering? Does he fear that touching his own emotionally laden responses will somehow diminish his professionalism or display a weakness as another form of "bloody mess"? Must he damn the flood, or can he find relief somewhere, with a colleague, a mentor or a counsellor? There is a famous image of Achilles tending to Patroclus' wounds (figure 6-1) showing that even the most savage of warriors can find moments of deep compassion.

Conclusion

Today's medical students and young doctors prize differing values from those shaping previous generations - by not being afraid to say "I don't know" and that I can live with ambiguity; and by treating medicine as a job rather than a vocation. This does not mean that they do not take the job seriously and act professionally; but they generally eschew the tradition of heroism. In an era of standardisation (all must satisfy common, assessable competences), in which collaboration is preferred to competition, and patients have become experts in their own illnesses thanks to the ready availability of information, have we moved beyond Wheeler's assertion that doctors are heroes because patients need them to be? Indeed, "hero" can also offer an embarrassing tag. Where clinical teams look after patients collectively, so all must have prizes, and autonomy generally works against the grain of collective activity. Medical educators now vigorously promote this new landscape of democratic medicine and healthcare (Bleakley 2014).

The new heroes in medicine are perhaps anti-heroes. They are the collective picket line demonstrating against unfair work conditions and cuts to health services. It is not that the hero (and heroine) is going away – it is an archetype – rather, the hero is presenting in new and radical forms. Our aim in this, and the previous, chapter has been to use Homer as a background against which we can "think otherwise" about the hero, to articulate an understanding of this contemporary transformation of heroism as it applies to medical culture.

Heroes exhibit qualities strikingly echoed by some modern doctors and there is a likeness too in the social contexts that allow their behaviour to flourish. In the course of this and the previous chapter, we have seen two types of medical hero, or at least two very different qualities that might be considered heroic. One is the person who cares for others, knowing they put their own life at risk; the other, the person who stands out for a quality that they take to extreme – anger, devotion to work, opposition to power. The first quality is alien to Homer. If a hero is defined as someone who risks himself to help somebody else, then the heroes of Greek mythology qualify only in a limited sense.

A Greek hero will straddle the body of a wounded or dead comrade to effect his rescue, but does not go as a disinterested party to do good. For example, Aeneas straddles the body of the dead Pandarus and is himself wounded (by one of the great rocks described above). Only protection from his goddess mother Aphrodite saves his life (*Iliad* 5. 297-310). Later, Ajax rescues Teucer, (*Iliad* 8.330-4); Antilochus rescues Hypsenor (*Iliad* 13. 418-23); and, in a long passage, Menelaus protects the body of

Patroclus (*Iliad* 17.1-59). Here, the hero is the person who exhibits extraordinary levels of care and attention – but the Homeric hero does not go as a disinterested party to do good.

In her book *Heroes*, Lucy Hughes-Hallett (2005, p.8) asks "What makes a hero? And what are heroes for?" We have attempted to answer the first question and, with it, to justify claiming that some healthcare staff, and particularly some doctors, take on and occasionally seek the mantle of hero. The second question is important because there are good arguments for doing away with heroes. Meier (2011, p.94), in their support, argues that: "confronted with the futility of much human endeavour, they summoned up the possibility of human greatness" and, though today's heroes may not be so great, "the distinction is only one of proportion". In contrast, Bertolt Brecht (1995, 75-6), in his play "The Life of Galileo", has Galileo contradict another character, who says "Unhappy the land that has no heroes!" Galileo replies: "No. Unhappy the land that needs heroes." Similarly, Hughes-Hallett (2004, p.3, p.14) is sceptical about the need for heroes. She ends the introduction to her book:

> On 12th September 2011 a group of people were photographed near the ruins of the World Trade Center holding up a banner reading "We Need Heroes Now". This book is ... an attempt to examine that need, to acknowledge its urgency, and to warn against it.

Her reason is that:

> An exaggerated veneration for an exceptional individual poses an insidious temptation. It allows worshippers to abnegate responsibility looking to the great man for salvation or for fulfilment that they should more properly be working to accomplish for themselves.

Hughes-Hallett then progresses the Hegelian Master-Slave dialectic: patients need doctors and the populace needs heroes, but this is the first step in the populace absorbing heroism into the social body. Heroism is then democratised – something that would seem strange to the current of the *Iliad*, but fits perfectly with the embrace of collaborative endeavour at the end of the *Odyssey*. Patients too have come to absorb doctors into the social body and de-heroise medicine through demanding greater transparency and better communication. Patient-centredness has morphed in some areas of healthcare to patient-directedness (such as self-help groups on the Internet for specialist conditions; or the "Hearing Voices" network, reclaiming "schizophrenia" as a viable part of the spectrum of human experience that should not carry a stigma).

Through small group work with our students, we have often tackled issues relating to the qualities of a "good doctor". After the familiar suggestions of knowledgeable, hardworking, empathic, able to communicate well, and so on, one student suggested "dangerous". Obviously, he explained, not dangerous clinically, but edgy, demanding, working and thinking at the limits and against the grain. He was thinking of the sort of doctor who would resist the Agamemnon of his or her day, perhaps as a conscientious whistleblower.

A past president of the Royal College of Physicians, Professor Carol Black, argued that increased numbers of women doctors could cause the medical profession to lose power and influence (Hall 2004). We have predicted a move to an environment where female qualities of teamwork and cooperation predominate and this is to be applauded. We have framed this as part of the democratising of medicine in which the hero and heroic, as both emotional and knowledge capital, are reclaimed and shared by patients. Might we, though, miss our dangerous loner? One woman doctor in training has no doubts: "Perpetuating superhero imagery is deterring the future of our specialty ... may I suggest we admit our weaknesses, talk openly about our job, invite our juniors to shadow us, and take off our capes for good?" (Whiting 2016).

We have then, in this chapter, moved against the classical hero, describing (i) heroines, (ii) "shared" or "distributed" heroism as extraordinary collective work and activity in a democratic re-distribution of "hero capital", and (iii) anti-heroism, as ways that the hero may be re-presented and refreshed in contemporary medicine. Some may say that we have acted illegitimately, moving out of the realm of heroes altogether. We ask the reader to consider: as the sea change in medical culture that we describe earlier in this chapter progresses, let us see how the hero adapts. We cannot kill the hero - by definition "he" is invincible. But we will see how the hero gains voice in new, and perhaps surprising, ways in 21st century medicine.

CHAPTER THREE

PUTTING IT BLUNTLY

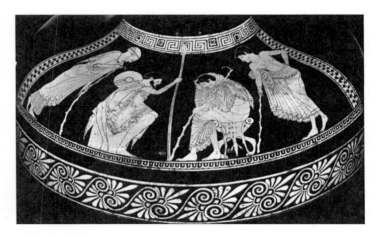

Figure 3-1: The Embassy scene

"I must speak out bluntly what I think and how it shall come to pass"
(Achilles in *Iliad* 9. 309–10).

Can "thinking otherwise" with Homer really help doctors to improve communication?

In current undergraduate medical curricula, much emphasis is placed on learning the skills of communication. This chapter "thinks otherwise" through Homer's *Iliad* as a way to address current dilemmas in communication skills training in medical education. We argue that how such skills are conceptualised and learned can be mechanistic, shallow and simplistic. Indeed, we recoil at the very idea that "communication" is a "skill". It is surely far deeper and more complex than the mechanical.

Homer was regarded in the Greek and Roman world as the father of rhetoric – the "communication skills" of the time. This reputation rested greatly on book 9 of the *Iliad*, most of which concerns an embassy from the Greek leaders to the now bitter, wrathful Achilles.

The mission of the three emissaries is to persuade Achilles to return to the ranks of the Greeks, who are being routed since his refusal to fight. They are sent to appease Achilles and to persuade him to return to the fray. We learn how the outcome of a conversation may be predetermined by the previous relationship of the speakers, and how a man beyond reason responds to reason; we should reflect that Homer's audience heard the piece knowing the outcome, giving it a tragic inevitability. Communication in medicine too is often in the tragic genre, paradoxically given an alliterative tag that borders on the lyrical: "breaking bad news".

We, the audience, cannot analyse Homeric discourse rationally, because in this, as in all communication, reason is disturbed by emotion. Treating communication as formulaic does not account for ambiguity, value conflicts, or unforeseen consequences, where medicine is a stochastic art - riddled with uncertainty. Teaching and learning communication skills through set, formulaic methods does not prepare medical students for the surprise elements in patient and colleague encounters as it bleaches out the key ingredients of idiosyncratic context and spontaneous emotional expression. Put another way, communication skills training makes a tragic mistake of treating a dynamic, complex, adaptive system (communication "on the go") as linear and open to an engineering analysis.

Much of Homer is formulaic, as we discuss in chapters four and five in particular, but this is a framework for recall of the narrative by the *rhapsodes* who sing the songs of Achilles and Odysseus. The narrative itself remains complex and open to improvisation as a response to context. Where students are taught formulaic methods of communication, such as how to break bad news, we see this as ill-preparedness for the liquidity of clinical work in which much communication with patients is spontaneous and unrehearsed. In contrast, it can be argued that a good deal of communication with colleagues remains formulaic as it is shaped by historical antecedents of how doctors should relate to other doctors and to other healthcare professionals hierarchically (for example, the ritual of the ward round – see chapter five).

Learning how to communicate now features prominently in the curricula of most health workers at undergraduate and postgraduate levels. How to elicit a history from a patient, to discuss treatment options, and to break bad news and deal with the distressed are regarded as clinical skills to be acquired through "cool" *in vitro* communication workshops - often in

"laboratories" under simulated conditions with simulated (actor) patients –
prior to "hot" *in vivo* clinical contact. Communication as script is scrapped
for impromptu coalface realities. This virtual rehearsal is made all the
more contradictory through the common use of videotape feedback and
analysis – all the while bleaching out the very issue that makes clinical
communication so challenging: the unexpected and emotionally coloured.

It is easy to forget that 40 years ago such educational methods would
have seemed extraordinary and unnecessary. Perhaps "communication"
was seen as unteachable. Certainly it would not be reduced to functional or
instrumental "skills". There are still plenty of students who doubt, in fact,
that this is a skills issue, believing that the ability to communicate is given,
and there is indeed some evidence that teaching communication skills in a
reductive way can be counter-productive (Willis et al 2003, Bleakley
2014), where such methods can paradoxically de-skill intuitive human
response, rather than afford a skill-set.

For Ivan Illich (2001), some educational methods parallel the de-
skilling of a human workforce, for example through the introduction of
specialties and specific technologies, stripping away the capital inherent in
the lay population. This includes the reduction of lively, complex human
interactions – conviviality – to instrumental competences, aligning humans
with machines and reducing: (i) the range of possible responses in
communication; (ii) the emotional and intuitive elements of communication;
and (iii) the complexity and liquidity of response to linear, pre-planned
and homogenised outcomes. While medicine and healthcare in general
properly claim territories and capital of skills and knowledge, areas such
as ethical and "professional" behaviour, such as communication, share a
good deal in common with lay social encounters and need not be
privatised by any specific profession.

In the ancient world, Homer was regarded as the father of many
branches of knowledge—rhetoric, tragedy, philosophy, and theology. This
chapter presents Homer as the unlikely father of "communication skills"
too. What has he to tell us across three millennia about talking and
listening to patients, their relatives and our colleagues? And what may we
learn from Homer that distinguishes him from other authors? We
concentrate on one book of the *Iliad*, book 9, to argue that the speeches
and silences of Agamemnon, Odysseus and Achilles show or conceal the
same hopes, fears and anxieties as those our patients experience. With this
familiarity, however, is mingled a strangeness of language, attitude and
belief.

It is this commingling of the familiar and strange, the civilised and
barbaric, in one of the greatest of literary works, that lets Homer teach us

across nearly 3000 years. We should learn from the close parallels, entwined with what is foreign, even repugnant, that any attempt to regiment the teaching of communication skills renders them banal and oversimplified. How context shapes and shades communication is learned with great force from a story that juxtaposes the familiar and domestic with events barbaric and fantastic; and that engages our emotions with immediacy in a language supposedly dead and a vocabulary archaic even when first written.

Book 9 of the *Iliad* is not essential to its action but is critical as an examination of the psychology of Achilles and the morality of his implacable anger, or rather "rage" (*menis*). There may well have been an earlier version of the *Iliad* that was simply a saga of war. There is evidence in this book of much original, unusual composition. A high proportion is direct speech as opposed to the author's narrative. It is tempting to attribute this special flavour to the genius of the "Homer" who crafted the final version of the story that has come down to us; tempting to suppose that he wanted to reshape the story and give it an ethical dimension that was entirely new to its audience. It is a special book:

> [Book 9] must have been created by the poet we call Homer, who would not have found the sort of pre-existing material for it which existed, say, for a standard battle scene. Both times we find direct speech deployed with great power (Griffin 2004).

The following is a précis of the events up to and including book 9, which provide most of the material on which our arguments are based. These arguments centre on learning how to communicate from an episode of miscommunication, itself set in an epic arising from an utter failure of communication. This failure arises partly from poor communication within a group and partly from a failure to move from entrenched positions. Both will strike a chord with anyone working in healthcare.

Up to now we have used the current convention "communication skills" to describe the very complex meeting of contextually-sensitive, historically- and culturally-tuned, ethically-sensitive, verbal and non-verbal utterances and performances that we characteristically reduce to the instrumental descriptor "skills" (just as we reduce "education" to "training"). Communication is perhaps better described as a performative "capability". We will continue to use the descriptor "skill" throughout this chapter as a convention. The reader should know that in our own minds, as we use this descriptor, we also bracket it out, or suspend its "closure" as the best term to use.

By the way, we have nothing against skills. Skills can be complicated, but they are not complex – for example, there are limits to their transferability. The word "skill" originates in 12th century Middle English and Old Norse, meaning "discernment". This is now obsolete, but is actually far closer to our understanding of what a "communication skill" in medicine can be. That a doctor *discerns* a patient's mood (and hopefully responds sensitively and appropriately) seems to us to be much closer to what actually happens in clinical communication than a practiced but disconnected response that may signal a hollow encounter.

The Embassy

Agamemnon, the Greek leader, has taken the woman Briseis, a treasured war-prize of Achilles, from him. Achilles was barely restrained by the goddess Athene from killing Agamemnon and has now sworn to take no further part in the fighting. He is by far the greatest fighter of the Greeks and his absence will be a disaster, causing many deaths. He departs to his section of the Greek camp with his army, and his anger festers.

The Trojans, assisted by Zeus, face the Greeks in open battle and beat them back to the Greek camp just shy of their beached vessels. As night falls, the Greek leaders debate how to avert inevitable disaster the next day and recommend to Agamemnon that he send an embassy to Achilles, offering gifts by way of apology to entice him back to action. Agamemnon reluctantly agrees, recognising his error and detailing the gifts he is prepared to offer by way of restitution. Three ambassadors of very different character are selected — Phoenix, an old retainer of Achilles' father; Odysseus, skilled in counsel; and Ajax, a straight-talking soldier.

Achilles greets the ambassadors warmly, calling them "old friends". They are taken into his shelter and given food and drink. In an enigmatic start to the debate, Ajax nods to Phoenix to lead off, but Odysseus intercepts the glance and begins. He makes a speech of 80 lines, the central part of which - nearly half - is a repetition of Agamemnon's offer of goods of restitution. He begins with brief thanks for their meal, then moves on to the military defeat that has occurred and the worse that threatens, emphasising the successes of Hector—guaranteed to irritate Achilles, for Hector is the only Trojan on a par with him. He urges Achilles to get back to battle now—there will be no point after their ships are burned. Achilles' own father warned him to govern his pride (or "great-hearted spirit"). Then he lists Agamemnon's promised gifts. He ends by asking him to take pity on the beaten Greeks, who would heap glory on him if he returns, especially if he kills Hector. Given the reputation for both Odysseus' wisdom and cunning, it is a remarkably underwhelming speech. It reminds us of many occasions when we have seen very talented and inventive clinicians giving underwhelming presentations to hospital CEOs or key management committees; or under-selling themselves in bids for research grant awards.

Achilles' reply is half as long again as Odysseus'—much longer, given that it lacks the repetitive offer of gifts in Odysseus'. It is an argument of passion rather than logic, of a young man consumed by notions of honour and dishonour. He replies to the last of Odysseus' arguments by saying that there is no point in being brave and active: the cowardly and the brave are rewarded alike; when he sacked many towns around Troy, the lion's share of the booty went to Agamemnon. He goes on to question whether the sons of Atreus (Agamemnon and Menelaus) are the only men who love their wives. Agamemnon robbed him of the woman he loved. He will pack up his booty and return home. Not all the gifts in the world could win him back; first, Agamemnon must pay in kind for the humiliation he has endured. Let them relay that back to the Greek leaders forthwith.

There is a shocked silence. Phoenix bursts into tears and asks what is to become of him, Phoenix, if Achilles returns home. Phoenix then gives a lengthy account of how he had to leave his own home, was welcomed and honoured by Achilles' father and became Achilles' nurse and mentor. This gives him the moral power to tell Achilles to abandon his pride and inflexibility. He tells—part metaphor, part theology—how Prayers, the daughters of Zeus, follow Sin (or *Atē*) around the world. ("Sin" is a poor translation of the Greek *atē*).[1]

The man who fails to listen to these daughters of Zeus is himself punished by *atē*. Let Achilles be placated by the generous offer of Agamemnon and the entreaties of his friends. Phoenix goes on to tell a long story about an earlier hero, Meleager, as an example of another inflexible, angered hero. Meleager had refused all gifts and entreaties until his town was in flames. He then, of his own conscience, came out and beat off the attackers, winning neither honour nor goods.

Achilles' reply is brief. He has no need of honour from the Achaeans. Phoenix should not curry favour with Agamemnon by trying to persuade him. Let Phoenix stay the night and sail home with him in the morning. Achilles then signals to his comrade Patroclus to make up a bed for Phoenix, expecting the other two to take the hint to leave.

Ajax, rather than speaking to Achilles, says to Odysseus that they should report their failure at once to the Greek leaders; and, continuing as if they had already left Achilles, condemns him as cruel and arrogant for spurning his comrades: even the family of a murdered man accepts blood money from the killer. Then he addresses Achilles directly: the gods have made him implacable over a single girl and here is Agamemnon offering him seven more. He should remember his friends and his obligations as a host. Achilles very briefly repeats his fury over the way he has been dishonoured. He will not return to war before Hector has set fire to the Greek ships. Ajax and Odysseus then depart, leaving Phoenix behind.

Perhaps Ajax, Phoenix and Odysseus fail to persuade Achilles because their arguments are poor or their collective rhetoric is blunt, while their deliveries are graceless and without form. In other words, they fall to the lowest common denominator, equivalent to pedagogies that resort to reductive, instrumental skills training. This is laziness. It is as if they have resorted to blindly following an introductory text rather than following their hearts, allowing improvisation and speaking with sensitivity to context. They neither compose nor are composed, but bluster and fumble their way through the equivalent of three weak business conference presentations. Of course, in the narrative, this sets up Achilles for a magnificent and unexpected rejoinder. Homer's narrative offers a situated de-skilling of Ajax, Phoenix and Odysseus, exposing the vulnerabilities of the best of men.

Embassy scenarios in the clinic and on the ward

"Communication skills" in medicine are usually understood to mean communication between healthcare worker and patient. We would like to interpret the term more broadly—communicating with patients, other professionals and the public, through the written and spoken word. Communication is a dynamic and complex activity system, an embodied cognition situated historically and culturally as discourse. As we suggest above, to disaggregate individual "skills" from this complex is a dangerous business, potentially reducing communication to only the communicator and an instrumental act. We use this scene from the *Iliad* almost as a metaphor for our own communications. In many of our interactions we listen and interpret confidently and comfortably, but we can be jolted out of our preconceptions by physical or verbal incongruity. So, in this passage, we have to set the rationality of the argument of the protagonists against the savagery of the battle scenes, the boasting of heroes over the corpses of the vanquished and the petty vindictiveness of the gods.

We will consider five dimensions to doctor-patient communication in the clinic and the ward: (i) preparing for consultations, (ii) cultural contexts, (iii) ambiguity and complexity, (iv) teaching communication, and (v) communication failure.

Preparing for consultations

In a chapter devoted to the angry, aggressive patient, Coid (1991) emphasises the importance of preparation, getting right those factors that are outside the consultation itself – preconceived attitudes, having the right colleagues with one, and body language. When the Greek leaders meet before the Embassy, two of them make clear their condemnation of Agamemnon. By implication, the ambassadors approach their interview in sympathy with the anger of Achilles. The three colleagues were chosen with care by the venerable counsellor, Nestor, and he ensures that they are fully prepared before they leave:

> Nestor the Gerenian charioteer gave them many instructions,/ Looking to each man, but especially to Odysseus, / To try to persuade the noble Achilles (*Iliad* 9. 179–81).

We are not given the reasons for their selection, but they are self-evident. Phoenix helped to raise Achilles from childhood. Ajax is a comrade in arms, almost an equal in battle. Odysseus is essential because he is a great speaker; Helen described his eloquence in an earlier book:

> But when he let forth his great voice from his breast/ And words like to winter snowflakes,/ No other mortal might then contend with Odysseus (*Iliad* 3. 221–3).

Odysseus is also renowned for his cunning. *Polumetis*—"of many counsels"—is one of the epithets most commonly applied to him. The arrival of the three colleagues is reminiscent of the "three wise men" system – described in chapter two - once used in the UK National Health Service as a mechanism for resolving professional and management difficulties with consultant doctors (DHSS 1986). To have these rather shadowy figures - chosen more for eminence than wisdom (very like Greek heroes) - arrive on your doorstep must have engendered similar feelings in their victim as in Achilles. As with many modern encounters, Achilles, Odysseus and Ajax all carry a baggage of emotion, reputation and history with them into the meeting. At one point, Achilles says: "The man is as hateful to me as the gates of Hell/ Who hides one thing in his heart and says another" (*Iliad* 3. 312–3). Directed at no one in particular, this is an Achilles' aphorism or wise saying about duplicity in another. On first impression, this refers to the hated Agamemnon, but there is an implicit reference to Odysseus "of many counsels".

As for body language, the interview starts strangely, with Odysseus intercepting a nod from Ajax to Phoenix intended to encourage the latter to speak first. But Odysseus pre-empts Phoenix. Why? What is the tacit underpinning to the explicit nod and its interception? We are not told. The *Iliad* has many touches of theatre like this but it is the sort of incident that might foul an interview.

Cultural contexts

An examination of consultations between students and patients led to a summary of the components of good and bad communication styles (Robert et al 2003). Good communication involved attentive responding, joint problem solving, and face saving (directed at the patient); poor communication was characterised by inappropriate responses, schema-driven progression (that is, moving the conversation on to fulfil the speaker's own agenda), and insensitivity to the patient's level of understanding. The authors also felt that the consultations often hinged around one or more critical moments or remarks. A final element was the set of assumptions that the interviewers brought with them to the encounter. The authors might have been describing this book of Homer.

The ambassadors exhibit great powers of listening, but there is more listening than hearing. They are goal-driven and approach the meeting with a fixed agenda that cannot mould itself in response to Achilles' passionate rejection (Scodel 2008). It is interesting above all to see "face saving" emerging from a discourse analysis of modern patient consultations. Face was everything to a Greek hero. The loss of face that Achilles suffered from Agamemnon's taking of Briseis is the main problem with which the ambassadors have to grapple in this book (as well as the source of the wrath that is central to the theme of the *Iliad*).

In his reply to Odysseus' offer, Achilles himself says: "Agamemnon will not persuade my spirit until he has repaid me all the bitter humiliation" (*Iliad* 9. 387). The implication is that Agamemnon can repay only through his own humiliation; any gifts offered through Odysseus can never be adequate recompense. This is the crux of the argument and it is ignored. Achilles himself is not playing by the rules because, in an honour society (Benedict 1946), both sides must save face and he is wishing humiliation on Agamemnon. Hainsworth (1993) states that the language is deliberately obscure at this point. Otherwise, Achilles might be too obviously at fault.

However, this is an instrumental reading of the *Iliad*. It is easy to be seduced by the simplicity of models of communication skills. We might learn more from broader reflections about the sensitivity engendered by close reading of a great and, to us, strange epic. Reading the *Iliad* for this purpose rather than just for pleasure is like opening a Russian doll—there is always one more level of interpretation.

Pendleton and colleagues (Pendleton et al 2004) recognise the importance of the cultural context within which consultations are embedded: "Doctors and patients and the nature of the consultations between them are profoundly influenced by the social and cultural context in which they take place". Examining discourse so far removed from our own should make us reflect on not how strange it is, but how strange our own might be. Making the familiar strange is the first rule of post-modern thinking and a key part of "thinking otherwise".

Angry patients make for complex consultations. Maguire and Pitceathly (2004) tell us that doctors tend to distance themselves from these encounters partly to protect their own emotions and partly because they believe they are protecting the patient. This belief is mistaken, because an exploration of the anger can reveal causes of which patients are themselves unaware. The ambassadors attempt no such exploration. Probably they feel its causes are obvious, since all of them were present at the original quarrel.

Harris (2001) argues that the story of Meleager's anger clearly recognises and parallels that of Achilles. It is, however, an unsubtle sermon, not likely to appease—the speech of a man going into a meeting with an agenda. But anger is rarely simple and cannot be isolated from both cultural and motivational settings. Although it has been mentioned only once so far in the *Iliad*, Homer's audience would have been aware of the choice Achilles has already made between a long but obscure life with a loving family, or death at Troy that will bring everlasting fame. In his angry reply to Odysseus, Achilles refers to this choice explicitly for the only time in the *Iliad*:

> My mother, the goddess Thetis of the silver feet, tells me/ That two fates await me on the path to death./ If I stay and fight at the city of the Trojans,/ There will be no homecoming for me but I shall have glory imperishable./ If I return to the beloved home of my fathers,/ My goodly fame shall perish, though I shall have long life/ And no swift end of death shall come near me (*Iliad* 9. 410–6).

This sense of the futility of his sacrifice is an obvious spur to his anger but is not acknowledged by his colleagues. Indeed there is a striking absence of reply by any of them to the individual points that Achilles makes. Schein (1984) describes the complexity of Achilles' reply, which swings between rational argument and passionate outburst. It is a denial of the very heroic principles upon which Achilles' life is based, a denial that makes it a very modern argument and juxtaposes the strange and the familiar within Homer's storytelling. The language and imagery that Achilles uses emphasise how alone he is, how set apart from other mortals. It is a wonderful speech, which his colleagues completely ignore or misunderstand.

Ambiguity and complexity

The three ambassadors are chosen for the different attributes that they bring. For a Greek audience, this understates it. Ajax and Odysseus would have been archetypes of the qualities for which they were renowned. Ajax goes into the interview as great warrior, bearer of a massive shield, slow in attack but indomitable in defence, a simple thinker. Odysseus, as we have seen, is the wily tactician and eloquent persuader. Such archetypes are characteristic of Homer. We look to the modern novel for psychological subtlety and complexity. Not so in communication skills training, where facilitators of professional or student groups are taught to deal with the Achilles and Agamemnons of those groups in terms that translate archetypes into stereotypes.

For example, Hackett and Martin (1993) categorise participants as "the mummy", "the windbag", "the rambler", and "the homesteader"; while Hanson (1981) employs the stereotypes of "the turtle", "the bull in a china shop", and "the interviewer". An archetype stimulates deep thinking because it is invariably both complex and ambiguous. Stereotypes are purposely simplified to get things tied up, explained. Archetypes are crafted, where stereotypes are out of a mould or manufactured. Perhaps the three wise men – Ajax, Phoenix and Odysseus - fail to impress where they appear as caricatures. It is like the PBL facilitator who habitually responds to medical students' questions with further questions, producing a low, barely audible, collective moan; or worse, an awkward silence.

There is rigidity about communication skills training, as if it is all about transmitting what is common, reproducible, transferable, and dependable. Kurtz and colleagues (Kurtz et al 1998) make no bones about this, saying: "communication is not a personality trait but a series of learned skills", the justification being that "the acquisition of skills can open the path to changes in attitude". Robert and colleagues (Robert et al 2003) clearly felt qualms about this approach, commenting that: "a more fine-grained understanding of the attributes of good and poor medical communication is needed to improve communications teaching".

Stereotyping is just one area of communication skills training that will lead us to a mechanistic, oversimplified approach.

Stereotypes, it seems, are rarely stable or sustainable. Characters remain complex. Odysseus becomes a devious and ruthless manipulator in another story, Sophocles' *Philoctetes*. In the *Iliad*, Homer, too, is capable of complexity. Just a few hundred lines beyond book 9, Odysseus shares in the irrational and savage killing of a Trojan spy. Ajax, after the Trojan War, is driven mad and commits suicide when he fails to win the armour of the dead Achilles, and so forth.

Teaching communication

The Greek equivalent of "communication skills" would have been rhetoric, which was one of the cornerstones of ancient Greek education. Homer was regarded as the father of rhetoric, a reputation that depended in large part on the Embassy scene of the *Iliad*. Ancient rhetoric had a purpose different from modern communication skills, being designed above all to persuade, by both reason and emotion. There was a real need to develop rhetorical skills in the ancient world. The young democracies arose in city-states small enough to let every citizen have his (definitely "his"!) say quite literally on matters political and legal. With no skill, a citizen would be disadvantaged materially and could find himself banished or even executed if at the wrong end of a lawsuit (recall the fate of Socrates). It is a sort of democratic process—the need to give patients more "voice"—that drives communication skills training now.

We should remember, then, that training in rhetoric fell into the hands of the Sophists, much despised by Plato as purveyors of technique without knowledge, particularly moral knowledge. Our contemporary training of communication skills follows the orthodoxy of our day. It is not in some absolute sense "right". Indeed, it is rare to see study of rhetorical devices on communication skills curricula, although study of communication through rhetoric has revealed that surface "communications" can dissimulate, distracting from, or negating, deeper motives (Bleakley 2006a, b).

The speeches of this book, particularly that of Odysseus, were regarded as exemplars from which later rhetoric developed. One feature that must strike a modern reader is the degree of straight talking, something that has recently been lauded as necessary in politics, mistakenly called "pragmatism", placed in opposition to a misunderstood "political correctness" associated with "liberal, establishment politics", and producing a "post-truth" climate whose natural habitat is Twitter.

At the beginning of the book, when the embassy is being planned, Diomedes tells Agamemnon that Zeus may have given him power but failed to give him courage. During the Embassy, Odysseus tells Achilles that he has forgotten his father's injunction to keep his temper, Phoenix tells him he should not have a merciless heart and Ajax refers to him as merciless and wicked—all apparently without offending Achilles, who shows a robustness in receiving criticism now lost. Achilles himself at the beginning of the *Iliad* calls Agamemnon a "drunken sot, with the eyes of a dog and the courage of a deer" (*Iliad* 1. 225) – brave, even reckless, words to one's commander-in-chief.

This straight talking is at odds with current concepts of "feedback" to students and peers. These recommend that critical comments should be introduced only after consideration of what was good; blunt talk is likely to be considered unprofessional. Straight talking developed into the skilful and eloquent vituperation of Demosthenes and Cicero. Both in Homer and in later Greece and Rome, those skills were not without risk. Orators put their lives at risk from their powerful opponents.

Communication failure

The action of the *Iliad* is predetermined: Achilles knows he will die soon; we know that he will rebuff his colleagues so that the tragic sequence of events can unfold and "the will of Zeus be brought to pass". The literature on communication skills has little to say about the consequences of failure. They are well illustrated by many anecdotes in the "Fillers" sections of the *British Medical Journal*, or by standing in the queue at your butcher's. We leave many patients and colleagues and meetings with a feeling that failure was inevitable. Perhaps we should read our own communication failures as part of a wider story, learn from them, and take that store of wisdom to future encounters. Book 9 of the *Iliad* functions to develop not the action but the ethics of the poem. In the passionate speeches of Achilles we see him first realising the emptiness of the heroic ideal, a theme to which he returns at the end of the *Iliad* after killing Hector.

Communication skills too can be taught as if they were unhinged from emotion – as exercises in rational planning - but it is emotion that disrupts the pre-planned clinical encounter. We can learn much about how emotions colour communication from the Embassy scene.

There is, however, a huge gulf of understanding of the origin of emotional life between Homer and our 21st century lives. We tend to think of emotions as personal and interior. As Ruth Padel's (1992, 1995) meticulous analysis of the language of the ancient world shows, "emotion" is something that visits us, from outside, and lodges in us. A fear, an ecstasy, a chilling anxiety, was often personified as a god, a force or an animal-like presence, which gripped you, or entered the liver, heart or lungs to make an impression. The expression of emotion then followed.

When standing on the edge of a cliff, where we would say that the fear of falling is "in" us, the ancient Greeks would say that the fear is "in" the potential fall. Emotion is already shared, collaborative, distributed. Surely this has something to tell us about "communication skills" for clinical teamwork? In a team setting, how is an "atmosphere" or "climate" initiated, distributed, maintained, resisted and felt collaboratively (Lewis et al 2005)? Is this not key to effective teamwork around patients?

Part of the "fine-grained understanding" that Robert and colleagues (Robert et al 2003) speak of might come from considering how the reader of the *Iliad* is aware of both strangeness and familiarity: strange in its language, which predates classical Greek by several hundred years; strange in the part played by the gods— immortal, mighty and largely irresponsible; strange in the habits and beliefs of the human protagonists; and strange as it must be after three millennia. Yet modern readers constantly identify with its themes and find echoes to take into their own encounters. The human condition illustrated by Homer is uncomfortably familiar.

For example, we 21st century readers, steeped in the romance of recent centuries, feel our hearts go out to Achilles mourning his lost love. But just before the end of book 9, the episode with Achilles ends with Achilles, Phoenix and Patroclus settling down for the night. Achilles—he who minutes before had described passionately how he was robbed of the woman he loved, who because of the wrath he attributed to that love is prepared to let Greeks die and the Greek army come to the brink of defeat—seeks solace in the arms of Diomede of the lovely cheeks. This Diomede, and Briseis the woman stolen from him, are both prizes of war—in 21st century terms, victims of rape. We need to pause often in our interpretations of any narrative to detect the lenses through which the story is refracted. We are all too familiar with contemporary episodes of women taken captive as sex slaves for the conquering army.

Above all, let us avoid reduction of the complex to the simplistic and formulaic, as communication skills training can so easily do; and let us pause on how reading Homer can shift gears in our perceptions and thinking, to "think otherwise". We forget that even our talk about ownership of emotions is historically and culturally formed, so that it seems strange to think with Homer that emotions visit us. Stepping outside of our habits is the first step to appreciating what is "other" to us, or alien.

But this move of "relativising" could be the first step in communication skills education for doctors. It is medical education as re-skilling, not de-skilling.

Notes

1. A discussion of its meaning in this context is given by Hainsworth (2000) and there is a wider discussion in the first chapter of Dodds (1951).

CHAPTER FOUR

LOST IN TRANSLATION

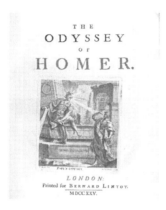

Figure 4-1: Pope's *Odyssey*

"Translation it is that openeth the window, to let in the light"
(Preface to *King James Bible*).

Receiving a history

"Taking a history" is the process of a doctor rephrasing the story a patient tells into medical terms. Our students at Peninsula College of Medicine and Dentistry, UK were encouraged not to "take" a history, but to "receive" it, an innovation emphasising the importance of listening, of respecting the voice of the patient. However, intervention even at this first level of translation is often lost at a second level, when the history is converted into a written, permanent record that enters the patient's notes. Here, the patient's voice is usually lost in translation and the patient's notes are absorbed to become part of the fabric of the medical community.

    "Taking" a history can have serious unintended consequences. It is an old saw in medicine that most of the diagnosis can be found in the patient's story. William Osler's most famous saying was "listen to your patient, he is telling you the diagnosis". Yet, between 10-15% of patients seen in primary care specialties (family medicine, internal medicine and paediatrics) are misdiagnosed, and misdiagnosis is a leading cause of malpractice claims in the USA (Sanders 2010). Lucian Leape and colleagues (Leape et al 1991) studied more than 30,000 hospitalised patients' records to claim that diagnostic errors accounted for 17% of adverse events; and these figures have been confirmed in more recent studies (Boodman 2013). Misdiagnosis does not matter when the patient gets better, or gets worse but returns to the doctor; however, some misdiagnoses can lead to adverse effects.

Recognising the importance of listening closely to patients' stories, narrative medicine has become the dominant form of the medical humanities. Literature is a great source for learning not only empathy, but also ethics. Contemporary narrativists in the medical humanities however warn us against over-interpretation of patients' stories. Johanna Shapiro (2011) fears narrative medicine becoming inflated through smart textual approaches that question the authenticity or reliability of patients' stories, and calls for "narrative humility" from researchers. Humanities-based researchers who study medical culture *in vitro*, but have little or no experience of that culture *in vivo*, may offer inflated theoretical notions about how both the lay public and clinicians think narratively, also perhaps ignoring Galen Strawson's (2004) important warning that some of us do not think narratively, and that the narrative movement has developed into a form of imperialism.

Delese Wear and Julie Aultman (2005) warn that exposing medical students to discomfiting literature can produce defensiveness and resistance to confronting issues central to good medical practice such as inequality and oppression. Students may readily tolerate benign plots and characters, but transgressive and challenging plots and characters at first produce resistance rather than empathy. This does not mean that we should avoid use of challenging literature in medical education, but rather that we are aware of potential resistance, narrative imperialism, and over-smart or inflated narrativist approaches. Each of these is an issue of translation from medical practice to patient experience using literary media and metaphors.

In a broad-brush challenge, Claire Hooker and Estelle Noonan (2011) point to the medical humanities' largely unexamined Western imperialistic tendencies, an issue that we explore later, in relation to the translator as potential coloniser. We can develop this idea. Where narrative is framed as story understood by privileged Westerners, "other" cultures have other ways of framing, telling, and listening to story. Of course, the lay patient is "other" to the professional doctor – they already inhabit different territories. Listening is the first part of the process of translation, but doctors have to record what happens; and, in teaching students and juniors, relay what they have gleaned from listening to patients, medical colleagues, and other healthcare professionals. Further, this happens both formally (case notes, case meetings, ward rounds), and informally (corridor conversations, coffee room chat, slips of confidentiality at social events).

We recognise, then, the value of narrative approaches to communication in medicine – particularly doctor-patient encounters, and we frame this as an issue of translation. We also recognise that translation may not happen within a narrative mindset or frame.

Translation matters

The interaction between patient and doctor may or may not be viewed narratively, but is a transaction that involves translation, where: "the physician's concern is to translate the subjective experience of illness into the recognizable discourse of medicine" (Hunter 1991, p.53), and "Diagnosis is a thoroughly semiotic activity: an analysis of one symbol system followed by its translation into another" (Kleinman 1988, p.10). Much may be lost in translation during this transaction (Roter and Hall 2006). Translation too, as T.S. Eliot in "Little Gidding" tells us, is sensitive to historical context: "For last year's words belong to last year's language and next year's words await another voice".

While clinical encounters have been studied as social transactions - interpersonal communications or teamwork effects – they have not been looked at specifically from the point of view of translation studies. Here, we mobilise study of translations of Homer as a lens through which we can rethink, in particular, doctor-patient encounters. In "thinking otherwise" with Homer about translation, we may gain a new perspective on doctor-patient communication, one that insists we think metaphorically.

First, however, what of literal translation in medicine, where the patient does not speak the first language of the hospital? Pauline Chen (2009), in the context of a North American healthcare system in which many patients do not have English as their first language, notes that, despite the availability of translators, doctors will often forge ahead with treatment, rationalising that contacting a translator will eat up valuable time. Chen quotes studies showing that this can be a misjudgement. Good communication between doctor and patient is part of the treatment process, from diagnosis through prognosis and treatment.

Even when a translator is called in, there can be issues. Bleakley (2017) notes that while translation in medicine is often thought of as a literal process, translators often work with metaphors - where there is not a straightforward correspondence between, say, a first hospital language of English and a patient's first language where the patient does not speak English. Such situations are becoming increasingly common as there is greater flow of people across borders, either by choice or forced as refugees of war or political crisis.

"Translation" itself is a metaphor and the waters of translation are already murky. Teodora Manea is a philosopher and medical ethicist who also works as a medical translator across three languages – English (her adopted language), Romanian (her first language) and German. In conversation with her, we learned much about the process of translation. Imagine a non-English-speaking patient arriving at an Accident and Emergency department with acute abdominal pain, at a loss as to how to describe the onset, location and severity of the pain. The doctor is unable to explain that he suspects that this is a gallstone that has migrated from the gallbladder and is lodging in the bile duct. How might "gallstone" translate into terms a layperson might understand? This is not big enough to be a stone, or even a pebble, and "grit" does not do the job. The conversation, with the patient in increasing pain, reaches an impasse. The work of the translator is to explain to the patient whatever the doctor says, with clarity. This is achieved largely through metaphor, but the terrain is slippery.

Metaphors are embedded in specific languages and are not universal; and to attempt to literally translate a metaphor from one language to another is a compound error. While medical interpreting assumes bridging between the host's and the patient's languages, and positions the interpreter as invisible, the reality is that interpretation happens in a live context where the interpreter is an agent and not just a facilitator, and "bridging" is disrupted by issues of what is lost in translation.

Illustrative examples quickly bring this alive. Teo discussed with us a male patient in cardiology undergoing an angiogram, in which a catheter is introduced into an artery in the groin area. "Groin" is derived from the Old English *grynde* meaning an "abyss", "hollow" or a "depression" – this is some way from the actual "fold" between the thigh and abdomen. "Groin" is already a troublesome word. Doctors refer to the "inguinal" area - that is of no help to the patient's understanding - but describing the groin as "between the legs" muddies the waters even more.

In languages other than English, the equivalent to "groin" can refer to architectural features such as the edge between intersecting vaults. In

German, the nearest equivalent is *leiste* that literally means a "thin, long piece of wood", or a "strip". A metaphor in German for the inguinal region is then a "narrow bar" – literally fine, but in English this could mean a tight passageway in a pub, or a thin piece of metal; and now we are miles away from the groin. In Romanian, there is no specific term for groin, and the next usual approximation will be "between legs". Along with the unspecificity of the language, the (older) male patient and (younger) female interpreter interaction complicated the dialogue even further.

Translation in medicine is usually thought of differently from metaphor in communication: either the literal need for translators where patients do not speak the first language of the hospital, as above; or "translational medicine" - the process of turning medical research into artifacts (medical devices, drugs) and practices that can be used in the treatment of patients. "Translation" is also commonly used to refer to putting theory or ideas into practice, or applying research findings.

Yet, even in the technical realm, translation needs metaphor. In fact, the Greek *metaphorá* (μεταφορά) means "to carry across". A metaphor carries meaning from one thing to another ("it's all Greek to me"). "Translation" comes from the Latin *translatio*, having the same meaning as the Greek *metaphorá* - to carry across. While medicine is constantly translating technically, we can only get to grips with technical issues, such as the chemistry of nucleic acids and proteins, through metaphor. So, the coded information of DNA is read and transcribed by "messenger" RNA, which translates it into amino acids that are the building blocks of proteins. This is by means of transfer-RNA ("transfer" is also from the same Latin root as "translate"). Translation is a metaphorical practice. Let us expand on this.

Issues of translation in healthcare contexts

There are four commonly encountered issues of translation in healthcare. First, the literal problem of translation, where healthcare workers globally struggle to understand patients whose language is not their own, as already noted. There is a persistent idea that translation should be literal, or faithful to the original. We have seen that even in "literal" translation we quickly enter waters muddied by metaphor. While patient-centred medicine encourages understanding of, and respect for, the patient's perspective, it is hard to see how doctors can remain faithful to every account that a patient brings. "Close reading" and interpretation of the "patient as text" comes with the job (Bleakley et al 2011). Patients' accounts are not necessarily trustworthy, and dialogue between doctor and patient is a process of negotiation of meanings. Clinical encounters are dramatic performances – doctors and patients in the process of "impression management" (Goffman 1959). Medical encounters such as consultations, and especially emergency visits, are elastic, not straightforward, often shot through with ambiguity.

Second, are translations between patients and healthcare providers. This area has been introduced above. A meta-review by Roter and Hall (2006) on studies of communication in medicine reveals generally poor translations by doctors of patients' stories leading to misunderstandings, misdiagnoses, and inappropriate treatments. This is acute in psychiatry, where, for example, the more bizarre and florid symptoms of psychosis are often like a language from another country that does not literally exist.

While orthodox treatments eschew issues of translation by attempting to normalise bizarre expressions through chemical and psychological treatments, more radical methods have attempted to translate across borders. For example, the schizophrenic communities set up by Felix Guattari in France and Ronald Laing in the UK explicitly set out to understand the world of psychosis not by translating that language into the reductive terminology of the current *Diagnostic and Statistical Manual of Mental Disorders V*, but by inhabiting the territory and language games of psychosis as a legitimate, indeed, poetic expression.

Laing (1972) then translates both neurotic and psychotic symptoms as a series of "knots" or complex encounters expressed as poems. Again, communication is neither literal nor direct, but metaphorical and staged. The "Hearing Voices" patient-directed movement (https://www.hearing-voices.org), supported particularly by more radical clinical psychologists, refuses labels such as "schizophrenia" and takes auditory hallucinations as a legitimate – albeit often deeply disturbing - experience to be appreciated rather than translated back into "normality" through psychiatric intervention. People with experience of hearing voices ask for translation against the grain – from the "normal" to their worlds.

It is debatable whether or not Laing and associates were guilty of romanticising the suffering of so-called psychotic people, and this reminds us again that translation is not necessarily benign. Indeed, where the "anti-psychiatrists" claimed that conventional psychiatric treatments offered an imperialism, a conquering and control of a state (of mind), the radical interventions (or conscious non-interventions) of the anti-psychiatrists might also be seen as a form of imperialism, potentially colonising the vulnerable.

Third, is the issue of translation across healthcare colleagues – between healthcare staff and health and social care support professions; and within medicine, between medical specialties. Given the increasing use of symbols, abbreviations and acronyms in the medical record, it already often looks like another language, inviting loss of nuances of meaning in the process of translation. Mis-translation and loss in translation are commonly encountered between professions even when working in the same team, but more commonly between teams. For example, where nurses typically work to "time", allocated democratically between patients, surgeons typically work to "task" – finishing whatever needs to be done however long it takes. Psychiatrists working with clinical psychologists find that the latter are sceptical of drug therapies as they are more psychologically oriented therapeutically, refusing to medicalise the patient. This approach is not readily translated across the medical blood-brain barrier, where drug therapies are currency.

In terms of within-medicine cross-specialty communication, a study of the rhetoric used in referral letters for the same patient reveals issues of mistranslations of meaning (Lingard et al 2004). A surgeon treating a knife wound writes an innocuous letter to a patient's GP informing her of optimal follow-up treatment, where a psychiatrist writes about the same patient informing the GP that the fight the patient got in to that caused the knife wound was probably due to instability in withdrawing from a long-term antipsychotic medication.

Fourth, (mis)translations between colleagues reveal that patients' "conditions" are enacted differently across different specialties. For example, Annemarie Mol (2002) shows that cardiologists, vascular surgeons, nurses, radiologists, pathologists, laboratory scientists, and patients enact atherosclerosis – hardening of the arteries – differently. The condition is not understood technically in differing ways, rather it is experienced differently, offering a variety of ontologies. Thus "a plaque cut out of an atherosclerotic artery is not the same entity as the problem a patient with atherosclerosis talks about in the consulting room, even though they are both called by the same name" (Mol 2002, p.vii Preface).

In the following section we grapple with how "thinking with Homer" might illuminate such issues of translation in medical contexts. We argue that translation studies themselves can throw light in particular on the critical first step of medicine's translation of person into patient. We examine translations of Homer using them as templates to open up the question of how translation studies can be applied to medicine and medical education, particularly to better understand the process of taking (or receiving) a history. Our method is to investigate both likenesses and striking contrasts between medicine and literary translation. We recognise that this engages us in meta-translation. We do not wish to move too far

away from patients' and doctors' experiences and so will ground our brief
analyses in medical encounters.

Translating Homer

There are hundreds of translations of Homer. Let us take a scene from the
beginning of the *Iliad*, where Achilles quarrels with Agamemnon, setting
the tone and theme for the rest of the epic (*Iliad* 1. 225-32). Achilles is
about to draw his sword and kill Agamemnon, but the goddess Athene
stops him. Rieu (1950) is one of the best-known translators of the modern
era (although his translation is now nearly 60 years old). This is his prose
version of the quarrel:

> Not that Achilles was appeased. He rounded on Atreides (Agamemnon)
> once again with bitter taunts. "You drunken sot," he cried, "with the eyes
> of a dog and the courage of a doe! You never have the pluck to arm
> yourself and go into battle with men or to join the other captains in an
> ambush – you would sooner die. It pays you better to stay in camp, filching
> the prizes of anyone that contradicts you, and flourishing at your peoples'
> cost because they are too feeble to resist".

Here is Chapman (2000) (the Chapman who so moved John Keats with the
elegance of his free translation of Homer):

> Thou ever-steep'd in wine,
> Dog's face, with heart but of a hart that nor in th' open eye
> Of fight dar'st thrust into the press, nor with our noblest lie
> In secret ambush. These works seem too full of death for thee:
> Tis safer far in th'open host to dare an injury
> To any crosser of thy lust. Thou subject-eating king!
> Base spirits thou govern'st, or this wrong had been the last foul thing
> Thou ever author'dst.

And this is the same passage translated by Robert Fagles (1999), one of
the most popular, if deliberately academic, of recent versions of Homer
and taken up as the Penguin Classics version:

> Staggering drunk, with your dog's eyes, your fawn's heart!
> Never once did you arm with the troops and go to battle
> Or risk an ambush packed with Achaea's picked men –
> You lack the courage, you can see death coming.
> Safer by far, you find, to foray all through camp;
> Commandeering the prize of any man who speaks against you.

King who devours his people! Worthless husks, the men you rule –
If not Atreides, this outrage would have been your last.

And finally, this is the version of the poet Christopher Logue (1992) from
his series of poems collected as "War Music", where Logue does not work
from the original Greek but offers a version of an English translation from
the Greek, thus layering the process of "translation":

"Mouth! King Mouth!"
Then stopped. Then from the middle sand said:
 "Heroes, behold your king –
Slow as an arrow fired feathers first
To puff another's worth,
But watchful as a cockroach of his own.
 Behold his cause –
Me first, me second,
And if by chance there is a little left – me third.
 Behold his deeds –
Fair ransom scanted, and its donor spurned.
The upshot – plague.
 O Agamemnon, O King Great I Am,
The Greeks who follow you, who speak for you,
Who stand among the blades for you,
Prostitute loyalty."

These four translations raise many of the issues that run through
translation studies. While the scene is the same, fundamentally different
things happen in each. This can be compared with Mol's (2002) reading of
the differing ontologies of atherosclerosis.

Rieu has translated poetry into prose, a translation that many have
considered prosaic. The version of Fagles is a well-known modern
translation. It is in verse and sticks closely to the Greek original. One
wonders whether the verse is more in form than spirit. It reads like prose
sliced into lines of roughly even length and the metre is hard to find. It
certainly does not capture the relentless beat of Homer's hexameters,
clearly reflected in Chapman's verse. Chapman gives greater gravity to the
epic tragedy by using iambic heptameters – "fourteeners" – a rhythm
evocative of trotting horses, as in the last line of the *Iliad*: "And so horse-
taming Hector's rites gave up his soul to rest".

He gives a lighter, but more grounding, rhythm to the *Odyssey* (which
is part comic in genre) through iambic pentameters: "Now when with rosy
fingers, th'early born/ And thrown through all the air, appear'd the morn".
This is the rhythm used by Shakespeare, based on the heartbeat (lub-dup,

lub-dup, lub-dup, lub-dup, lub-dup): "Shall I compare thee to a summer's day?/ Thou art more lovely and more temperate" (Sonnet 18).

The modern poet Christopher Logue is perhaps the most exciting of the four translators. He is bold in his recreation of the story, moving a long way from the Greek, and it can be difficult to recognise many of the passages in the original. Again, Logue did not read Homer in the original Greek; his poetry is taken from translations and so is a translation of a translation. Logue lands square in the territory of the patient whose first language was not English, who could not get "groin" so the best approximation was "between your legs" – an unfortunate mis-description, full of possibility for misunderstanding and circulating in a world of metaphor. Logue too takes Homer from one metaphorical level to a deeper one, where the action accrues mystery. This, in medicine, is territory for either brilliant diagnosis or fatal misdiagnosis, away from the mundane and easily read.

What further relevance does this have to the medical encounter? Let us turn to a patient history for some illumination:

> I was out shopping when my vision suddenly went very strange. It became fuzzy and blurred in my right eye; the image got all mixed up and then briefly moved to blurring on the left side. There was an impression of double vision. I had something similar about a year ago, but that was with slight weakness on my right side and the visual disturbance was not the same.

This might appear in the patient's record as a truncated translation: "sudden onset of blurred, ?double vision. h/o previous TIA-like attack" (where h/o is "history of", and TIA is transient ischaemic attack – a sort of minor stroke). The patient's story and that in the medical record might be taken as the two ends of the translation spectrum. (In fact, no patient is as fluent as this example. The account would be punctuated by "ums" and "ers", repetitions, corrections; and possibly embroidery, mis-memory, and motivated forgetting – and almost certainly interruptions by the doctor). What are the issues here for doctors as translators? We consider four: faithfulness to the original, identity, power, and contingency.

Faithfulness to the original

Translators are clear on the difference between transcribing legal documents, when faithfulness to the original is paramount, and translating, say, a speech, when the motive behind the words may justify moving a considerable way from the literal. Where does the patient's narrative or

n\
re\
mo\
lang\
H\
literal\
freque\
malprac\
we have\
account).

Transl\
constitutes\
of translatin\
traditore an\
Eysteinsson 2\
based on "tran\
earlier, derives\
carry across"; *tr*\
give over" and he\
– "to lead over"). \

Chapter Four

74

the originals. For I thought I ought to give the reader \
words, but their weight". Translation - from patie\
The doctor's translation then follo\
colleagues, and in texts – may \
recommendations, and that "weight" is more\
ways, and through medical tre\
translation professional identit\
retains one is soci\
into which the \
reinforcing into \
induction t\
layperson \
full pro\
pre\

Translation stu ......nges from those\
adhering closely t   that give a much freer\
interpretation (Furba   ... Haywood (2012) illustrates this\
spectrum from the "i   .. to the "ideomatizing" through an Italian\
sentence - *Le piace molto la novella del Boccaccio*. The "interlinear" is the
literal or faithful translation: "To her pleases much the story of the
Boccaccio". This awkward version can be improved, as: "She likes the
story by Boccaccio very much". The "ideomatizing", however, would
move further to: "She's mad about the Boccaccio", an interpretation of the
original. Note that Haywood misses the extremely literal translation or
transcription of the linguistic researcher, who may leave marks for pauses
and "ums" and "ers".

The issue of being faithful is not a simple one. In 1861, Matthew
Arnold (1905, p.10) gave a famous series of public lectures while
Professor of Poetry at Oxford University - *On Translating Homer*. He
asked the prior question of precisely what we mean by "faithfulness".
Most translators inevitably resort to metaphor and rhetoric for explanation.
Cicero (1903, 5.14), in rendering the speeches of Demosthenes into Latin,
was clear that his duties lay as much with his role of orator as of translator.
Cicero rejects literal translation for "weight" or quality: "I did not think it
necessary to translate word for word, but have kept the spirit and force of

t to record, to different
w both Arnold's and Cicero's
can be interpreted in a number of
important than the literal. Standard
pes is one of the ways in which medicine
as a community of practice. It is a language
alised with extreme gravity or sense of purpose,
eighty responsibilities that medicine brings. This
a community of practice is itself a translation, from
medical student to trainee doctor (or proto-professional) to
essional or registered doctor; and then on to specialist. A life
ously understood and given meaning through lay concerns is now
translated into professional expectations as deepening of expertise. But
learning medicine, as medical education now so firmly grasps, is not
simply about knowledge, skills and values, but rather identity formation.

Doctors have to *reduce* the patient's story for functional reasons -
otherwise there is simply too much information. Such reduction need not
be instrumental, in the vein of the reduction of complex communication to
functional skills, discussed in the previous chapter. It can be creative and
imaginative. Renaissance alchemists would have described creative
reduction as a process of "burning down to dry essences". We talk of
"cutting to the chase" and "getting to the point". Surgeons stereotypically
like to avoid unnecessary "fluff". This reduction of the patient's story too
is not merely practical – rather, it is aesthetic, within the genre of
Minimalism, only saying what needs to be said, but with elegance, polish
and flair.

But this is a deliberate, reflexive move and most doctors reduce the
patient's story – translating into medical lingo - out of habit. It is simply
"what we do around here". It may easily happen, however, that a critical
piece of information is not recognised and is lost in that shortening.

So, translation is not necessarily reductive but can be inventive.
Insertion and addition may occur for reasons, for example, of clarity, or
emphasis through pun. In Chapman's translation earlier, for example,
"heart but of a hart" is a fair word for word rendering of the original, but
introduces a pun not present in Homer. Doctors should be aware of the
subtle meanings of such punning. Analogy, for example, is used widely in
pattern recognition diagnoses as a kind of punning, sometimes outwardly
cruel in its twinning of the desired and the undesired - for example
"chocolate cyst" in an ovary, "apple core lesion" for colonic cancer

(Bleakley 2017). Translation occurs across registers involving differing senses – from the written and spoken to verbal languages; from mouth, ear and hand to eye.

As for the spirit of the original, Arnold's distillation of this spirit of Homer is widely quoted and used still as a yardstick to assess translations:

> … that he is eminently rapid; that he is eminently plain and direct, both in the evolution of his thought and in the expression of it … that he is eminently plain and direct in the substance of his thought, that is, in his matter and ideas; and, finally, that he is eminently noble. [1]

Arnold himself describes these as qualities typifying Homer, rather than the spirit of Homer. Of our examples above, one might argue that Logue's interpretation of a translation best captures these qualities of vigour, movement and passion, and Rieu's the least. But Logue is a highly imaginative, "embodied" or sensual poet. Most doctors would argue that not only is the medical narrative devoid of this vigour and passion, but that such qualities have no place in a medical context. We disagree, as our parallel drawn between medical histories and Minimalist art above suggests. The point is to turn an instrumental account into an aesthetically pleasing or challenging one, or to give form to the formless. What is aesthetic by definition grips, engages and educates the senses. This is surely the whole point of introducing the humanities into medical education. A story of crushing central chest pain can be very vivid even on the 100th retelling and the medical rendering may be an emotional catalyst for thought and action.

Identity

We introduced identity above. The identity of the doctor can be thought of as multiple – for example, doctor as scientist, professional, humanist, team player, manager, and educator (Bleakley et al 2011, pp.63-79) - but what of doctor as "translator" (active identity) and as "translated" (passive identity)? The translator's identity is nebulous, probably best captured by the title of Venuti's (2002) book *The Translator's Invisibility* – an invisibility noted by Dryden (1697/ 2016): "But slaves we are, and labour on another man's plantation; we dress the vineyard, but the wine is the owner's … we are not thanked; for the proud reader will only say the poor drudge has done his duty". The doctor is, as translator, then one stage removed from the action, as it were, that resides within the patient's experience.

But of course that experience is given greater meaning and direction or consequence by the doctor's intervention. As "translated", the doctor's passive identity is two stages removed from the patient. Here, the doctor must suffer representation (or more often misrepresentation) as character in film, television and literature. These days, such media representations are often "pulp" or "soap" as for example TV medi-soaps. While such TV programmes do offer a public service – there are helplines to call if content raises issues for the viewer – it is the health issue that is highlighted and not the character or identity of the doctor, that may be maligned or misrepresented in the effort to "entertain" rather than "infotain". The translator here gains greater invisibility as serial translation seeks to democratise medicine - but may ironically lose actual medicine to an imagined medicine in the translation.

The variety in the translations of Homer is extreme but shows that this is not an unimportant matter. This invisibility is dangerous. It suggests the foreign text can pass into another target language pure and unmediated. The medical translator, probably the most junior of the team, is likely to be similarly invisible. As with other translators, she may be unaware of the constraints that identity formation can impose. Nearly every aspect of the written medical history is formulaic: the order of events, the lay-out, the use of abbreviations, and the extent that the patient's voice can be quoted are all defined. This can be helpful to the novice to avoid omitting important information and to other doctors in helping the rapid assimilation of detail.

Rabin (1958, pp.123-45) describes how translation is dependent on the extent of previous translation, because it builds a stock of tropes that deal with translation problems. The canon of practice, however, especially in medicine, is mostly unconscious and unrecognised. It may then limit expression and censor the transmission of information. Again, it is a cliché in medicine that the diagnosis rests in the patient's story. A critical diagnostic clue may therefore be lost with the omission of that item in the history.

Perhaps the most striking equivalence between translator and doctor is in the ethics of practice – obvious in medicine, less so in translation, at least for the non-translator. But for translators, it is critical and a theme that recurs. Spivak (1993, p.183), for example, the main translator of the celebrated late deconstructionist philosopher Jacques Derrida into English, says:

> First, then, the translator must surrender to the text ... no amount of tough talk can get around the fact that translation is the most intimate act of reading. Unless the translator has earned the right to become the intimate

reader, she cannot surrender to the text, cannot respond to the special call of the text.

Venuti (1993) talks of:

> The violence of translation (residing) in its very purpose and activity ... Translation is the forcible replacement of the linguistic and cultural difference of the foreign text with a text that will be intelligible to the target-language reader.

The medical translator reacts strongly to the notion that she is engaged in anything aggressive or violent. The ethics of her practice would currently encompass confidentiality and the qualities needed for close and empathic listening. Translation studies should open medical eyes to the possibilities of aggression and acquisitiveness, and deeper consideration of a process that has, to some extent, to be intrusive. The intrusive nature of the physical examination of the patient, particularly intimate examination, has been stressed in medical education for decades. The metaphorical language in translation studies of intrusion and aggression is another way in which light can be shed on the everyday activity of "taking a history" – implying extraction rather than willing sharing (again, "receiving a history").

Translation of the patient's condition into medical understanding is then a performative issue – such as the "ownership" of a bodily area exposed to physical examination. As Michel Foucault (1973) famously argued in *The Birth of the Clinic,* when doctors made home visits the physical examination was not translated across to medicine in terms of ownership, but was an issue of capital owned by the patient within the family home. With the advent of the clinic in the hospital, ownership of the physical examination passes over to medicine, where translation of the patient's bodily state flows towards medical ownership. Intimate body parts are catalogued and logged in what are called "the patient's notes" but are actually the "doctor's notes".

The participant most likely to be rendered invisible in the medical scenario is then the patient, the source text. It is interesting to look for parallels in Homer. Logue's translations, for example, are far from the original, but the source in Homer can generally be identified. There is a clear gap between Logue and Homer nevertheless. This echoes the gap between doctor and patient, narrowed considerably in sensitive and meaningful translations of patients' symptoms into doctors' diagnoses and subsequent interventions, but maintained by their respective differences in identity and dramaturgical performances. Best translations occur where doctors and patients have respective insight into each other's performances as they tolerate, indeed enjoy, the opportunity for displaying both technical expertise and humanity within the encounter. Again, good communication makes for better healing in a direct sense, but also indirectly as it reduces the possibility of error.

Medical rituals can act as translation "intermediaries" (Latour 2007) - mere repositories of habits - rather than "mediators", frustrating potential innovations in practices. Why medical error continues at such a high, and unacceptable, rate as a consequence of poor clinical teamwork and failing to listen closely to patients' stories may be because new networks are not being initiated as translations fail across actors stuck in habitual practices. While the patient is the source text, he or she has not been exposed to "close reading", and varieties of translations have not been closely examined.

Power

Translation is an instrument of power in the hands of the translator, who can exercise a kind of violence. Venuti (2002, pp.208-23) notes "the power of translation to (re)constitute and cheapen foreign texts" and "to trivialise and exclude foreign cultures". In a psychoanalytic reading, Venuti argues that Robert Graves' translation of the Roman writer Suetonius entirely misrepresents the Latin original, where:

> Graves' interpretation ... assimilates an ancient Latin text to contemporary British values. He punctures the myth of Caesar by equating the Roman dictatorship with sexual perversion, and this reflects post-war homophobia that linked homosexuality with a fear of totalitarian government, communism, and political subversion through espionage.

Goethe (2006, p.200) noted such potential cultural imperialism two centuries ago:

> There are two maxims in translation: one requires that the author of a foreign nation be brought across to us in such a way that we can look on him as ours; the other requires that we should go across to what is foreign and adapt ourselves to its conditions, its use of language, its peculiarities.

What does the doctor think she is doing in these terms? How much is she straining to avoid the "abusive fidelity" that, Venuti (2002) argues, masks much of cultural dominance? Should she bring the patient's account over into the target language of medicine, or travel over to the patient to preserve the "foreignness" of that language from the reference point of the "medicalised"? The language of the medical history may be so far from what the patient says that this discussion may seem irrelevant, but should the doctor strive to maintain a close correspondence between the two? In terms of our discussion, is the characteristic medicalisation of the patient's account "abusive fidelity"? Certainly, the feel of the original account is usually lost completely as emotional content and context are both lost entirely in formal translation to a medical record, but may be impressed in the memory of the doctor as an informal record or a "complementary fidelity".

Daniela Maria Martole (2009, p.149) notes that:

> Modern translation theories have been oscillating between two main tendencies, clearly formulated ever since 1813 by the German theologian and philosopher Friedrich Schleiermacher in his lecture "On the Different Methods of Translating".

On the one hand, the translator can move the author towards the reader as a "domesticating" or "ethnocentric reduction" of the text; or, the reader can be moved into the foreign territory of the author, who remains undisturbed, as a "foreignising" or "abusive fidelity". We have considered both trajectories here, but note that in the historical and current climate of medicine, "foreignising" of the patient has been the dominant method. Indeed, there is hegemony at work, despite the advertised "patient-centred" intentions of medicine.

We call for a greater "domestication" of medical lingo and "standard" (i.e. habitual) practices as part of an authentic democratising of medicine through medical education. We have a model in translations of Homer. Christopher Logue's poetic leap of faith brings Homer home to an interested audience without ancient Greek, and without loss of quality, dynamism and meaning. While Logue shows infidelity in the face of the literal lines of Homer's *Iliad*, he shows impressive and insightful fidelity to the poetic spirit of Homer.

Contingency

By "contingency" we mean circumstances such as time, place and specialty, largely outside the control of the translator, and doctor as translator, that influence their textual practices. The era in which Homer was translated makes striking and obvious differences to the translation. The Penguin Classics translations by Rieu had an overtly democratising purpose.[2] It is interesting to ponder the "best way" of translating Homer, if one were attempting a new version outside the limitations of culture. If one cuts short a long argument and accepts that poetry must be rendered by poetry and that Greek dactyls must be rendered by English iambics, there remains an interesting argument about whether an archaic rendering is not closest to how Homer was received in the classical world. The *Iliad* had to be contemporary at some point, but even when first written down around the 7th century BCE, it was already quite old, sounding perhaps rather Shakespearian then, and certainly in the later Athens of Plato and Aristotle. The translations of Chapman and Pope may therefore give us the closest feel of Homer as his audience (of the 4th and 5th centuries BCE) received the epic song cycles.

Our doctor is equally constrained by the context in which she works. Different fashions of the layout of the hospital record have prevailed over the years; even keeping a record in primary care in the UK was not universal in Britain 50 years ago. The computerised medical record of the future will transform how the patient story is preserved. Further, as we argue throughout this book, medical education is undergoing a sea change in which communication with patients and colleagues is considered to be paramount. This is based on two sets of evidence: first, communication with patients is a health intervention in its own right; and second, poor communication in clinical teams creates ground for potential error. Patient satisfaction and safety are both paramount in contemporary healthcare.

The issue of specialty pertains to both translator and doctor. Christopher Logue was a poet, whose possible interest in democratisation would not extend to a prose translation, while prose underlay the principles of Rieu. Fagles sounds like a classicist and translator rather than a poet, for reasons given earlier. The type and quality of translation depend then on the background and expertise of the translator. In medicine, the specialty again affects how the patient's story is recorded and how it is translated rhetorically between specialty interests (Lingard et al 2004). The narrative of the immediate problem, the "past medical history", and the social circumstances are more likely to be recorded by the psychiatrist than the surgeon (though the last will be closely recorded by other specialists within the surgical department, such as the occupational therapist and physiotherapist).

The issue of the social circumstances of translator/doctor or, on a broader canvas, the cultural milieu in which they operate has already been touched on in the section on identity. There, the accent was on the appropriate language of translation - whether it should reflect the strangeness of the original or be brought entirely into the fluency of the target language. Here we deal with language *and* culture rather than language *in* culture. For the doctor, the difference is between capturing the nuances of a patient's description and recognising the different constructs of health and disease within which they might operate – we know of a local Cornish farmer, for example, who treats his abnormal heart rhythms by jumping off the barn roof onto his heels or grasping the electrified fence keeping in his cattle! His translation of medical advice is, to use Martola's (2009) term again - via Friedrich Schleiermacher - entirely "domesticated", an "ethnocentric reduction" to the local and particular.

Conclusion

It is of academic interest to consider the taking/receiving and recording of a medical history, but we would prefer to see a practical advantage to patients and their care. We do not intend to paralyse activity by overanalysing. Translators themselves recognise this risk and accept that they must be practical:

> Translators are never, and should never be forced to be ... neutral, impersonal transferring devices. Translators' personal experiences - emotions, motivations, attitudes, and associations - are not only allowable in the formation of a working TL (target language) text, they are indispensable. (Robinson 1991, p.260).

Our purpose, however, has also been to not set out a specific programme for translation in medicine - to legislate on best practice. Rather, we have drawn on translation studies - applied to Homer in particular – first, to raise awareness about the importance of translation; second, to draw attention to the value of recognising and articulating translations where these form networks or support for practice innovation; and third, we show how faithfulness to the original, and factors such as identity, power and contingency are key and contested factors in translation in medicine. We encourage doctors to not take translation for granted but to consider its complexities, as they take on the identity of doctor as translator. Patients take their illnesses seriously; doctors take their interactions with patients seriously; and the power of translation can do justice to both. "Thinking otherwise" with Homer can shed new light on the power of translation.

Notes

1. Furman (1992, pp.38-9) quotes, but is not as critical as we would be, Arnold's requirement that Homer's translator should "try to satisfy scholars". This demand would surely be a deterrent to most readers.

2. Rieu's son and Peter Jones revised his translation of the *Odyssey*. Dominic Rieu
is illuminating in his preface on how the manners of the time affected his father's
translation: "Requests and instructions in the poem are always given crisply;
E.V.R. almost invariably prefaces them with a "kindly" or "Be good enough to".
(Peter Jones asked me: "Was your father a courteous man?" Answer: "Yes".)"
(Rieu 1991, p.viii).

CHAPTER FIVE

SING, MUSE

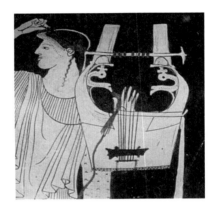

Figure 5-1: The singer of tales

Medical history as oral tradition

In the previous chapter, we discussed medicalisation of the person (first into "patient", and then "case") as an issue of translation, warning against both mistranslation (that can end in misdiagnosis), and translation poverty (the complex person reduced to presenting symptom through a medical frame). However, we noted that the translation of person to case could be re-visioned: as an aesthetic act of Minimalism and not just a plain reduction. Minimalism, as we discuss below, is a fully intentional and imaginative stripping down to bare essences – a re-presentation of the complex in bare, skeletal elegance (Meyer 2004).

In this chapter, we progress the original work of Richard Ratzan (1992), who argued that the traditional presentation of the medical case history is a legitimate form of oral recital (in Homer and Ratzan's term "winged words" – a translation of *epea pteroenta* in the Greek). This, in the Janus-faced tradition of Homeric poetry – on the one hand strongly coded, rule-bound and formulaic, and on the other, open to creative interpretation according to audience response. Ratzan drew on the groundbreaking work of the American student of epic poetry Milman Parry (1902-1935), who showed that Homeric poetry was based on a tradition of oral performance governed by extensive use of formulae or fixed expressions. This framework considerably lightened the load on the memory of the performers while providing room for improvisation.

As Albert Lord (1912-1991) (2003, p.4), Parry's assistant, said: "The singer of tales is at once the tradition and an individual creator". Ratzan, however, only looks backward to Homer to justify his claim, while we suggest also looking around, to modern contemporary aesthetic forms such as Minimalism, to find a genre or aesthetic home for the "reflexive" case presentation and its creative possibilities in performance.

Further, we argue that a genre shift, from the purely functional to the aesthetic of Minimalism, challenges a typical objection from within medical humanities and ethics that the case presentation is both depersonalising and dehumanising for patients - where the "case history" acts as an irreversible translation device from the patient's felt "illness" to a medicalised "disease" (Kleinman 1988). Rather, in acting as a medium for identity construction of the doctor as professional performance artist, we suggest that learning how to recite the case history does not just provide a means for forming a professional identity within the medical culture, but sensitises doctors towards the public, as audience, offering a radical version of "patient-centredness".

The history of the development of oral poetry shows that performers must be able to translate readily between select audiences (the court, senior doctors) and public audiences (coffee houses, the ward). In other words, the doctor herself must be Janus-faced, looking inward to satisfy medical culture's demands for a polished performance, and looking outwards as a sensitivity towards maintaining the interest and understanding of an audience of patients and other clinicians and healthcare staff. The latter is achieved as the patient is (re)enacted through the intra-professional recitation, a unique and aesthetically valuable form of embodiment through expert practice. For example:

> Mister Smith is a sixty-year-old man who came to A&E with crushing, central chest pain, which radiated down the arm and up into the neck. The pain came on out of the blue while working in the garden. There has been no previous episode. His ECG showed ST elevation ...

This is a fairly typical medical history that a junior doctor might relate to a senior member of the clinical team. We argue that this and other ways in which healthcare professionals communicate have many central characteristics of Homer's *Iliad* and *Odyssey*, showing features typical of oral narrative traditions that are an integral part of oral cultures. Narrative traditions play an important part in both medical memory and identity construction and serve to compare those traditions with Homer's. We recognise that a return to Homer to think otherwise about medical habits and traditions can be seen as nested in two encompassing activities. First, considering the structure of medical speech as performative (enactments or practices), adding to a recent interest in ontology (states of being) in medical practice, rather than epistemology (conditions of knowing) (Mol 2002). And second, employing Homer's epic poems as touchstones to explore communication both within and between communities of experts, novices and laypersons.

The *Iliad* and *Odyssey* are each long poems of some 15,000 and 12,000 lines respectively. If we started to recite the *Iliad* at the start of the working week, we would be finished on Wednesday or Thursday, depending on the stamina of the audience.[1] Both epics were written down around 750 BC and describe events occurring 300 - 400 years before. Various aspects of the composition of the texts, both at the level of words and phrases and at the level of major themes, puzzled scholars through the 18th and 19th centuries. They began to address the problem when it was realised that the poems predated writing; they were part of an oral tradition - epic stories handed down from one generation to another. Only the "spoken" (or, in fact, sung) word was available, where "oral epic song is narrative poetry composed in a manner evolved over many generations by singers of tales who did not know how to write" (Lord 2003, p.4).

Critical to this definition is that Greek epic poetry was not simply recited *but constructed and created during recital*. Improvisation was key to good performance, while performance memory was structured by formulaic scaffolding, explained below. In ancient Greek, singers and poets share the same descriptor - *aodoi* - the modern equivalent of which would be "performing (or performance) artists". The recitation of the epics was known as much for creation as recreation, where a formulaic epic narrative would be re-storied through leaps of the singer's imagination, against a predictable hexameter, six-beats to the line rhythm. So the singer was also called *rhapsodos*, literally "a stitcher together of songs" (Dalby 2006, pp.174-5).

"Stitching together" is a metaphor that runs through Homer like a message in Blackpool rock, to refer to crafts as diverse as boatbuilding and weaving; and to the act of poetry itself as a stitching together of words (Dougherty 2001). There is much improvisation in this, but what is improvised is built on formulae – just as a jazz musician improvises around scales. Odysseus is the master of "stitching together" where his forte is adaptability.

Medical students too learn how to stitch together a performance such as a case presentation on a ward round in formulaic ways; and gain expertise in diagnosis by stitching together scientific knowledge with practical clinical knowledge in tacit "illness scripts". Only as expertise is established through practice can improvisation occur and this is based around a known set of chords, scales or tonal progressions gained through exposure to patients whose illnesses are fitted into pre-existing classifications. Students build up "illness scripts" (Lubarsky 2015) - highly condensed mental notes summarising key conditions that become supplemented or fleshed out by meeting patients. Presenting symptoms are in time subject to pattern recognition as the primary diagnostic method. This can be summarised as a stitching together of knowledge and practice,

Milman Parry (1971, p.272) defines "formula" as: "a group of words which is regularly employed under the same metrical conditions to express a given essential idea". For example, the same words are often combined throughout the poem to form pairs of noun and epithet, or even longer combinations, sometimes running to complete sentences.

Achilles, around whose wrath and appeasement the *Iliad* revolves, very often has the epithet "swift-footed" attached to his name. When dawn breaks, personified as a goddess, she often has the lovely epithet "rosy-fingered" attached to her. Indeed, the whole line for the breaking dawn is used about 20 times in the *Odyssey*: "When the child of morning, rosy-fingered dawn appeared". The extent to which the poet called on and reused such a stock of words, phrases, and sentences only became clear on detailed examination, through the work of Parry and Lord.

Below, the first lines of the *Iliad* have been used to demonstrate this - the following is Lord's version (2003, p.143), itself based on Parry's (1971, p.301):

μηνιν αειδε, θεα, Πηληιαδεω Αχιληος

ουλομενην, η μυρι' Αχαιοις αλγε' εθηκε,

_____ -----------------------
πολλας δ' ιφθιμους ψυχας Αιδι προιαψεν

----------------------------------_____

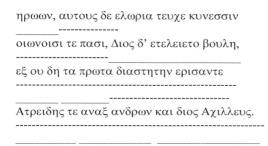

ηρωων, αυτους δε ελωρια τευχε κυνεσσιν

οιωνοισι τε πασι, Διος δ' ετελειετο βουλη,

εξ ου δη τα πρωτα διαστητην ερισαντε

Ατρειδης τε αναξ ανδρων και διος Αχιλλευς.

"Wrath; sing, Muse, of Peleus' son Achilles,
The baleful wrath that brought countless sufferings to the Achaeans,
And many brave souls sent to Hades
Of heroes, and made prey of them for dogs
And carrion birds; so brought the will of Zeus to pass,
When first in strife apart stood
Atreus' son, king of men, and godlike Achilles"

The unbroken lines represent formulae - that is, collections of words that appear verbatim elsewhere in the epic. The broken lines are also formulaic - parts of them, or the words in different form, appear elsewhere. For example, "Αιδι προιαψεν" (*Aidi proiapsen*) means "sent to Hades", a common activity around the walls of Troy as men fell in brutal, hand-to-hand combat. When the poet has in mind to kill off one of his fighters in a battle scene, this gives him his line ending. Each time Achilles appears in the tale, the metrics of his name - ti-tum-tum - allow it to be placed almost anywhere in the line. There is then a set of formulae that allows the poet to fill the rest of the line, while he plans how to move the story forward.

Parry and Lord extended their research to oral poetic traditions modern at the time, in particular in Yugoslavia between the First and Second World Wars (Lord 2003). They found an equivalent use of formulae. Their work showed that the formulae were not simply *aide-memoires* to allow the poet to remember the poem and recount the tale verbatim. Rather, they were metrical combinations that allowed the poet to compose on the spot. Again, oral poetry is not simply recited, but constructed and created during recital, while containing a strong formulaic element. The point is that the formula provides the basis for improvisation, again, just as a jazz musician will use a well-practised structure of chord changes or harmonic patterns from which to express something novel in an extended solo.

Each telling of the *Iliad* was then a new and different poem. That is a wonderful concept, difficult for us to understand. Most modern speakers would not give even a short talk without notes or Powerpoint backup. The singer of the *Iliad* sang for six hours a day for three or four days. In the Yugoslavian tradition, the singer-poet tailored the story to the audience. If they were restive, a shorter story would suffice. The issue is probably more subtle and complex than this. It is easy to imagine that a particular poet might become revered and his style imitated more closely than others, so that a greater degree of fixity of the text emerged. Kirk (1960), for example, distinguished between the kinds of singers that we noted earlier: the older *aoidoi* (singers in oral society), and the *rhapsodes* – literally, again, "stitchers-together of songs" – members of the literate world drawing on and reinventing ancient craft.

Songs in hospital

"Songs" appear in hospital as routine medical work. Previous chapters note that routinisation in hospitals has embraced long-standing rituals that echo Homeric accounts: particularly, the exercise of hospitality and the nature of heroic interventions. Seen from a Homeric perspective, this may turn ordinary labour into the extraordinary stitching-together-of-songs as recitals. There is a parallel with different medical scenarios. We started with a typical account of a patient's illness that a junior doctor might relate on a ward round. This is not a new parallel. Again, Ratzan (1992) saw this two decades ago.

Drawing on the *Iliad*, he compares the oral tradition with the medical Grand Round in terms of "professional, social, and pedagogical significance", where "a singer of medical tales recites a medical case history that is judged by its skill in transmitting the story and, in some venues, by its performative excellence".[2] The parallel is therefore attractive because these are ritualised occasions and the experience of both Parry and Lord was that the Yugoslavian epics were typically sung on ceremonial occasions such as weddings and religious festivals.

Our original contribution builds on Ratzan's insight to show that the stripped-back case presentation, often critiqued as purely functional and as a translation of the patient's illness capital into medical disease capital, can be reconfigured. This formulation of the "case", as our parallel with Ratzan's work shows, can be fruitfully compared with Homeric poetic-song formulations, and that is clearly of great interest to us given the focus of this book.

Also, moving beyond habitual, unthinking performance (all script and no postscript), the primary medical "song" of the hospital, the case presentation, can be considered reflexively. That is, it is deconstructed for its habitual form and purpose, and then reconstructed diligently and critically or with reflection as to its form and guiding values. This is the work of the medical educator. In our argument, the shift in reconstruction of the case presentation hospital song is from the functional to the aesthetic. The burning down to dry essences of the person, first to "patient" and then to "case", may re-present the person through a Minimalist aesthetic, by-passing de-personalisation. We introduced this model in the previous chapter and will now develop it.

The Grand Round presentation is too serious to risk all on memory and the medical history will usually be summarised in writing for the presenter. Not so the "business ward round" ("specialty" or "unit" round in North America), when the presentation is often truly oral and from memory. (These are regular meetings when some or all of the team discuss and visit their patients).

Are there other examples? Oral recital is not confined to medical work, but embraces healthcare more generally, involving, for example, multidisciplinary team meetings, such as briefing and debriefing in operating theatre teams and patient care reviews in community mental health teams. We would argue that the handover between nursing shifts falls into this category, as do telephone conversations between healthcare staff, some aspects of clinico-pathological conferences, and handover and triage on Accident and Emergency units. Also, in Nendaz's and Bordage's (2002) model of clinical reasoning, students are asked to represent the problem in a brief and medicalised language which is itself very formulaic and which is intended to help them arrive at differential diagnoses. At our medical school, each student is assessed weekly on a case presentation that he or she is encouraged to deliver in formulaic style.

The medical history and genre

We started with a typical case presentation. Let us look at it with the eyes of a Parry or a Lord:

> Mister Smith is a sixty-year-old man, who was admitted to the ward from casualty with crushing, central chest pain. There was no radiation down the left arm or up into the neck. The pain came on suddenly while he was working in the garden There has been no previous episode. His ECG showed ST elevation, etc.

We could argue about the details of whether a phrase is a formula or formulaic. The point is that these are also *aide-memoires* that allow the junior doctor rapidly to present each of the 15 or more patients whose story she heard the previous night. The formulae will pertain particularly to medicine; surgical or psychiatric patients will need their own set of formulae, just as the different stories of the *Iliad* and the *Odyssey* do. The power of the case presentation rests with its brevity and pointedness and the - often striking - link of word and image (given extra power where it is pathologised, such as "crushing pain").

While Homeric poetry is composed in hexameter verse: "regular, rhythmical lines that always have six beats and thirteen to seventeen syllables" (Dalby 2006, p.16), the case above could readily be transposed, "sung" as Shakespearean iambic pentameter with five beats (doubled) to the line:

> Mister Smith is a sixty-year-old man,
> Who was admitted to the ward from
> Casualty with crushing, central chest pain.
> There was no radiation down the left arm
> Or up into the neck. The pain came on
> Suddenly while working in the garden
> There has been no previous episode.
> His ECG showed ST elevation.

Our point is that rhythmic form is the standard weave of the song or recitation, upon which the details are embroidered. The case presentation is a mantra whose repetition does not lead to spiritual transformation but creation of professional identity as an expert practitioner. The case presentation can be seen as an elegant convention: systematic; based on brevity, clarity and concision:

> A 62 year old man came to the Emergency Department complaining of mid-sternal pain, shortness of breath and nausea.
> "Mr K is a 23 year old who had an episode of bleeding two weeks ago. He was urinating and noticed blood in the urine."
> "Mrs B presented at the A&E department with severe pain in the upper abdomen radiating to the back".

There is apparent objectivity, or singular lack of affect, that irons out an initially disturbing account ("noticed blood in the urine"). But this is sense-based, ontological, where description prevails over analysis. If there is a characteristic style, then it is the brevity and smoothness of the presentation. Aesthetically, this can be compared with the presentation of smooth, industrially precise surfaces that characterises Minimalism in its sculptural forms since its heyday in the 1960s (Meyer 2004). However, smoothness of surfaces does not signify lack of deep affect in response. Just as highly stylised Minimalist art viewed in an antiseptic white cube gallery can get the heart rate of an enthusiast racing, so Ratzan (1992) notes that the heart rates of junior doctors increase as they enact the performance of the case presentation in a "highly charged atmosphere". The white cube of the gallery is now the white cube of the clinic or ward, and the art is performance. The performance must be of a high quality – lives, and the quality of lives, are at stake

We must not, however, think that re-casting the case as polished Minimalism offers a form of logic for that case. We insist that the reflexive translation into Minimalist form is also a way of embracing uncertainty. Mimimalist art can be puzzling and ambiguous. For example, Minimalist sculpture, such as the infamous line of 120 firebricks by Carl Andre bought by the Tate Gallery in London ("Equivalent VIII") in 1972, conceived in 1966, is characterised as "what you see is what you see", "self presentation", or "things in themselves". In other words, the artwork is self-explanatory. This of course is true at the immediate perceptual level, but nonsense conceptually. The work has all kinds of conceptual implications, possibilities and readings. There is depth in surfaces for example.

This is true also of a "case", because every person's symptoms are unique even as they are classifiable into groups. The man with blood in his urine may have noticed this on several occasions over days, or only once; the blood may have been a trace, or very obvious visually, seen in the urine flow as well as in the pan; there may have been some pain, and certainly a degree of strain, in passing urine where this was associated with prostatic hyperplasia – an enlarged prostate. The reactions of each person will be different, as will their stories of symptom presentation, even as the underlying condition may be shared.

There is then complexity, ambiguity and uncertainty in the case and this transfers across to the pared-down case presentation. Minimalism shares this distinguishing feature. One of the most famous Minimalist poems, by the American paediatrician William Carlos Williams, plainly describes a friend's farmyard with white chickens and a "red wheelbarrow" glazed with rainwater. The poem begins, however: "so much depends/ upon" the red wheelbarrow. Now we are cast into the realm of uncertainty or ambiguity. Just what depends upon this functional tool? Further, Williams turns the ordinary into the special, a gift that poets share with good doctors, who make their patients feel special. The doctor who makes the correct diagnosis that leads to the cure is, in the patient's eyes, always special, even where the diagnosis may seem pedestrian to the doctor. The pedestrian – like Williams' wheelbarrow – is "glazed".

What the poem does not tell us (and this is the point of stripping out context) is that Williams was in a heightened emotional state when he wrote it, having stayed up late the night before visiting a very sick child in his practice. Williams himself wrote that the poem emerged out of deep affection and respect for a black man who worked at the farm where the red wheelbarrow was spied – a man who had to work in sub-zero temperatures with farm implements and equipment.

Lorelei Lingard and colleagues (Lingard et al 2003) argue that there are identifiable genres of case presentation – in particular the difference between the medical "school genre", where students seek to present without interruption, and the "workplace genre", where seasoned practitioners seek to use case presentations as a way of constructing shared professional knowledge. The case presentation is formed according to context.

Again, the way the story is recounted, or "sung", also declares and defines an identity construction. The expert sews-the-song-together (*rhapsodos*), often bringing together several stories in a grand story. Novices must learn this poetic technique and ritual, and those who do this well impress expert teachers and also shift identity, from "medical student" to "trainee doctor". Those who sew-the-song-together in clinical settings under clinical supervision enacting the "school genre" rather than the "workplace genre" will be seen as less capable by those supervising experts. Canny medical students soon learn the ropes as far as the differing demands of these shifting contexts are concerned.

The aesthetic worth of the case presentation

Let us recap the argument for the aesthetic worth of the case presentation. Narrativists who have turned their attention to the ways that stories are told in medical encounters consistently note the bias in the medical narrative towards objectivity, to include objectification of the patient (Hunter 1991, Montgomery 2006). This serves, they suggest, to encapsulate and stabilise the objects of interest, placing symptom before person and medicalisation before existential lifeworld accounts of the patient. The process of the medical case history has long been seen as boiling the rich soup of the patient's narrative to the hard tack that medics can stomach, a necessary reduction (Kleinman 1988, Donnelly 1988). But this has always been an instrumental reading, or a utilitarian justification. We are advocates of the art of medicine and suggest that good medical practice has style, presence, refinement, or quality. Medicine practiced well is aesthetic, rounded, reaching beyond the functional.

"Aesthetic" at root means "sense impression", so an aesthetic medicine is sensible or makes the best uses of the senses, as it is also sensitive, relating to patients' needs. Further "aesthetic" does not imply embroidered, ornate or Baroque (grand, exaggerated and exuberant). In boiling away excess or reducing to bare essences, medicine can be refined. Let us give more examples to support our notion that the typical case recitation fits (and adds to) the genre of Minimalism, a form of objectivism whose aesthetic is the pared-down and the polished surface. Here is a radiologist reading X-ray images:

> This is a double contrast barium enema. There is an area of narrowing in the sigmoid. The undercut edges give an apple core appearance. This is colonic carcinoma.
> This is a chest X-ray of an adult patient. Calcification is rounded and peripheral. With this degree of symmetry and also eggshell calcification in the right para-aortic region, the most likely diagnosis is sarcoid.
> (With permission of Dr Richard Farrow).

In both cases pattern recognition is at work, through use of metaphor or resemblance ("apple core lesion" and "eggshell calcification"). This is an expert with many years' experience. The language is stripped back, precise, polished through the generations of cultural (medical specialty and sub-specialty) oral narrative practice, or "song". This is a recital in the tradition of oral performers of epics. The subject matter is epic – life-threatening disease in one case (colon cancer).

In terms of the power of embodied metaphors, these descriptions offer a kind of minimalist poetry but perhaps without the essential ingredient of the ambiguity that William Carlos Williams' poem introduced, discussed above. However, perhaps the complexity is given with the subject matter. Ian Hamilton Finlay (2002), from *The Blue Sail,* claims that surface - or what is "given off" - is all, where a hay-barge is described on a "sea-lane", as giving off a "scent/ of hot/ sweet hay/ and salt".

The poem is purely descriptive, yet intensely atmospheric. Indeed, it works because of the sudden shift of register from vision to smell. We look at the words printed on the page and we hear a song as we recite the words to ourselves or speak them out loud to a gathered audience. The poem then shifts us to another sense register in which we must draw on memory. And then the ambiguity kicks in. The smell is of "hot sweet hay" and "salt". What a strange combination. But then we recall that the hay is on a barge in a "sea lane". The salt is the smell of the sea.

The radiologist's comments too are both descriptive and charged, but go further in offering a diagnosis. As the Minimalist sculptor Robert

Morris (Marzona and Grosenick 2004), suggests: "simplicity of form is not necessarily simplicity of experience"; and Susan Sontag (2009) echoes this sentiment in *Against Interpretation*, her infamous challenge to hermeneutics:

> ... ours is a culture based on excess, on overproduction; the result is a steady loss of sharpness in our sensory experience ... What is important now is to recover our senses. We must learn to *see* more, to *hear* more, to *feel* more ... Our task is to cut back content so that we can see the thing at all.

What better advice for diagnosticians, whose business is close noticing? And does the oral poet not sing to his audience for precisely the same reason - to educate both the senses and sensibility, to bring a new level of awareness? The powerful link between word and image engineered by the precise form of the medical case account satisfies the demands to educate what Rudolf Arnheim (2004) calls our "visual thinking", where "The discipline of intelligent vision cannot be confined to the art studio; (but) it can succeed (in other disciplines) only if the visual sense is not blunted and confused in other areas of the curriculum". Here is a precise lesson for medical education as it learns from the arts and humanities.

Readers at this point may feel that we are offering an apology for a reductive, albeit polished, method that fails the patient as complex person, as narrativists have claimed. However, we argue that such method cast as Minimalism is not at all cold-hearted, but rather offers *warm appreciation prior to cold explanation*. The isolated symptom is not of course the whole person, and must be contextualised; but the symptom too should be addressed in its self-display as we isolate and magnify its properties, as in dissection.

There is a danger in such appreciation turning into morbid fascination, a charge often brought against medicine, but our point is nevertheless made, that medical aesthetics is prior to medical ethics in its need to describe symptom prior to diagnosis. A burning down to dry essences as method (the word "clinical" is used in everyday speech to describe this) disguises perceptual riches of close noticing and attention that constitute the deep structure of medicine's Minimalist poetics of practice as a code of close observation.

To return to Homer, when a character has spoken in the *Iliad*, Homer's next line creates itself, with a formula to fit every circumstance:

τον δ' απαμειβομενος προσεφη ποδας ωκυς Αχιλλευς
την δ'   λευκωλενος Ηρη
τους δ'   πολυμητις Οδυσσευς

Answering him spoke forth swift footed Achilles
Answering her spoke forth white armed Hera.
Answering them spoke forth Odysseus of many counsels.

So the doctor can call on formulae to move through familiar territory as s/he also makes sense of an unknown bodily event:

Examination of the … system …….. within normal limits.
U's and E's ……………………… unremarkable.
Full blood count ………………… no abnormality.

The start of each sentence can reach any of the three endings given a suitable bridge. Equally important is that, in addition to the formula theory that affects word combinations and sentences, whole themes recur throughout both the *Iliad* and the *Odyssey* (Foley 1988). Arranging a truce, preparing a meal, offering a sacrifice, or sticking a spear in a member of the opposing camp occur several, often many times. Such iterations, as protocols, are expected to progress in a certain way and a certain order whether in Homer or in healthcare.

Just as the pilot and co-pilot must run through the safety checklist prior to take-off to avoid potential disaster, no matter how many times each of them has flown this particular plane, so the litany of the World Health Organisation's Surgical Safety Checklist must be repeated for each patient at each operation to avoid error such as "wrong patient operated on", "wrong side operated on", "equipment not available", "we didn't know she had a latex allergy", "the blood was not ordered", "the X-rays are not here" and so forth (Gawande 2010).

The effect of oral traditions

Before considering where this comparison of oral traditions might lead, we should consider the limits to the argument. We make the point later that ours is a literate world. Oral traditions now are very different and we have moved, with the advent first of writing and then electronic information, to what was already described three decades ago as a "secondary orality", a product of the era of word-processing and the World Wide Web (Ong 1982, p.136). Yet many characteristics remain the same. There is a risk of regarding primary orality as primitive or folksy. Ong (1982, pp.12-13) draws a parallel, for the literate world considering the oral, of describing a horse to those who know cars but have never seen a horse. A horse is then a wheelless car, running on hay rather than petrol, and so on, where: "In the end, horses are only what they are not".

The format in which doctors narrate in the special circumstances described is formulaic. Why does it have this fixity, this tradition? First, it aids memory. It is hard enough to remember the patient's story without also having to think about the format and language with which to recount it. George Bordage (Nendaz and Bordage 2002) introduced the term "semantic qualifiers" to describe the transformation of the patient's story into simpler abstracts or structures, employed as cultural code and capital within medical circles and translated back into varieties of medical tales. This aligns with current models of expert clinical reasoning, drawing on findings from cognitive psychology research, as a mix of the intuitive and the rational (Eva 2005). "Intuitive" refers to enactment of tacit knowledge – again, "clinical scripts" as memorised series of patient presentations linked to scientific knowledge or "concept maps", the latter elaborated through recall and stimulated by pattern recognition.

So, the pain that came on suddenly in my knee and that I have had a couple of times before becomes "acute, recurrent, large joint pain". Students armed with this language remember the patient's story more easily, realise similarities with other stories and so move to a diagnosis. In (al)chemical terms, there is first *reductio* (from the complex story to the abstract signifiers), and then *iteratio* (repetition). Note that the abstraction is still an embodied metaphor, a series of potent images stalking the student's mind or imagination ("acute", "recurrent" linked to "pain").

Where chemistry is literally formulaic: A+B+C=X; alchemy (proto-chemistry) is the power of the image to provoke and be remembered. Francis Yates in *The Art of Memory* (Yates 2001) reminds us that memory is stimulated through powerful sense-based associations, such as those between words and images and is laid down through iteration or repetition. "Rote" is not a good word to describe what is deliberate and focused practice. For medical education in diagnostic acumen, students do not simply need repeated exposure to patient "cases", but deliberate structuring of such exposure. Structuring takes the local context into account and then resonates with the bard's/ singer's/ poet's/ performer's/ diagnostician's movement between convention and invention according to the nature of the audience.

There is a risk of exaggerating the importance of memory for our modern singer, given the ready availability of a written record. It cannot be exaggerated for the ancients. So critical was memory in a pre-literate society that the ancient Greeks' Mnemosyne, Memory personified, was seen as one of eleven children from the union of Gaia (Earth) and Uranus (Heaven), and a titaness (Notopoulos 1938; Hesiod 2008, lines 132-8). In a society that could not record, the poet was one of the few preservers of collective memories, of recording the law, and of disseminating ideas. Others might be priests, wise men and wise women. S/he was the living record of society and its mores (Havelock 1986, pp.73-8).

In ancient Greek society, his or her performance created an identity - an *enactment* of identity (although not necessarily giving great status, if the one contemporary account we have of a bard in the *Odyssey* is accurate). This is an irony, as the bard sings largely of the honour of the hero, whose honour, as we have seen in chapters one and two, is achieved by being talked of in admiration long after death, achieving a kind of immortality.

Mnemosyne becomes a very minor figure in later, literate society, but her symbolic importance lived on in her daughters, the nine Muses, who are invoked at the beginning of both the *Iliad* and the *Odyssey*. Our own capacity for memorisation is dismal by contrast. The Greeks put the blame for this squarely on the advent of writing. Plato (1971, p.563), in the *Phaedrus*, tells the story of an Egyptian sage introducing writing to his king. It will, he says, make the Egyptians wiser and will improve their memories. The king disagrees. Writing will: "produce forgetfulness ... because they will not practice their memory ... . You have produced an elixir not of memory but of reminding". Yet the immensely elaborate mental mechanisms to aid memory put in place in the ancient world owed everything to later-developed visual memory and nothing to pre-literate culture (Havelock 1986).

Earlier, we noted (and answered) the objections of narrativists to the reduction of the patient's story to a formulaic medical "case". Similarly, classical scholars argued whether Homer's formulae produced a dulling effect. Some thought he was protected from a similar process by the richness of the epithets available to him such as "grey-eyed Athene", "ox-eyed Hera", and "Agamemnon king of men". These are all evocative, but do they remain so when Athene is grey-eyed for the 14th time in the *Iliad*?

"Crushing, central chest pain" is hugely dramatic; it is just that doctors have read it in textbooks, heard it as students and used it often early in their careers. Parry takes an objective view (Parry 1971, pp.426-7) where he accepts that formulaic epithets can be disappointing, but in general "They flow unceasingly through the changing moods of the poetry, inobtrusively blending with it, and yet, by their indifference to the story, giving a permanent, unchanging sense of strength and beauty". Perhaps too, Lord's view of his singer of tales applies even more to the medic: "expression is his business, not originality, which, indeed, is a concept quite foreign to him and one he would avoid, if he understood it" (Lord 2003, pp.44-45). In how many medical schools will students be taught that their growing diagnostic capability is a thing of beauty and not just function?

If we accept an element of performance in the recounting of the patient's story, we must not forget the importance of the audience (Bauman 1977). Lord (2003) stresses how great an effect they might have on the performance - how their restlessness may shorten the delivery, or their enthusiasm may lead to a richer embroidering of themes. So the medical singer's audience may affect the details and elaboration of the account and ultimately the care of the patient. This offers a radically new version of patient-centredness, where the junior doctor or medical student presenting the case has already talked with the patient (as audience), and now, in front of her seniors, is re-presenting the patient in consciously Minimalist style. Paradoxically, the rehearsal may occur after the public performance, where "backstage" for patients is now "frontstage" for physicians, but the play's concern is the (re)embodiment of the patient. This is medicine as reflexive performance.

The creation of identity

As we have said, each telling of an epic poem was in part a new poem, an act of creation. The bard was not just remembering 15,000 lines using the techniques described, repeating them verbatim, but quite the reverse. Each recital created the story anew. As s/he sang, so s/he made the poem – s/he was not only the singer, but also the song (on female bards, see Dalby 2006).

The poems of ancient Greece were performed in Panathenaic Games, in symposia and in public places, and were also sung to select audiences - the king and his court. Similarly, traditional song-poems of Yugoslavia were sung in coffee houses to an inclusive public audience, but also exclusively to male guests at a Moslem wedding. While medical tales are told to a select and critical audience, often in the case of junior doctors an audience ready to pounce on mistakes, the public audience (patients) is enacted and embodied in the process (and not just kept in mind). This recreation of the patient is slyly criticised by Ratzan (1992) as disembodying the patient through the case history conventions, to be presented as a "skeleton".

The pun is good as the case history must be in skeleton form, but we argue again that considered Minimalist form and style must not be mistaken for a disembodiment. Stripping back to dry essences - as William Carlos Williams or Ian Hamilton Finlay do in their poetry; Donald Judd, Robert Morris and Carl Andre do in sculpture; and Eva Hesse does in painting - is not the same as disembodying, depersonalising or dehumanising. It is perhaps more likely that this depersonalisation will occur in Lingard and colleagues' "school genre" form of presentation than in the "workplace genre", where the former presentation is dis-located rather than dis-embodied (Lingard et al 2003).

The outcome of the clinical presentation, again, is an identity construction as "aesthetic forming", where "doctor" is formed in difference from "patient", but in *respect for, and tolerance of, that difference* (Bleakley et al 2011). Paradoxically, this has often involved ritual humiliation in medicine (see chapter eleven), where respect and tolerance are not enjoyed in the enactment of professional hierarchy; but times are changing. This also describes a classic apprenticeship. In an oral society, everything is so learned; study, as we understand it, is not possible. The embryonic Slavic poet first listens and absorbs the rhythms, metre, themes and formulas. Then he starts to piece together parts of the poems; finally, he sings the full song before a critical audience - an audience capable of greasing his bow and instrument strings when he left the room if his performance was dull.

What of our young, trainee doctor? Her identity is in part formed by the performance of the ward round and in other public arenas. The performance takes place within strict limits learned by first listening as a student, then, just like the Slavic bards, performing before a critical audience. This absorption of words, phrases and expressions is not just a question of learning and memorising, but more an active soaking up, grounded in performance, that Nagler (1967) long ago described as a "gestalt", a holistic grasp of the occasion. This, again, is the ground for identity construction, the means by which a medical self, an identity of "diagnostician" in particular, is formed, both aesthetically and ethically (Bleakley 2014). There is undeniably a lingering historical form of heroism in this self-forming and it will be interesting to see if this is tempered in an age in which the gender balance has shifted to more women entering medicine, a theme considered particularly in chapters one and two.

The doctor is currently trained (rather than educated) to recast the patient's story into a medical mould; she is a critical intermediary between the illness that patients bring into hospital and the disease they take home (Kleinman 1988). We have described elements of this speech act - a set of linguistic transformations, or compressions, from lay talk to stylised medical talk - as ontological practices that serve to construct identities. This compression limits the doctor to a greater extent than the bard. The form in which the tale is couched is highly traditional and both styles very conservative. There are specifics of the patient's illness, the physical findings and laboratory tests that have to be included and to be accurate. Other material - such as illness in the family or whether anyone is looking after the cat - are embellishments whose inclusion will depend on local attitudes. They will depend too on the character of the doctor. Expression of the social aspects of medicine depends on education, temperament, beliefs and audience. The cat may be written in the record but it takes on a different life when it is spoken out loud.

From a previous generation, Parry (1971, p.270) suggests that: "Just so, writing may influence the text of a poem ... but will not have any (influence) upon the style, nor upon the form, nor upon its life in the group of poets and the social group of which its author was a part". The singer in the *Odyssey* reduces Odysseus to tears when he unwittingly sings of the quarrel between Achilles and Odysseus (*Odyssey* 8. 62-96).

The spoken word moves us in a way that writing cannot, although followers of Jacques Derrida would disagree, where Derrida famously sets out how speech has gained dominance over writing in the Metropolitan West, so that we are a logocentric, or word-centred, and writing-impoverished culture (Derrida 1997). Poetry and philosophy for Derrida are acts of mark-making rather than sound, practices that literally make an impression (in the soft clay). This, says Derrida, is because writing gives you time to think. Speech is too hasty and unprepared. But this returns us to the interesting dilemma in the pre-literate Homeric tradition. Speech for the singer is well rehearsed, built on a template that includes repetition and iteration. But there is also continuous reinvention, room for improvisation and spontaneity.

Speech, suggests Derrida, aims more at the control of others than collaborative exchange. Those in authority, such as surgeons, may think that they talk with their teams, but they are more likely to talk *at* them, giving instructions and advice rather than asking open-ended questions or soliciting the views of others. Hospital songs too, by the nature of their forms, can be authoritative, rather than facilitative of collaboration - telling, rather than conversing to share differences.

Another feature of orality is that its thinking is concrete rather than abstract. Ong (1982, p.49) discusses the work of the Russian developmental psychologist and linguist Alexander Luria with illiterate subjects and concludes that: "oral cultures tend to use concepts in situational, operational frames of reference that are minimally abstract in the sense that they remain close to the living human lifeworld". We cannot say that orality produces the same effect among doctors because they exist in a literate culture, but there are interesting parallels with the medical mindset.

Telling the same story to different audiences

The junior doctor will tell the patient history more than once to different audiences. A different doctor on the same team might also repeat the same history. Is it the same? Is it the patient's story? Does it matter? Is the distinction between the medical song and the patient's song that we made above valid? Parry and Lord had the opportunity to ask their Yugoslavian singers to repeat the same tale twice, sometimes with an interval of years between; or to listen to a tale sung by another and then sing it themselves. They asked the bard if they were the same tale.

> Q: Was it the same song, word for word and line for line?
> A: The same song, word for word and line for line.

All versions were recorded. To the literate recorder, they were quite different: to the singer, they were the same (Lord 2003). With or without the help of the written record (the patients' notes), the telling of the history differs with each teller and telling. To the Slavic singer, tradition and the stability of the story are everything, but this does not mean that the words are fixed. He probably has a quite different notion of what a "word" and "line" are (Kirk 1960). In professional settings, we regard writing as dominant and the written record as the definitive version of events. In a court of law, the medical record will be the gold standard, though it will probably not be the memory of either party. Imagine a society where laws reside in the memory of a few bards; where lawyers do not exist and cannot be imagined.

There are two issues here: first the recasting by the doctor of the patient's tale. As Kleinman (1988, p.207) suggests: "The physician and family caregiver are situated in the gap between the copy and the original. There is a great danger when they recognize only the original". This is an issue of translation, which we discussed in the previous chapter. The other issue is a concern with truth and accuracy - the primacy that the professional world gives to writing over speech, the opposite of the patient's world, where everyday speech genres are privileged over writing.

It is a cliché now to recognise the doctor's story as radically different from the patient's. The issues rest on what is happening about the story's reformulations (in both directions) and how far it does and should go. How far should the patient's account be believed in the first place? (How often is "admits to two glasses of wine per day" written rather than "drinks two glasses of wine"; or "denies alcohol" rather than "does not drink"?) (Donnelly 1988, Montgomery 2006).

The next crisis

One of the great pleasures of studying Homer is to try to conceive what it is like not to be illiterate but to have no letters - to have only (why only?) the spoken word. What, for example does it do to individual and collective memory? We literally have no concept of how it feels to remember, think, make laws, come to agreements in an oral society. What happened after the alphabet arrived, during the difficult childhood and adolescence of writing? Because we write, we may think we have some idea of what was gained but do we have any notion of what was lost? What would happen if our doctor could not record the patient's story but had to process it all internally? And to look forward to the next great event in medical recording, what will happen when we have the electronic patient record? How much patient narrative or account should be a part of this? The information technology ideal is, of course, none. While we have argued for the value of conscious or reflexive Minimalism as a style and form for re-presenting patients, we do not equate this with a collapse of the patient into the virtual.

We have examined what happens at the writing down of the patient's story through the lens of translation studies in chapter four. The moment at which the *Iliad* and the *Odyssey* were captured and fixed as text, simply the mechanics of this, is fascinating to contemplate. We can only really interpret this through our own cultural biases (Bakker 1997). We need the same leap of imagination to think forward to the implications of the future online patient as we do to go back to the first edition of Homer.

If we lose now from transforming Mr Smith's agonising chest pain - with all that it means to him and his loved ones - into a myocardial infarct, what is lost when he becomes a T2800 M58000 (the code for an infarct in SNOMED, the Systematised Nomenclature of Medicine)? Havelock referred presciently to the move from orality to literacy as a "crisis" (Havelock 1986, p.17). We are about to turn patients into avatars. Is that our crisis in medicine?

Notes

1. Some idea of the sound of such a recitation can be found by browsing YouTube. The great difference between performances shows how little we know of pronunciation, delivery or musical accompaniment.

2. In the UK, the Grand Round is a meeting for all grades of medical staff at which one or more patients of particular interest or complexity are discussed. Typically, a junior member of the team describes the patient's illness, and senior members and the audience discuss points of interest and educational importance.

CHAPTER SIX

COMPASSION

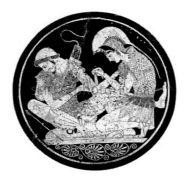

Figure 6-1: Achilles tends the wounds of Patroclus

Communication: skill, or style for life?

In chapter three, we argued that communication skills teaching in medical education can reduce a complex process to instrumental tips. We illustrated this with the famous Embassy scene from the *Iliad* in which Achilles is visited by Odysseus (the wily strategist), Ajax (the blunt warrior) and Phoenix (the wise older man), who hope to persuade him to return to the fray after his refusal to fight the Trojans in the wake of an angry exchange with Agamemnon, in which the commander of the Greek army pulls rank on his best fighter. None of the "three wise men" are able to persuade Achilles to return to battle. Their communication styles reveal serious flaws.

Communication is now widely regarded within medical education as a component of medical professionalism, a learned set of skills and attitudes exhibited in performance, and open to objective measurement or assessment (Stern 2006). Communication includes not only doctor-patient interactions, but also working with colleagues (usually in team settings), educating students, and communicating generally with the public. Policy documents typically prescribe how doctors should behave and communicate as professionals, and list the virtues that inform these behaviours. For example, the UK General Medical Council's regularly updated *Good Medical Practice* includes "probity" (being honest and trustworthy) amongst its recommendations, suggesting that "probity" and "acting with integrity" are "at the heart of medical professionalism" (GMC 2006, p.27).

We agree that communication and professionalism are vital to the practice of medicine, but where medical students' learning of communication has been reduced to performance of atomised, instrumental skills (competences), the complexity of real clinical encounters can be lost. Transfer from the protected learning space (often in simulated encounters with actor patients) to messy clinical contexts is compromised.

Such encounters are contextually sensitive, and imply ethical responses. Educationally, they could also be grounded more in reflection on life experiences than feedback from actor patients in simulated settings. We argue that communication skills are usually considered a-historically, and as given - transparent and unproblematic - activities. Thinking otherwise with Homer can provide a rich background against which to interrogate contemporary versions of interpersonal communication as part of a doctor's professionalism.

There are many "God terms", to use Kenneth Burke's (1966) descriptor for a dominant or exclusive rhetorical notion, in the world of communication skills training - not just in medical education but across the healthcare, caring and helping professions generally (especially in psychotherapy and counselling training). Perhaps the most overused or pervasive is "empathy".

At the time of writing there are more than 1,500 books available on empathy (Baggini 2017) – a veritable business, selling something on which we cannot agree a common definition and which, despite the best attempts of neuroscientists, has no identifiable brain "empathy circuit" that can be mapped through fMRI scanning. Part of the problem is that one school sees empathy as an emotional identification with another (for example, another's suffering), while another school emphasises cognitive identification – a rational understanding of another (for example, another's way of thinking or reasoning) (Bazaigette 2017, Bloom 2017, Sahaklan and Gottwald 2017). Mapping brain functioning is then complicated by prior definitions of what states of mind or states of emotional response you are looking for.

Paul Bloom (2017) describes a "rational compassion" of the sort that doctors might employ, where there is emotional distance between doctor and patient, yet the doctor still "feels" for the patient. He makes a comparison between this state of being and that of Mahayana Buddhist "compassion" described as "great compassion" and distinguished from a more trivial "sentimental compassion" that is also fleeting. "Great compassion" is an enduring state of authentic care for others and for life in general that is characterised by enthusiastic detachment, a concern that does not drain us, as "sentimental compassion" does.

In the orthodoxy of the "helping professions", to not consider empathy as central to your work is a heresy. Following particularly from Carl Rogers' (1951) necessary conditions for a person-centred professional relationship – empathy, congruence and unconditional positive regard – empathy has become the cornerstone of patient-centred clinical practice too.

But, again, what precisely, is meant by "empathy", and is it a modern notion that upon close inspection actually has feet of clay? Through a return to Homer, we problematise the modern notion of empathy, comparing it to pity and compassion as understood in both the ancient and modern worlds.

By questioning what we see as a false division between the cognitive act of empathy and the affective state of compassion, and by recovering a more poignant, ancient use of the now abused (and sometimes abusive) term "pity", we show how the Classics can enrich the communication agenda of contemporary medicine. We suggest that knowledge of an epic story such as the *Iliad*, from the point of view of its tragic content, may provide a script that prepares us for a deeper appreciation of the suffering of patients. This is an axiom of the "literature and medicine" school.

In problematising empathy, we necessarily demand complexity and ambiguity in an era where many medical educationists concerned with professionalism demand simplification, clarity, instrumentalism, empiricism, and measure. We call for a return of empathy to its grounding in the senses, where empathy can be read metaphorically rather than literally, as a challenge to the reductionist approaches characterised by instrumentalism. Finally, we argue for a reading of empathy as a verb rather than a noun, so that empathy is context-specific, as act or performance, rather than personality condition.

Homer's use of "pity" in the *Iliad* offers a striking reminder of the value of critically reviewing the status of words such as "empathy", that have become part of the unexamined fabric of communication skills teaching, again inflated in untouchable "God terms". We examine scenes in the *Iliad* that elicit pity in the characters and the audience, offering a mix of the entirely familiar (a soldier saying farewell to his wife and child), and the bizarre (another soldier-hero fighting a river god); of gentleness and savagery; of the homely and the foreign. Attempting to project ourselves into the mindset of Homer's audience broadens our understanding of how words and actions are intimately linked. Again, it also reminds us that meanings are contingent on the age and peoples that form them.

Pity in Homer

At the end of Book 6 of the *Iliad*, there occurs a famous scene in which Andromache, the wife of Hector, pleads with him to stay within the city walls and not take the attack to the enemy:

> Hector smiled, looking at his son in silence.
> But Andromache stood beside him, her tears flowing.
> She put her hand in his and called him and spoke to him.
> "My lord, your passion will destroy you, and you take no pity
> On our little child, nor me, ill-fated, your widow
> Soon to be." (*Iliad* 6. 404-409).

And then at the end of a long speech:

> "Hector, indeed you are father to me and dear mother
> And brother and strong husband.
> Come now, take pity and stay here on the rampart
> That you may not leave your child an orphan and your wife a widow".
> (*Iliad* 6. 429-32).

Hector replies that he would feel shame to avoid the fighting and goes on:

> "For I know this well in my mind and in my heart,
> That the day will come when holy Ilium (Troy) will perish,
> And Priam, and the people of Priam of the strong ash spear.
> But it is not so much the pain of the Trojans yet to come
> That troubles me, nor Hecuba herself, nor Priam the king ...
> As the thought of you, when some bronze-armoured Achaean
> Takes you off in tears, robbing your days of freedom ... ,
> But may a mound of earth cover my dead body before I
> Hear your cries and know they drag you captive."
> (*Iliad* 6. 447-65).

This is followed by an iconic scene, loved by the ancients, where Hector stretches out his arms to his son but the baby shrinks away from him, scared by the horse's hair plume on his helmet. Hector laughs and removes his helmet, takes his son and invokes

"Zeus, and you other immortals, may this boy, my son,
Be as I am, pre-eminent in war among the Trojans,
Great in strength, as I am, and rule over Troy with strength;
And some day may they say: 'This man is better by far than his father'"
(*Iliad* 6. 466-79).

He hands the child back to his mother, who takes him "weeping and smiling at once". Her husband, "noticing this, took pity on her", and says that "no man will kill him unless it is fated, but no man may avoid his fate". And then, in very simple language:

So saying, glorious Hector took his plumed helmet;
And his beloved wife returned home
Turning often to look back
(*Iliad* 6. 482-96).

And that ends the scene between them. She will not see her husband alive again, although this episode occurs early in the *Iliad*. We, the audience, know that. We are already familiar with the story, and that is the point. Experienced doctors make good clinical judgements with ease because they access stored "scripts" from previous, similar, encounters. This principle stands for communication exchanges also. But "scripts" are also at hand in literature, and perhaps the most common argument for the value of studying literature for practising medicine is that stories prepare you for patients' plots and characters; and genres, such as tragedy, offer archetypal scripts (Kleinman 1988). Exposed to such scripts as the parting of Hector and Andromache, pity is, as it were, hard-wired.

Homer's audience, indeed any later Greek or Roman audience, would have known the Troy story intimately; known therefore that it is scripted that Hector will die at the hands of Achilles, and that Troy will fall. For them, and for us, knowing that Hector's words accurately foretell the fate of Andromache and that the baby will be thrown to his death from the walls of Troy deepens the poignancy of the scene above. Such foreknowledge by the audience is characteristic of Greek tragedy (of which Homer was regarded as the father). Generally speaking, we moderns prefer not to know how things will turn out. The pity of the ancient audience is greater because they know what will happen to Hector and his family – the arc of the tragedy. It is a feeling familiar to those caring for patients - pity for someone of whose fate we have an understanding broader than, or certainly different from, theirs, given by the work doctors do. Entering the experience of the other, which we take to be an essential characteristic of empathy, is, in such a case, a valuable but different process, because the other, the patient, does not always know his or her fate. The doctor knows the potential arc of the course of an illness that the patient suffers. This, again, is the arc of tragedy and its knowledge precedes instrumental empathy.

Communication, virtue, virtuosity

Consider the adaptability in communication that a community-based practitioner must develop: in multicultural settings, with children, with the elderly and confused, and with persons across a spectrum of disabilities, including mental health issues. This same doctor will also engage with the "autonomous patient" (Coulter 2002) who properly rejects paternalism, with patients' advocates including family members, and with the savvy internet-informed patient. How shall we best prepare medical students for such intense relationships? It is important that we do this well, as there is a growing body of evidence demonstrating that the quality of the relationship between doctor and patient has an effect on health outcomes beyond, simply, patient satisfaction (Roter and Hall 2006).

While communication skills are included in learning outcomes across the spectrum of medical curricula globally, and are at the heart of recommendations concerning good medical practice, just how to best teach such skills is debated (GMC 2006, 2007). There is an emerging trend towards use of "safe" simulated settings with both actor patients and expert patients, involving videotaped encounters and direct feedback in custom-built clinical skills laboratories or communication suites. Proponents argue that this offers both "standardisation" of experience and possibility of standardised assessment (Klamen and Williams 2006, pp.53-74).

Assessment is usually through a station of an Objective Structured Clinical Examination (OSCE). In such undergraduate assessment contexts, typically a set of skills, such as "shows empathy", "maintains eye contact", "communicates information clearly and precisely" are atomised as "competences", serve as learning outcomes, and offer assessment criteria. This instrumental approach is now seamless with postgraduate education. For example, the UK General Medical Council's *The New Doctor* specifically lists competences to be achieved for a Foundation (Junior) doctor to progress to registration, including demonstrating "empathy and the ability to form constructive therapeutic relationships with patients" (GMC 2007, p.86).

However, "empathy", as we suggest, is a problematic term. As Veloski and Hojat (2006, pp.119-20) warn: "the theoretical investigation of physician empathy has been hampered by ambiguity in its conceptualization and definition", where "there is no agreed-upon definition of the term". Worse, empathy may be an operational term for a psychological state that "may not even exist" (ibid.). Empathy then becomes not something to define but a metaphor to help us understand a mental and emotional event. Indeed, a key contemporary text on empathy in medicine, *Empathy and the Practice of Medicine: Beyond Pills and the Scalpel* is, paradoxically, replete with the authors' uses of metaphors to describe empathy in a collection that is otherwise characterised by the desire to represent empathy as an empirical phenomenon (Spiro et al 1993). Metaphors of transportation, site, and resonance are common, and commonly occur together, describing placing oneself in the lived experience of the patient's illness, and entering the perceptual world of the other. But these are cognitive events of understanding and insight, rather than heartfelt compassion.

In a book-length empathic treatment of "sympathy", Lauren Wispé (1991, p.78) discloses the core metaphor for empathy as that of travel, or crossing over. This raises questions concerning the motives for that travel, from anthropological study, to the morbid curiosity of the tourist, to the desire for conquest and control of the imperialist or colonist. Is empathy by doctors an authentic entry into the feeling state of patients, or can it be a paternalistic and imperialistic occupation of the patients' lifeworld? Indeed, as Jane MacNaughton (2009) strongly argues, is empathy actually possible at all? Of course we can share a range of feelings and experiences with others, but we cannot, by definition, know the unique other.

For MacNaughton (2009), empathy is a "dangerous" practice. Not just a "god term", but also perhaps a malevolent influence. The doctor-patient relationship is an "I/ Thou" relationship in which one can respect the other with authenticity, but it would be inauthentic to imagine that one can enter and inhabit the other's experience, by definition private and singular. Attempts at inhabiting the experience of the other are fraught with dangers of colonising. We can feel *for*, but not *with*, another.

Pinker (2012, pp.689-713), writing about a broader stage of the decline of violence throughout the world and across the centuries, is sceptical of regarding empathy as the cure for all ills:

> The decline of violence may owe something to an expansion of empathy, but it also owes much to harder-boiled faculties like prudence, reason, fairness, self-control, norms and taboos, and conceptions of human rights.

Going one further, Paul Bloom (2017) believes there is much wrong with empathy: that it is used ambiguously, as we have already noted; that it is biased towards those we favour; that it is directed to individuals rather than groups; and that it may be abused, leading us to wish to retaliate against those who harm people with whom we empathise.

Empathy is fraught with conceptual ambiguity, placing us in the same position as the circular operational definitions of ambiguous psychological notions such as "intelligence" – that "intelligence is what intelligence tests measure". Empathy may be what empathy scales measure, or is a *construct*, a useful heuristic, rather than a tangible state of being. Yet, we undeniably feel in the presence of suffering in common humanity, and here, we argue that a better descriptor for this feeling may be "pity", as described by Homer. Substituting pity for empathy is not merely a semantic sleight of hand. Pity also goes beyond MacNaughton's suggestion that the best we can do is offer sympathy.

The dictionary definitions of empathy and pity reinforce our argument that empathy is a modern, operational term, grounded in technical-rational thinking; where pity is an ancient term grounded in the senses. *The Shorter Oxford English Dictionary* defines empathy as: "The power of projecting one's personality into, and so fully understanding, the object of contemplation". In contrast, pity is defined as "A feeling of tenderness aroused by the suffering or misfortune of another, and prompting a desire for its relief". The first definition implies mastery, indeed occupation; the second, a contemplation and appropriate action, importantly qualified by the descriptor "tenderness". This is a more feminine response of *discrimination* – hence our claim that this is grounded in the senses.

You would think that the dictionary definition of pity is hard to beat, but the word has been corrupted in modern usage, as a kind of sneering. The novelist Graham Greene, in *The Heart of the Matter,* describes Scobie, the main character of the book, as "a weak man with good intentions doomed by his big sense of pity". In the preface he makes a distinction between "pity" and "compassion", sceptical of the former but approving of the latter:

> I had meant the story of Scobie to enlarge a theme which I had touched on in *The Ministry of Fear*, the disastrous effect on human beings of pity as distinct from compassion. I had written in *The Ministry of Fear*: "Pity is cruel. Pity destroys. Love isn't safe when pity's prowling around." The character of Scobie was intended to show that pity can be the expression of an almost monstrous pride. (In Bergonzi 2006, p.124).

In a medical context, Michael LaCombe (1993, pp.54-66), writing in the persona of a senior devil to a junior colleague, recommends using pity to pervert empathy: "permit them to see their patients as simpering fools, helpless wrecks of humanity with whom they could never identify. Let this pity grow, spread like a cancer within them, and you need not worry". Such an understanding of pity is idiosyncratic. It requires a distancing from the object and a feeling of superiority that, we suspect, most would not think was implicit in the term. We have indeed tipped over into instrumental empathy. Definitions matter. Or perhaps this is a matter of understanding and experience rather than definition.

The roots of empathy and compassion appear superficially similar: - pathy and –passion derive, one Greek, the other Latin, from words apparently to do with suffering. Their difference lies in their prefixes – suffering "in" (*em*) or "with" (*com*). In fact, the Latin word *patior,* from which "passion" derives, had a meaning largely confined to suffering or tolerating unpleasant experiences, whereas *pathos* was a much more neutral word meaning experiences both good and bad. *Chambers Dictionary* unconsciously reflects this ambiguity by translating the "-pathy" of empathy as "feeling", and of sympathy as "suffering".

The word sympathy existed in classical Greek times with a meaning very similar to that of today. Empathy, in classical Greece, meant a state of emotional engagement, positive or negative (the opposite of apathy). "Pity" derives from the same word as "piety", the Latin *pietas*. In Old and Middle English, the two senses were intermingled, only separating in the 16th century, when both words took on negative meanings – as a kind of knowing superiority.

Paradoxically, when empathy entered modernist thinking, it was wholly grounded in aesthetics, but has since lost this foothold. Although Jodi Halpern (2001) finds echoes of the term in Hippocrates, it is a 20th century invention, formally coined by the German psychologist Titchener in 1909 as a translation of the German *einfühlung* - literally meaning "aesthetic sympathy". Indeed, Titchener's description only provides further ambiguity, where he says of empathising with another's expressions or qualities, such as pride, that he "feels them in the mind's muscle" (in Wispé 1991, p.78). The metaphor is again one of movement, of crossing over, of a paradoxical "at-a-distance" proprioception, but now we are in the body of the mind, an unfamiliar territory for many contemporary cognitive models of empathy that reduce cognition to brain functions based on engineering metaphors, emphasising, for example, "wiring", "connections" and "transmissions".

The German philosopher Theodore Lipps (1851-1914), who had a formative influence on Freud's model of the unconscious, used *einfühlung* as early as 1903, originally in aesthetics, to describe a process of the observer "entering into" a work of art, and it is only later that such language was used by him to describe entering into the mind of a person.

Importantly, in these early formulations, the passions are clearly engaged, and this differs greatly from contemporary definitions of empathy as the cognitive or knowing partner to affective "compassion". Our conclusion is that there is not only conceptual confusion concerning "empathy", but that the word as currently defined ignores its derivation, in that *pathos*, and especially *empathia* in its original Greek meaning, is a state of *emotional* engagement and not one of cognitive knowing. It is certainly not one of practiced, instrumental "skill" (as learned in "empathy workshops" – territory familiar to one of us (AB) who attended such workshops, designed by Carl Rogers and run by his daughter Natalie Rogers, in the early 1980s, while training as a psychotherapist).

As the General Medical Council (GMC) in the UK and similar medical governing bodies worldwide emphasise virtues such as empathy, probity and integrity as essential to the practice of medicine, we should examine virtue, as did the ancient Greeks. We follow the well-trodden path that there is a direct link between ancient Greek and current Western thinking (Fredrick 2002). Discussions of virtue thread through Plato, particularly *Meno*, *Protagoras*, *Republic*, and *Laws*. *Meno*, a dialogue between Socrates and the young aristocrat Meno, opens with Meno's question to Socrates: "is virtue something that can be taught? Or does it come by practice? Or is it neither teaching nor practice that gives it to a man but natural aptitude or something else?" (Plato 1956).

Socrates' rhetorical strategy is to not answer the question, but to direct attention to the key prior question: "what is virtue?" In answer to this, Socrates says: "The fact is that far from knowing whether it can be taught, I have no idea what virtue itself is" (ibid., p.115). This resonates with contemporary scepticism over measuring "empathy" before we have a clear notion of what empathy is. This is a matter of "proof of concept".

Over 2,400 years after Plato, Louise Arnold and David Stern (2006, 19) graphically model medical "professionalism" as a classical Greek temple, where the supporting base (as three steps) is composed of "clinical competence" (knowledge of medicine), "communication skills", and "ethical and legal understanding". The roof is "professionalism", and the pillars supporting the roof are four virtues: "excellence", "humanism", "accountability", and "altruism." The authors explicitly equate professionalism with "virtue" (ibid., p.20). "Excellence", currently a buzzword in medical education policy documents, is characterised by "a commitment to exceed ordinary standards" (ibid., p.21). Here, a return to classical Greece will help us to further define "excellence", and also sharpen our understanding of "virtue". This, in turn, will lead to a better understanding, and appreciation, of "empathy".

In describing the relationship between rhetoric and athletics in ancient Greece, Debra Hawhee (2004, p.17) notes a tradition of naming specific virtues, such as courage, but also of articulating an overall "virtuosity" (*aretē*). Hawhee describes Greek athletic competition as a form of "rhetorical practice and pedagogy" in which competitors persuaded, or won over, the audience through their bodily prowess or virtuosity. In early Greek athletics, winners were judged by their ability to enter the field of play (*agōn*) as a warrior enters battle, showing the virtues of courage, honourable engagement, and physical prowess. However, as athletic contests matured, virtuosity was judged as excellent where it explicitly avoided moralising, or piety.

This subtle shift framed virtuosity as a highly focused or concentrated activity combining physical prowess (skill) with wisdom of the body (*mētis*) that is best translated as "adaptability", and an art of timing or exploiting opportunity (*kairos*). This combination goes well beyond mere competence, turning sport into performance art. In the field of play that is the *agōn* of communication in medical practice, excellence might better be termed virtuosity, where virtuosity is a combination of skill (in reading, and responding to, cues), adaptability, and the art of timing.

Let us explore this a little further with emphasis upon empathy. While technical virtuosity – for example as surgeon, diagnostician, or psychiatrist – is easy to grasp, how might we frame virtuosity in the non-technical realms, such as communication and its subset of empathy? Arnold and Stern (2006, p.21) describe empathy as a subset of "humanism" - one of their pillars of virtue – along with respect, compassion, honour, and integrity. Further, these virtues must be enacted (or performed) for them to have any meaning, and this enactment is embodied in communication that is clinically informed and ethical. These authors distinguish empathy from compassion, where empathy is defined as a cognitive "ability to understand another person's perspectives, inner experiences, and feelings without intensive emotional involvement", plus "the capacity to communicate that understanding" (ibid., pp.23-24).

Compassion, in contrast, refers to the affective dimension of being "moved by the suffering or distress of another and by the desire to relieve it" (ibid., p.24). As we shall see, when Homer describes what we might now call the skilful employment of empathy, he uses the term "pity", which artfully collapses the modern technical (and arbitrary) distinction between cognitive and affective components.

Our shift from the virtue of the communicator to virtuosity in communication serves an important function – it links us back to Classical thought in two senses. First, in Homeric Greek language (and then thinking), there is no sense of personal agency as intention. Medical students come with the modernist cultural baggage of "introspection", "autonomy" and "self-regulation", descriptors that would have had no meaning in Homeric Greek.

Empathy is considered as something that comes from within oneself and is projected onto another, as the dictionary definition suggests. In Homeric Greek, there is no "I" who is "empathic", and then no projection outwards of empathy from within the self to another. Rather, pity is embodied in an action, or is a verb, and is contextual. That is, pity is distributed - embodied in a social occasion or as an immersive engagement with the natural environment. Ruth Padel (1992, 1995), in discussing images of suffering in ancient Greek literature, does what medical educators now encourage – she shows that a value or a virtue can only be understood in terms of a performance. It is not what the medical student thinks that matters, but how she acts. Further, the act is not mediated through the inner world of the student, but through the total context of the student's engagement with the world at any one time. Again, virtues are immersive expressions and not personal projections.

To elaborate this point against the modern dominance of subjectivity, in Homeric Greek, many verbs, often those describing what goes on in the head, do not exist in the active form. There is no first person active voice ("I understand you"). Rather, these notions are expressed as a "middle voice" verb, which is "very close to passive, what is done to you by an outside agent" (Padel 1995, p.23). Not "I am disappointed", but "disappointment is upon me", and this is known in the form of the resultant activity – disappointment as performance. If empathy, recast as pity, is considered as a verb rather than a personality trait, it is interesting to consider its meaning in this middle voice.

This unhooks us from our obsession with "character training" as professionalism in medical education. Rather, we are now interested in how medical students act with patients as a contextually-sensitive performance in which "compassion" is a distributed phenomenon and not capital owned by individuals. Thinking otherwise with Homer can then re-cast "patient centredness" as a verb and not as a slice of communication capital that, paradoxically, objectifies the patient. Instrumental application of empathy as a "thing" learned in workshops can end up like a magical lubricant owned by the professional that is applied to the dysfunctional machinery of the patient.

While we have warned against cultivation of personality type in favour of consistently observable activities of patient-centredness, a return to Classical thought also helps us to reframe the virtuous personality in terms of a social identity. Let us return to the conceptual model of professionalism proposed by Arnold and Stern (2006). As described above, a supporting pillar, or virtue, central to professional behaviour is humanism, which includes empathy and compassion. Humanism is defined as "a sincere concern for and interest in humanity" (ibid., p.22), without which, how could doctors treat a variety of patients with concern? We will not pursue here the difficulties presented by that weasel word "sincere", connected as it is with probity or honesty. Rather, we are interested in the implications of "humanism" and its relationship to identity.

In an effort to provide an alternative to the Western humanistic tradition's way of thinking about selfhood and identity, Michel Foucault (2005) made a close study of late Greek and early Roman texts that describe a "care of the self". These texts do not address a core (immature) self that must realise its potential, but rather show how an ethical self can be developed, constructed, or produced as a social performance in particular contexts. In the same way that athletes can attain virtuosity through practice and artful engagement, so persons can shape themselves aesthetically, or form character.

Such a background provides a new reading of medical education – not just as a technical "training" (again, a sad reduction to instrumental skills), but as an aesthetic self-forming, to shape a professional identity. Hawhee (2004, p.93) equates this process with *phusiopoiesis*. First described by the pre-Socratic philosopher Democritus, *phusiopoiesis* is the *"creation* of a person's nature" (ibid., p.93, our emphasis) grounded in poetics or aesthetics, not in simply functional behaviour.

Foucault (2005, pp.98-9) discusses texts by Philo of Alexandria (20 BCE–50 CE) and Epictetus (c.55-135) that suggest those interested in care of the soul, as well as care of the body, could form a "clinic" where you learn collectively how to do philosophy. We can readily translate this into contemporary medical education, where aspiring doctors learn both how to treat the body and how to set up the circumstances that will offer a healing or therapeutic *relationship* with patients. Importantly, at the same time, the medical student is doing work on identity, or forming a style of life.

In Foucault's reading (ibid., pp.339-40), Epictetus provides far more sophisticated advice on speaking and listening than most contemporary texts on the medical encounter. For example, Epictetus warns about being captivated by the speaker and not listening-through to what is underneath the surface talk. This recognises that talk is acting rhetorically, and certain persuasive elements must be recognised and challenged. Listening is also charged rhetorically. We can listen in various ways – hearing what we want to hear (rhetorical listening), missing the point (not listening well), or listening well (offering benefit both to speaker and listener), including knowing when to be silent. Speaking and listening are not instrumental but an art, requiring discrimination and diligent practice.

A return to pity

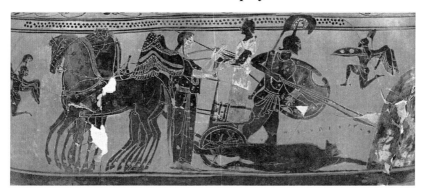

Figure 6-2: Achilles drags the body of Hector around the walls of Troy

Hector's foreboding of the fall of Troy is correct. But Homer's *Iliad* ends before the fall of Troy, with Hector's death. Achilles kills him in revenge for Hector's slaying of Patroclus, the beloved friend of Achilles. Achilles defiles Hector's body by dragging it around the walls of Troy and denying it burial. The climactic ending is the secret visit of Priam, the Trojan king, to the Greek camp to beg for the return of his son's body for burial. He starts by reminding Achilles of Achilles' own father, Peleus, and comparing Peleus' fate with his, Priam's, own:

> "Reverence the gods, Achilles, and take pity on me
> Remembering your father, yet I am still more pitiful.
> I have endured what no man else on earth has endured before.
> I have brought to my lips the hand of the man who killed my son."
> (*Iliad* 24, 486-506).

The Greek word *eleos*, used in this dialogue, can mean both "pity" and "mercy". *Kyrie eleison* means "Lord, have mercy on us" but also "Lord, pity us". In examining how wars are memorialised, Tatum (2004, p.165 and note) hesitates between the uses of pity or compassion to describe the feeling of Achilles for the old man. He appeals to "modern usage" to draw a distinction between the two words that we suspect does not exist for most contemporaries.

Since the death of Patroclus, Achilles has behaved like a savage, slaughtering the enemy in vast numbers even when they are disarmed and beg for mercy; he has sacrificed Trojan princes at the funeral pyre of Patroclus. Since his quarrel with Agamemnon at the beginning of the *Iliad*, Achilles' refusal to take part in the war has been morally suspect. With his later actions, he moved beyond the pale of acceptable morality. The above scene with Priam restores his humanity. He takes Priam by the hand and, knowing that his own death will come soon, tells Priam that suffering is the lot of man, that Zeus keeps two jars at his feet, evils in one and blessings in the other, which he distributes randomly to humans.

In this speech, says Macleod (1985, pp.8-11): "there is endurance and sadness, but no bitterness, no railing or cringing". And, "This is also the fullest and deepest expression in words of Achilles' pity for the suppliant; for pity, as Homer and the Greeks represent it, is a shared human weakness. And it is pity which is at the heart of Homer's conception of poetry". We must not judge Macleod's use of "weakness" as negative. By it, he means a shared human wound. Indeed, the common ownership of "pity" affords recognition of the fundamental nature of humanity – that we are flawed and liable to wound and be wounded. Achilles takes pity on Priam, and Hector's body is restored and receives burial.

Such was the spirit of compassion that infused this last book of the *Iliad* that some late commentators argued it could not belong to the original version. One powerful argument for its integrity is the apparently unconnected scene between Hector and Andromache described above. It contrasts Hector, a man with a wife and child, the main defender of his city, who undertakes a task to which he feels ethically bound, with the solitary, selfish Achilles, driven only by wrath and a desire for revenge (Macleod 1985, Schein 1984).

There are also deliberate echoes in this scene that take us back to the very beginning of the *Iliad* when Agamemnon harshly rebuffs the pleas of another father, and initiates events that lead to the deaths of Patroclus and Hector. The epic turns a great circle until a quarrel that started in Book 1 with a suppliant to a king, is resolved with a king who is now the suppliant. Both protagonists at the beginning (Agamemnon and Chryses) will survive the war; those at the end (Achilles and Priam) will die. Achilles is a better man than Agamemnon because he can regain his humanity and do what is right. The body is restored to Priam, who takes it back to Troy for cremation and burial. Agamemnon is cast as a man without pity and we, the audience, must pity Agamemnon for his character flaw.

The pity of the audience is elicited for a final time by the lamentations of the three women most important to Hector during life – his wife Andromache, his mother Hecuba, and Helen. It is striking that almost the last words of the epic are left to Helen. In a sense, she had nothing to do with him (as relative, wife or lover), but she is ultimately responsible for his death, because she left her husband to elope with Paris and brought the Greeks in pursuit to Troy. Hector and Priam are the only two of the city's inhabitants who have treated her with kindness and without reproach since she left her home. It leaves the epic on a note of ambiguity. We are left looking backwards and forwards to the wrongs done in the past and the many deaths to come in the future. Helen, the cause of the war, is one of the few to survive it.

Conclusions: empathy ancient and modern

Examination of the *Iliad*, a foundation stone of Western thought, reassures us with scenes like those recounted above, with which we can identify easily. Yet we should learn from Homer that such identification is facile. For example, it is commonly assumed that women are more empathic than men, and Hojat and colleagues confirm this as a significant difference in scores between male and female medical students (Hojat et al 2002a, 2002b). Yet Homer elaborates his view of pity and compassion largely through male characters. It can be argued that the sharp contrast between their heroic aggression and savagery and their familial tenderness makes the quality of pity more subtle, evanescent and complex.

We have already argued that listeners to Homer's stories in the oral tradition may have been sensitised to pity, as the story unfolds in a characteristic manner. Yet Hojat and colleagues (Hojat et al 2004), in a further chapter in their extensive research programme on empathy in medicine, suggest that medical students are de-sensitised, or lose empathy, as they move through medical school (yet they see more patients). This is often explained as a necessary development of defence against the sheer volume of distressing circumstances that the doctor will meet. But these studies come with a health warning – the data are based again on measurement of "empathy" without rigorous proof of concept, so that, again, the object "empathy" may be constructed by its measurement.

If we take the core of the meaning of empathy as engaging with, and understanding, the mind or purposes of another, it may seem unsurprising that there was no word to describe this over two millennia ago. More

importantly, the notion of entering the mind of another would, again, have
been incomprehensible to ancient Greece – at least for humans (Padel
1992, 1995). The Gods, or natural forces, may do this through dreams, and
do so in the *Iliad* (2. 1-75, for example). We should pay more attention to
the metaphors we use in describing empathy. What do we mean by
"entering" the mind of another, or "resonating" with it? We automatically
locate the mind, or consciousness, within the brain.

Where Homer located it would have depended on what precisely was
being described. "Thinking" is located in internal organs, the pericardium
or the diaphragm, linked through an overall receptive quality (*phrenes*)
(Padel 1992). In turn, *phrenes* act as containers for passion (*thumos*).
Thumos does come to mean the heart, but in general it is a mood or quality
that resides in organs rather than being one. The "mind" then did not arise
in the body, but entered organs as responses to events. Consciousness was
more nebulous - an airy substance located in blood or breath (Padel 1992).

Emotions were more complex still, located in the chest, heart, liver, or
breath (Onians 1988, pp.23-89). But is this any cruder or more primitive
than locating "mind" in brain - already complicated by recent work on the
enteric nervous system located in the gut (Furness et al 2014)? The
complexities of language, of course, will subvert such locations through
metaphor, for example Titchener's embodiment of mind in locating
empathy in the "mind's muscle" – a way of saying that we are *moved* by
things.

Recall the two events recounted earlier - the sacrifice of the princes,
and throwing Hector's baby son from the walls of Troy (the latter episode
not in the *Iliad* but known to the audience and haunting the scene with
Andromache described above). The *Iliad* is full of savagery – the killing of
enemies by painful and grotesque means; boasting over the corpse;
refusing to spare the life of a helpless foe. It is a small step to label those
who do savage deeds as savages, or primitives. Yet our own killing is
savage, but done by others, usually at a distance, usually unseen. Sheather
and Hawkins (2016) describe two things as standing out "from the
conflicts that have disfigured the world in recent years: the casting aside of
moral boundaries; and its subsequent normalisation".

In the film "Troy", Hollywood rewrites classical mythology to avoid
unpleasantness and sweeten a pill too bitter for modern audiences. In the
scene between Hector and Andromache, Hector shows her a secret way
out of Troy and, at the end of the film we see her and the baby escaping.
Hollywood does not want to know about its heroines led off to
concubinage, and babies hurled from city walls. Yet similar distressing
events are happening in war zones such as Aleppo as we write. We

generally recoil from such distressing scenes as outside observers and we feel compassion for victims. But this is not "trained". It is a gut response that might as well be described by the ancient Greek *thumos* – an indication that we can be roused to emotional response. Modern "empathy" does not help to better explore these gut, human feelings.

Our medical education approach to training empathy within the framework of professionalism has strayed too far from this direct, human response to tragedy. It is cultivated and dry, almost pompous. It is a kind of knowing that again is potentially invasive or colonising of another's experience, rather than appreciative of it. The best way to illustrate this is through a warning. "Empathy" has been colonised by the business world as a "business opportunity". Here is some blurb from the website http://www.empathytraining.co.uk: "So, imagine if you were really able to read people and turn them into business benefit by selling to them, or managing them, more effectively. Empathy is a powerful tool for you to do just that!" In our "post-truth" condition, politics too has been appropriated as just another business.

The company "empathytraining" gives a definition of "empathy": "understanding what makes people "tick" and dealing with them more effectively". As medical education becomes more management-oriented and less patient- and pedagogy-oriented, we are likely to see "quick fix" empathy training gaining a foothold in medical students' and doctors' education. Note the colonising language – "dealing effectively" with others sounds like one-way traffic. Dictators are good at "dealing effectively" with others; so are drug dealers and con-artists.

If this is the current of contemporary medical education, let us step out of the river and return to ancient Greece. Homer still resonates with us and can inform our ethical practice because the *Iliad* and *Odyssey* have poetic depth; meanwhile pity, sympathy, empathy, and compassion have been examined formally in medical education for only half a century (Wilmer 1968) and, in our view, in a surface manner now drifting into facile business-speak. "Pity" is not a sneering, but a shared ability for compassion. And patient care is grounded in compassion. Doctors might note the saying often, and probably wrongly (http://quoteinvestigator.com/2010/06/29/be-kind/), attributed to Plato: "Be kind; everyone you meet is fighting a hard battle."

CHAPTER SEVEN

LYRICISM

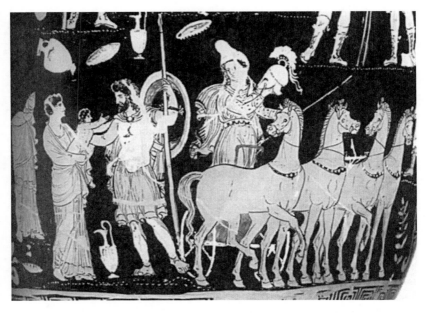

Figure 7-1: Hector's poignant farewell to the wife and child he will not see again

Waxing lyrical

In researching teamwork in the operating theatre, one of us (AB) observed intestinal surgery on a male patient suffering from Crohn's disease, carried out by a senior, male surgeon who would not mind being described as old school.

Crohn's disease, one form of Inflammatory Bowel Disease, offers a puzzle to scientific medicine. Its exact causes are unknown and there is no cure at present. The symptoms can be debilitating - mild to severe inflammation and thickening of the intestinal tract (anywhere from mouth to anus, although usually the large or small intestine) leading to general fatigue, abdominal cramps, diarrhoea and weight loss. Crohn's disease appears to result from an overactive immune response, and shows elements of an autoimmune disorder. Where lifestyle, diet and drug therapies fail, surgery offers a final option. A portion of the inflamed intestine is removed in a bowel resection, giving relief, but possibly not cure.

The surgeon in question was carrying out this operation and talking his assistant through the anatomy, when he suddenly stopped in mid-stream and asked the whole team to gather around the patient on his side of the table. The fact that the invitation was so cordial took some of the team by surprise, as they dutifully moved closer. The surgeon had gently lifted a portion of the intestine to reveal some fascia (connective tissue). A combination of the reflective surface from the liquidity of the tissue illuminated by surgical lights produced an extraordinary local rainbow effect. The gut fascia shimmered. The surgeon wanted to share this moment of wonder with the team, the revelation, or perhaps the conjuring, of this interior rainbow.

He seemed to be talking to the temporary phenomenon itself, in a moment of touching gratitude and celebration. It was like a modern conjuring of ancient Homeric *phrenes* - discussed in the previous chapter – the interior body medium through which "thinking" occurred, or which "gathered" thoughts to it. More so, this was a revelation for the team members. The scrub nurse said afterwards that she had never heard this particular surgeon "wax so lyrical", and that this tender moment really touched the team as a whole, who felt drawn together as a unit to experience this delicate and temporary wonder.

The operation, it should be noted, was deemed a success. Previously in decline in popularity amongst his colleagues, the surgeon's ratings soared, his display of "emotional intelligence" was favourably noted, and more, his lyrical interlude was read as a notable moment of patient-centredness for a surgical episode.

A man who had a similar operation for Crohn's disease has uploaded a You Tube video of a portion of the procedure, giving the following explanatory commentary (Hirschberg 2009):

> Taken in about 1995, I gave my surgeon my video camera and somehow convinced him to video tape (sic) my operation. The operation was to remove several diseased sections of colon/small bowel effected (sic) by my Crohn's Disease. This was actually the 2nd time my surgeon had opened me up like this and pulled a whole bunch of pieces out. I got to hold almost

the entire length of my large intestines in my hands (after the surgery was complete of course). I guess I'm a tinkerer to the end, even when it concerns my own body mechanics.
(https://www.youtube.com/watch?v=w89s28pkhrw).

What is striking about this commentary is its moments of lyricism amongst an otherwise matter of fact, mechanical view ("tinkerer", "body mechanics"). The tinkering patient continues in the same vein: "I love to know how stuff works. There's one shot I particularly like where you can hear the heart monitor beeping and you can see the intestines giggle subtlety (sic) with each beep". More, he then notes how the surgeon engages lyrically with the patient. In talking his assistant through technique, the surgeon addresses his teaching not to his assistant, but directly to the patient himself, as if he was awake, so that the patient says: "And I absolutely adore how they are explaining each step to ME (sic) in the first-person as the video proceeds while I'm laying there dead(ish) on the table".

In literature, the lyrical poem is characteristically autobiographical and expresses feelings, drawing out elements of beauty and form (Cowan 2012). At its best, such literature offers close observation of sensible events rather than abstractions. In these surgical cases, the lyrical is both embodied (the beauty of the patient's gut), and embedded - in immediate, lived tragedy (the gut is diseased).

Ironically, Crohn's disease signifies the opposite to the fine discrimination advertised by the lyrical genre. It seems as if the body has lost its ability to discriminate. Where the immune system normally fights off foreign invaders, in Crohn's disease there is a loss of discrimination between the normal, healthy life forms in the gut and foreign bodies. The body then attacks itself. This can be thought of as a form of auto-anaesthesis – the opposite of a discriminatory sensibility or the ability to choose between what is and what is not of value. An anaesthetic dulls, where the aesthetic event acutely raises awareness, or attunes the senses.

Crohn's disease then acts as a metaphor for what opposes the lyrical – thickening, irritability, and an inability to discriminate what is of value resulting in unintended self-harm, rather than autobiographical finesse. It is a burden for its sufferers, and a blessing to see that in both of these surgical examples lyricism, in a sense, was part of the intervention to relieve suffering.

In the case of the surgeon who drew attention to the chance appearance of the rainbow in the gut fascia, what impulse grabbed this normally taciturn man to announce such an embodiment of beauty and radiance in a frankly uncharacteristic moment of tenderness and lyricism? Such tender-minded behaviour is normally denied, or openly mocked, in the tough-minded climate of the operating theatre. Indeed, to whom was this surgeon speaking? Not, as it seems on first appearance, to the gathered audience of the surgical team and attendants, but rather to the self-display of the intestine itself, as an embodiment of lyricism.

This moment could be read as a recognition and celebration of the lyrical as the Cinderella partner to the more commonly noted epic, tragic and comic events by which medicine and surgery are more easily recognised. To a Homeric audience, our surgeon might seem to be possessed by the gods (*enthousiasmós*), literally overwhelmed by enthusiasm.

Medical genres

The lyrical is usually overshadowed, or indeed squeezed out, by the dominance of the epic, tragic and comic genres in medicine. That medicine is concerned with the epic is self-evident – the cycle of life from pre-births to comas and deaths; whole population epidemics; slow-burning viral disorders; large scale pharmaceutical interventions from birth control to anti-depressants; the new plagues linked to conspicuous consumption, where populations inflict diseases - such as type 2 diabetes - upon themselves through lifestyle, unable or unwilling to make changes; avoidable medical error as a major source of injury and death; and so forth.

Tragedy is everyday in medicine – "acute", "emergency" and "intensive" care; sudden and serious illness; genetic disorders; chronic conditions that wear down the body and spirit; spirited people who suffer from terminal illness yet live life to the full; patients in a coma with loved ones talking to them in blind hope; the desperation of those who wish to end their lives in dignity but are legally blocked from doing so; and so forth.

The widespread use of the comic genre as a mode of initiation or socialisation and identity construction has been the medical profession's long-standing secret and a source of interest and critique particularly for sociologists and psychoanalysts, but is now publicly advertised as a common theme for medical television soap operas. The comedy is dark – "black", or "gallows", humour (Piemonte 2015). The French surrealist André Breton first coined the term *humour noir* to describe gallows humour, where the topic is usually illness, suffering and death, often aimed at a specific victim.

Breton credits Jonathan Swift as the primary source for modern black humour, whose stock-in-trade includes taboo subjects usually associated with bodily functions. This connection with the suffering body makes it easy to see why black humour should be adopted in medicine, yet the motive is rarely to poke fun at the victim but rather to use such humour as a defence against carrying the full emotional impact of daily exposure to suffering, and to initiate clinicians into expert use of this ego defence.

Sigmund Freud (1928) famously defined all humour as an emotional anaesthetic, deflecting and absorbing the full impact of affect that would otherwise be too much to bear, where the ego "insists that it cannot be affected by the traumas of the external world". Black humour affords the biggest sponge, soaking up the emotional excess that would otherwise swamp us in times of trial.

Patients would be horrified to hear the banter - often at their expense - in the tearooms of intensive care teams or the changing rooms of surgical teams. In places close to death, such as intensive care units, accident and emergency departments, and surgical theatres, black or macabre humour is carefully hidden from patients' families and friends, as a "backstage" performance. In the public realm, sick jokes about tragedies generally backfire. The danger of accepting that we can laugh at the tragedy of others, or institutionalise this in public comedy, is that we become desensitised to the very thing we are trying to protect ourselves from through comedy.

Lyricism, however, serves a different function. The lyrical impulse draws our attention not only to delicacy, tenderness, and the joyous (*jouissance*), but also to verve, desire, eroticism, the fecund, abundance, and generation. Synonyms for "lyrical" include musical analogies such as choral, dulcet, harmonious, chiming, lilting, songlike, tuneful and rhythmic; others concern the tasteful, such as poetic, pleasing and rhapsodic. Such delicate flowers are hard to sustain in the face of the tragic, epic and dark comedic currents prevailing in medicine. Indeed, the rare beauty of the lyrical and poetic is more likely to be overshadowed by the sublime (Bleakley 1997), where the epic comes to absorb lyricism.

The sublime is the bigger and darker force in aesthetics – the awe and wonder felt in the presence of a thunderstorm. Traditionally associated with the "divine", the sublime appeals to the faux divinity characteristically attributed to the headline-grabbing heroic acts of big surgical or medical intervention. While the sublime is a headline grabber, most medicine takes place beyond or behind the front page. In this apparently mundane medicine, we may find that "small is beautiful", offering an everyday radiance of care - again, the tender and delicate, the sudden revelation of the embodied lyrical with which we opened this chapter. In what sense do we celebrate, or even encourage such lyricism in medicine?

We believe that we need to maintain the profile of lyrical work as a gesture of resistance against the dominance of the epic, tragic and dark comedic in medicine. There is a pragmatic reason for this. At the heart of good medical practice is an acute sensibility expressed through diagnostic acumen. This is the ability to take a good history, including a physical examination, and to subsequently make good clinical judgements. Around 15% of avoidable medical errors are due to misdiagnoses (Sanders 2010), where diagnostic acumen is a combination of a keen narrative sensibility (hearing patients' stories) (Charon 2011), and heightened use of the other senses such as sight (Bleakley et al 2003) and smell. As Abraham Verghese (1999, p.299) notes:

> Smells registered in a primitive part of the brain, the ancient limbic system. I liked to think that from there they echoed and led me to think "typhoid" or "rheumatic fever" without ever being able to explain why. I taught students to avoid the "blink-of-an-eye" diagnosis, the snap judgement. But secretly, I trusted my primitive brain, trusted the animal snout.

Repression of the lyrical equates to dulling or anaesthetising of the aesthetic possibilities of medical practice – a more acute and generous sensibility whose practical outcome is closer noticing for better diagnoses and overall humane care. Conversely, emphasis upon the lyrical may turn medicine from a tough-minded to a tender-minded practice in a tough-minded world, again challenging the classic emphasis of medicine on "cure" rather than "care". Follow this line of reasoning through, and we echo the argument of chapters one and two, where traditional, masculine heroic medicine transforms into a more feminine, collaborative practice.

The erosion of care

Improvement in doctors' ability to communicate well with patients and with colleagues is of pressing concern in medical education, as we have seen from previous chapters. This relates particularly to the continuing phenomenon of "communication hypocompetence" (Platt 1979). Where technical competence is generally good in graduates from medical schools, the non-technical areas of communication and teamwork present an ongoing concern, despite over 30 years' worth of attention to formally teaching communication in undergraduate curricula. The symptoms of our inability to produce doctors who can communicate effectively with patients and colleagues have produced an iatrogenic epidemic of epic proportions - that of unintended medical error (Bleakley 2014).

Medical error is a major source of injury and death. In 2000, an estimated 225,000 people died as a result of medical error in the USA (Starfield 2000). Indeed, in 2004 medical error was recorded as the third major cause of death after cancer and heart disease in the USA

(HealthGrades Quality Study 2004). Martin Makary and Michael Daniel have recently confirmed this in a 2016 *British Medical Journal* article (Makary and Daniel 2016), noting that "medical error" does not appear on death certificates or in rankings for the cause of death.

A similar iatrogenic epidemic can be noted in the UK, where estimates for deaths caused from medical error vary between 11,000 per annum to 72,000 per annum (Barron 2009). Vincent (2001) puts the figure at 40,000, while a more recent 2012 survey by Hogan and colleagues (Hogan et al 2012) suggests that there are 12,000 *preventable* deaths in UK hospitals every year due to problems in care. While this is more than three times the number of fatalities from road traffic accidents, we should not forget that there are 400 million successful patient episodes each year in the UK National Health Service. Clearly, however, we have to address this iatrogenic epidemic grounded in communication hypocompetence.

Medical students are usually keen to gain meaningful contact with patients, but even before graduating, they show signs of empathy decline (Pedersen 2010, Neumann et al 2011). The evidence base suggests that doctors as a whole are, relatively, fairly poor at communicating with patients (Roter and Hall 2006); communicating with colleagues in, and across, team settings (supposedly co-ordinating practice around patient care pathways) is particularly bad, where "70–80% of healthcare errors are caused by human factors associated with poor team communication and understanding" (Xyrichis and Ream 2008). This can be addressed by "improving communication and teamwork skills" (Agency for Healthcare Research and Quality 2008), again transforming heroic, competitive medicine into collaborative care.

Current forms of education into effective communication within structures of professionalism, now often learned in simulated settings, appear to be failing. Thus "Medical mistakes still occur at an alarming rate" and improvement is "slow and sporadic" (Graban 2011). We seem to forget that what Owen Barfield (1973) called "poetic diction" – the ability to turn a phrase beautifully according to context - is a health intervention in its own right. We then call for medicine to explicitly inhabit the lyrical genre, where grace, elegance, sensibility, sensitivity, and so forth, are seen as essential capabilities for the humane practitioner. Without the lyrical, medicine is impoverished, or instrumental.

We suggest that repression of the lyrical in medicine and medical education, for whatever reason, may be the cause of the well-documented phenomenon of empathy decline in medical students and junior doctors. "Empathy decline" (we use the term cautiously - see the previous chapter six for a critique of "empathy") is a technical term that dissimulates its complexities - the excessive dulling of sensibility, as overcompensation for potential emotional overload, in the face of the epic and tragic. Such dulling of sensibility may lead to erosion of care.

Our suggestion goes further – the erosion of care is not confined to a containment of emotional response, rather it includes the blunting of the senses, compromising perceptual acuity necessary for expert physical examination and diagnosis. We are not the first to notice such perceptual erosion – Abraham Verghese (https://www.ted.com/talks/abraham_verg hese_a_doctor_s_touch) has campaigned for many years to maintain quality of hands-on doctoring in an era of increasing reliance upon remote imaging and tests for diagnostic purposes. For Verghese, hands-on bedside technique is also a lyrical medicine, one of intent to care and engage. Verghese is both a respected physician and an accomplished writer, for whom the territories of lyrical composition and sense-based medicine are clearly complementary.

Our plea is then for an aesthetic medicine informed by the lyrical. By "aesthetic" medicine we do not mean "surgical enhancement". Freud's dictum that the repressed returns in a distorted form can be applied to medical practice and medical education, where repressed aesthetic (beauty) returns as its opposite form – anaesthetic, dulling, brutal and ugly. This runs throughout patient services – numbing schedules, top heavy clinics, impossible targets, heavy handed or cumbersome management, bad food, poor design in hospitals such as lack of natural light, uncared for buildings – to unfeeling or brusque face-to-face care and outright abuse (see chapter eleven). Of course, there are structural causes of such symptoms, including lack of financial resources.

Shall we then learn our lyricism from physician-authors such as Verghese? Certainly this provides a meaningful touchstone for medical students because such writers draw on their experiences of the ethical and sensible practice of medicine to illustrate their lyrical themes. But all lyrical writers ultimately owe a debt to Homer, for it is in Homer and the Homeric imagination that we find the primary examples of lyrical sensibility. Importantly, in Homer, the lyrical is embedded in the epic, tragic and comic – as is the practice of medicine – and is embodied, or illustrated in relation to the physical stresses and strains of the human body. Even in the most distressing descriptions of savagery in warfare, Homer manages to find a lyrical touch – here, with the guts showing in quite a different way to our surgical example opening this chapter. As they spill out of Polydorus at the point of death, he attempts to hold them back:

> Then Achilles went after the godlike Polydorus,
> son of Priam. His father did not allow him to fight

because he was the youngest of his children
and was the most loved; and he was the swiftest of foot.
Just then, showing off how swift he was in his foolishness,
He was rushing through the front lines of battle until he lost is life.
Achilles, swift and godlike, threw his spear into the middle
Of his back as he rushed by, where the golden buckles
Of his belt joined, and his breastplate doubled down on it.
The point of the spear went through by his navel
And he fell to his knees and screamed. A dark cloud
Covered him, holding his guts in as he fell (*Iliad* 20. 407-18).

The lyrical body in Homer

Where, in other chapters in this book, we return to Homer as a primary source, in this chapter we purposefully draw on a secondary source. This is a contemporary "excavation" of the battlefield of Homer's *Iliad* to reconsider the deaths of mainly minor figures – soldiers - as an atmospheric war memorial by the poet Alice Oswald (2011), who read Classics at Oxford. In *Memorial* Oswald offers a radical re-working of parts of Homer's *Iliad*. She bypasses the primary action of Homer's epic - the quarrel between Agamemnon and Achilles and its consequences - to foreground another layer. She reveals this sub-text as the poem's *enargeia* – a "bright and unbearable reality". This is a term used by the ancient Greeks to describe the autobiographical appearance of the gods rather than appearances in disguise, and is then a term describing epiphanies. In this excavation of the *Iliad* for its "atmosphere", Oswald reveals a particularly lyrical seam within the epic. A lyrical account is of course in its own right an epiphany – a realisation of the extraordinary in the ordinary.

Oswald focuses upon the deaths of soldiers as described by Homer, often as brief and gruesome sketches, literally to the point, as spears pierce flesh and organs are impacted, such as Polydorus' death above. Again, she sees this detail in the *Iliad* as forming a parallel world - that she describes as "a set of atmospheres" - to the main action or narrative impulse. This rhetorical move effectively erases the epic's narrative structure to, again, reveal its lyrical pockets of action. We learn from Oswald not just a revelation of content as "atmospheric", but a poetic technique that we can readily transpose onto reading medical culture, to ask unsettling questions - in particular about the strained relationship between communication and medical error.

Oswald then re-members dead soldiers and their means of dying through a contradiction: poetic listing; as if creating a war memorial. Lists are normally literal and do not need to be repeated by definition. Oswald's lists are at first sight epigrammatic and bear repetition to burn them into memory. But the epigrams soon dissolve in the liquid diction that is Oswald's hallmark. For example, the soldier Dolops dies from being speared, with "the beak of death" pushing "out through his own chest". These short descriptions offer highly compact biographies and intensely direct ways of knowing, leading us straight to the heart of the individual. Naming, or "personifying" (Hillman 1992), is compounded through similes, so that a death in battle is, in Oswald's reading of Homer, "Like a wind murmur", or "Like the war cries of cranes going south escaping the rain". Such similes, suggests Oswald, derive from pastoral lyric, "because their metre is sometimes compressed as if it originally formed part of a lyric poem".

Collectively, the descriptions of how these soldiers die that Homer offers add up to an atmosphere or climate that we can equate with medicine as well as war, with patients replacing soldiers. Medicine of course characteristically draws on militaristic metaphors such as the "war on disease" and "fighting infections" (Bleakley 2017). Paradoxically, medicine's Achilles' heel is its historical legacy of working within militaristic hierarchies and command chains, which frustrate the collaborative and democratic communication exchanges needed for effective teamwork around patients, and supportive communication with patients in consultations.

Just as war has its casualties, some caused by "friendly fire", and many of which are civilian ("collateral damage"), so medicine has its casualties – natural and unnatural deaths, including that spectre of the iatrogenic epidemic grounded in "communication hypocompetence" that we described earlier, and which can be thought of as medicine's own unfortunate "friendly fire".

Oswald's poetic strategy also foregrounds Homer's lyrical charge, a lyricism often overshadowed in the *Iliad* by its sweeping epic and tragic concerns (while the *Odyssey* more obviously has lyrical concerns, as well as its epic and tragic themes, and its occasional comic incidents). We suggest that this same poetic strategy can be applied to medicine and medical education. Students and junior doctors learn a good deal about the foreground of the epic, tragic and dark comic. We have argued that medicine is framed by the epic and heroic in order to keep the tragic at bay, hoping for the narrative arc of the epic to play out within each tragic "case" so that the patient experiences a victory and homecoming rather than an upset, a stain, a turn for the worse, or a death. The repressed tragic then returns in a distorted form, as tragedy engineered by medicine itself – iatrogenic illness and doctors in distress (Peterkin and Bleakley 2017).

However, what is missing in this analysis is the overall atmosphere or climate that is constituted by the deeply lyrical content of the passage of people's lives through the clinic, the hospital and the operating theatre. Let us take an illustrative example, transposing Oswald's poetic device on to medicine.

Oswald's poetic technique develops empathy (or rather the deeper and more universal sense of pity as compassion, as we argued in the previous chapter six) in the reader for the unknown fallen soldier, elsewhere a mortality statistic, through an autobiographical moment using lyrical form. So Iphinous falls on the battlefield; "springing into his chariot" he feels "a blow on his shoulder" and "dropped/ Like a leaf from a topmost twig". We come to know Iphinous, albeit briefly, through the lyrical association with a gently falling leaf, and in this brief elegy, gravity, honour and dignity are suddenly restored to the soldier. Within the noise of battle is a bubble of quiet within which we might hear a leaf fall.

An arrow hits another soldier, Gorgythion, that "flies" through him. Oswald compares his death to a "poppy being hammered by the rain" in June, so that it "Sinks its head down", as does Gorgythion. In a startling analogy – in the direction of the abstract lyrical to the concrete – Oswald compares the drooping of the poppy's head (blood red of course) with a typical soldier's death: "When a man's neck gives in/ And the bronze calyx of his helmet/ Sinks his head down." The lyrical comparison is drawn from culture rather than nature.

But the calyx, as every botanist and gardener knows (Oswald also learned the craft of gardening), is the name for the sepals of a flower that in turn enclose the petals; although calyx is used generally in biology to describe an enclosing, cup like structure, such as the renal calyces – "holding" chambers through which urine passes. Bringing together the bronze helmet and its specific calyx produces a lyrical marriage of culture and nature. We normally think of a helmet-shaped part to a flower, but not of a flower-part of a helmet. The horror of battlefield death is then paradoxically softened, but remains tart.

These pithy descriptions are also, in medical terms, "cases" - their causes of death now described poetically and sensibly, rather than technically and in dull prose (as in doctors' reports). A further example – "poor ARCHEPTOLEMOS" evokes the feeling of a very ill patient with fever in the intensive care unit - one minute there, the next, gone. The soldier's life burns away in a flash, like "fire with its loose hair flying", that is "unmasked light" with a characteristic "look" that "shocks everything to rubble" as it "rushes through a city", where "flames howl through the gaps" in the rubble. To the family, the patient who has burnt out is like the city demolished and they stand in the rubble, shocked and howling. Worse, if they discover that the death was a result of a medical error: a misdiagnosis, a team miscommunication, or an error in treatment.

To add insult to injury for family members, where tragic medical errors are made, apologies are sometimes not forthcoming, or communication with family members fails to fully disclose the error for fear of filing malpractice claims (Truog et al 2011). Oswald describes the death of Polydorus, where "somebody has to tell his father" who is "looking for his favourite son", exhausted; so that he "stares himself stronger" in the face of bad news "Clenching his whole face fistlike/ Around the stones of his eyes". We do not know if he is steeling himself, refusing the inevitable tears; or if he is staring down the bringer of bad news, in medicine usually the senior doctor. In this scenario too, desperately sad acceptance is sometimes displaced by immediate anger and possible abuse on the part of family members (see chapters eight and eleven), with the (again, usually senior) clinician who is "breaking bad news" in direct line of fire.

The tradition of "lament poetry", which Oswald reveals as the atmospheric caul hooding Homer's otherwise muscular epic, could readily be adopted as a core competency in learning communication skills in medical education (we use these contemporary instrumental words – "core competency" and "skills" - with a health warning, where they devalue the complexity of doctors communicating with patients and colleagues). Rather than reinforcing the tradition of poor, even disgraceful, dealing with disclosure when things go wrong in medical care, perhaps we can learn from lament poetry about lyrical communication – in other words, so-called "breaking bad news" that is sensitive, sensible and deeply felt. The content of the news doesn't change; the truth must be told, a death has occurred.

But the why and how, and the manner of telling, are critical, just as Oswald's re-telling of the *Iliad* is a necessary poetic gesture. This would constitute a medical language that speaks directly to the person concerned – the anaesthetised patient as if she were fully aware; the relatives of the dead in honest but caring and supportive terms; the everyday patient as person and equal; and the colleague as collaborator. If such bad news is broken with that degree of concern and honesty, it constitutes a poetic gesture, well beyond the purely informational and literally descriptive.

Finding a place for the lyrical

Part of the vitality of the *Iliad* and *Odyssey* rests in their re-telling. Audiences expected the bards to stay true to the oral tales first written down by Homer, but also craved the individual touches of bards who

improvised around familiar themes producing lyrical effects. As Christian
Meier (2011, p.197) notes, by around 600 BC in ancient Greece, festivals
were being held that featured competitions between singers, "where such
competitions clearly stimulated efforts to retell old myths in ever new,
better, and more beautiful forms". Lyricism was added to the epic cycles,
tragedy, and comedy.

It would be unfair to say that the lyrical has been abandoned, or driven
out of medicine altogether, through the dominance of other genres,
particularly the pincer effect of the epic and tragic. While the Greek idea
of the symposium (literally a "drinking party") is usually associated with
philosophical and political debate, special symposia included poetry
contests as platforms for development of lyrical forms of expression that
celebrated unique personhood and moral virtue.

In medicine, the Grand Round can be seen as a version of the poetry
symposium, encouraging eloquent and pithy "case" presentations (see
chapters four and five). Here, as in the ancient Greek festivals, the epic
song cycles with their familiar tropes such as aphorisms (wisdom
condensed into sayings) (Levine and Bleakley 2012), as medical lore, are
re-storied for contemporary times through lyrical inventions. The old
myths concerning symptom – grounded in tragedy and epic forms – are
embroidered or carefully compacted in lyrical forms as they are
personalised for this particular patient at this particular bedside. They are
mannered performances, where the practical and critical forms of
evidence-based medicine are given lyrical form as idiosyncratic, narrative-
based patient histories.

Coda

Alice Oswald's lyrical re-writing of Homer's war memorials may be seen
as a feminist reading, displacing active heroism with passive reception in
acts of dying re-told gracefully, to restore dignity to the dead. This concern
is mirrored generally in feminist readings of healthcare, with an emphasis
upon care rather than cure. We suggest that where lyricism remains
subservient to the dominant genres of the epic, tragic and dark comic, or
indeed is repressed, this has a serious consequence. Repression of the lyrical
may frustrate the exercise of a formed sensibility. The latter is expressed not
only in terms of an appreciation of the value of tender-minded care, but also
in clinical acumen as expertise in physical examination and diagnosis.
Perhaps so-called "empathy decline" in medical practice, that can be argued
to be an iatrogenic effect of medical education, is the primary symptom of a
loss of the lyrical imagination in medicine.

CHAPTER EIGHT

ANGER

WRITTEN IN COLLABORATION WITH DR DAVID LEVINE

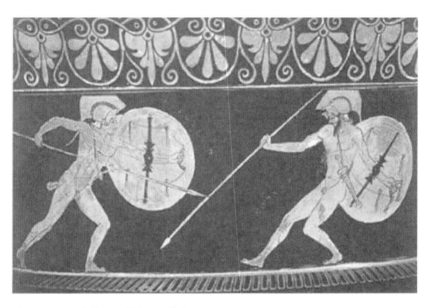

Figure 8-1: Achilles and Hector fight

"He drove forward with a yell"
(Achilles rejoins the fight against the Trojans, *Iliad* 19. 424).

Medicine as epic

Medicine and surgery are intrinsically stressful occupations. Moment-to-moment stressors in medical work are rarely catalogued but cumulatively important. For example, a recent UK study of the shift of a senior emergency medicine consultant showed that he was interrupted on average every ten minutes (Allard et al 2012). Some of these interruptions are vital, but most simply disrupt the flow and tempo of work and offer distraction rather than focus. Such unwanted interruptions can inhibit clinical reasoning and generate frustration. Interruptions may be considered minor stressors in relationship to medicine's main characteristic – living with uncertainty (Wellbery 2010).

Add to this: long hours requiring intense concentration in often poor working environments; maintaining a professional demeanour in the face of roller-coaster emotions; adapting to ad hoc clinical team settings; trying to adhere to guidelines, protocols and targets as idiosyncratic challenges unfold that demand improvisation; emergent paranoia as a reasonable response to management surveillance; and sometimes difficult patient encounters, and the reasons for mounting frustration are clear.

In contexts such as surgery or emergency medicine, frustration can be intensified particularly by equipment failures, and poor intra- and cross-team coordination. There is a range of emotional, physical and intellectual responses to cumulative stressors and these can be considered at the levels of the individual, the team and the culture. At the level of the culture, medicine has historically been performed in the genre of the epic as we argue in our Introduction and elsewhere.

As medicine has increasingly come under public scrutiny for transparency and is rapidly changing its constitution – for example with more women than men entering the profession and workplace, and collaborative, inter-professional teamwork preferred to autonomous practice – so the cult of heroic individualism is dissolving, and along with it the historical alignment of medicine with the epic genre. Despite this shift in genre, there are many issues that linger from medicine's historical relationship to the martial and heroic world that we address in this chapter. In particular, we consider how both the latent and explicit energies of frustration and anger in medicine may be productively channelled. First, let us consider the status of the historically belligerent culture of medicine, with its key metaphor of "medicine as war", a theme that runs throughout this book.

Medicine as war

It can be argued that the cultural psyche of the Metropolitan West is shaped as much by the Homeric epics, the *Iliad* and the *Odyssey,* as by biblical lore and the great humanistic texts of philosophical inquiry stemming from Plato and Aristotle. The *Iliad* is a war book, part of which the late poet Christopher Logue (2003) rewrites under the striking title "All Day Permanent Red" – a bloodbath, a crimson-stained earth, red mists descending. Medical historians have thoroughly mined Homer for the literal battlefield, such as descriptions of war wounds (Manring et al 2009). But medicine as a metaphorical battlefield has attracted less commentary, yet this metaphorical frame is probably the key signifier for contemporary medical culture, and is highly problematic (Bleakley 2017). Does medicine have to be aligned metaphorically with war and has this always been the case? What are alternative leading metaphors to medicine as war? And would changing metaphors change the culture and practice of medicine?

A metaphor works by transposition, where a particularly abstract or complex idea or object, such as the body, can be grasped in terms of a simpler or more familiar notion, such as "plumbing", or a "machine" – for example, the brain is (like) a computer (Lakoff and Johnson 1981). The metaphor mediates between what is unknown and what is known. Through metaphors of war, the complexities of medicine can be reduced for ease of comprehension. We can think of enemies (illnesses such as cancer, causes of illnesses such as bacteria and viruses) on battlefields (the hospital, the operating theatre, the clinic) being attacked by commanders (doctors) of armies (clinical teams) with sophisticated weapons (drugs, surgery). Medicine's "hospitality" (sharing the same etymological root as "hospital") has been forced to adapt to a tough-minded, masculine Procrustean bed. Arrigo (1999) describes medicine as "anchored by martial images and saturated in war-making discourse".

In Greek myth, Procrustes was a blacksmith who made an iron bed to which he fitted people by stretching them or cutting off their limbs. Does the bed of martial metaphors force the practices of doctors, healthcare practitioners, and above all patients, into fitting what can otherwise be seen as an arbitrary set of guiding metaphors? Phrases such as "war on cancer", and talk of *combating* illness, where *invading* bugs are the *enemy* in the *battlefield* of the patient's body, that is under *siege* but might be treated with *magic bullets* are taken for granted and then not actively changed in discourse, and discourse is the script shaping performance, or how medicine is practiced.

It is not only the language and metaphors of the activities and sites of war that might shape medical practice, but also the language of emotions accompanying strife, such as "exploding with rage". Hodgkin (1985) notes that medical training includes a hidden curriculum of metaphors concerning the temperature control of emotions – for example, when the patient is boiling, the doctor can reduce the emotional temperature through cold detachment.

Nominalists will argue that words are merely surface descriptors and that they do not shape practices. Most linguists, however, would disagree, suggesting that language matters, shaping not only our thoughts, but also our performances. Lakoff and Johnson (1981) have argued eloquently that metaphors become embodied in lifestyles. Metaphors are not just tropes (figures of speech) - rhetorical devices used to persuade - but figures of thought that shape activity as metaphors become embodied in valued cultural forms and patterns of work. "Medicine as war" can form belligerent postures, as practiced performance, such as the stereotypical "scalpel-throwing surgeons" discussed by Scheinbaum (2012), hopefully now becoming an extinct species.

This moves language beyond mere representation and depiction of objects, to language embodying objects in, and as, activity. Metaphors do not mirror reality but create realities – not simply describing, but inscribing and prescribing, behaviour.

It was not always the case that medicine was described martially (Fuks 2009, Lane et al 2013). Notions of "fighting disease" seem to have entered western medicine particularly through the works of Thomas Sydenham (Fuks 2009) in England in the mid-17th century. Prior to that, links between illness and violence metaphors referred to a moral struggle. Where medieval medical texts refer to "fighting" metaphors these are in the context of fighting sin, so that illness may be metaphorically contextualised as a moral problem. "Holy" and "healing" stem from the same root, where a holy body is a whole body, balanced and well.

Sydenham may have known the poet John Donne's sermons that included frequent use of "illness as violence" metaphors; and in his writing, such as "Devotions Upon Emergent Occasions", Donne describes his own illness in 1627 as resembling a "siege" and a "cannon shot". Donne thought he was dying from a fever "that blows up the heart", also describing an "illness that invades".

Sydenham described medical intervention as if he were vigorously using an assault weapon: "I attack the enemy within", where "A murderous array of disease has to be fought against, and the battle is not a battle for the sluggard". The most famous physician of his day, Sydenham summed up his approach as: "I steadily investigate the disease, I comprehend its character, and I proceed straight ahead, and in full confidence, towards its annihilation".

Sydenham's metaphors, however, did not constitute a dominant discourse at the time. Such a discourse was established in modern medicine two centuries later by Louis Pasteur's "biomilitarism". Montgomery (1996) notes that while early 19th century doctors used passive language such as plagues "laying" upon people, Pasteur mobilised an unashamedly active, militaristic language, where diseases "attacked" persons. Pasteur's description of germ theory overlaid a previous language of "excess of vital forces" within the body with one of invading armies laying siege to the body that becomes a battlefield. Over a century later, as Fuks (2009) suggests, "The war metaphor is so familiar and commonplace in our medical rhetoric that we easily lose sight of its militaristic origins and significance".

In other words, medicine as a battlefield is now a naturalised notion, but once had to be established with militaristic zeal. As Fuks further argues, the medical gaze can be equated with the martial gaze, as the battlefield changes through history from the sickroom of the 18th century, to the pathologist's bench of the 19th century, to the imaging room of the 20th century, and the DNA sequencer's computer screen of today.

A "war against cancer" was first described in a lead article in the *British Medical Journal* in 1904 (Reisfield and Wilson 2004). This rhetoric was extended to identify the "fight against cancer" as an issue of imperialist domination, where the disease itself was described as "darkest Africa" waiting to be discovered and conquered. Later, cancer cells were identified with Bolsheviks, as "anarchic", threatening the stability of the body (ibid.). Cancer has continued to attract militaristic and imperialistic language. In 1971, Richard Nixon, then President of the United States, delivered a famous speech declaring a "war" on cancer, where science would "conquer" the disease. At this time, bioscience was replete with martial terms such as "killer" cells and "invasive" species. However, to employ martial language against itself, there are casualties from this approach.

Is illness to be eradicated before it is understood? Symptoms may serve purposes. For example, being constantly "run down" and prone to minor infections may show that we are stressed from working too hard. Depression and anxiety – so readily treated by drugs – may be a sign of a manic culture, where the threshold for depression remains low. Where illness is a target and an enemy to be eradicated at all costs, the cost may be the patient, who suffers from the "friendly fire" of side effects as iatrogenic illness. Treating illness as an enemy can serve to depersonalise and deprive the patient, whose unique voice is lost to the generalised "target", and who may be reduced to helplessness, where the doctor plays the active hero role and the patient is a bystander as the illness dragon is engaged in battle, hopefully to be slain.

Hodgkin (1985) pointed out that "medicine as war" is readily twinned with "the body as a machine", further alienating patients through "mechanistic hubris" rather than recognising the organic individuality and humanity of each person. Hodgkin notes that fighting wars is primarily a masculine activity. Medicine as war may have been useful in reinforcing the demand for steel and stamina that doctors needed to work long hours within a militaristic hierarchy and code of honour, but such a culture - serving to work against the development of feeling tone and reflection in doctors' work - is outdated. At a personal level, it encourages great concern with reputation, the equivalent of the fighting Greek's honour (*timē*), a concern that can lead to the sort of violent outburst that Achilles demonstrates at the start of the *Iliad* (Scodel 2008).

Alternatives to medicine as war

In 1978, the novelist and social critic Susan Sontag wrote a groundbreaking book *Illness as Metaphor* (Sontag 2009a), in which she launched a – paradoxically - hostile, no-holds-barred invective against the use of metaphor to describe illness, but in particular against martial metaphors to describe cancer and its treatments. In short, she saw martial metaphors as stigmatising the patient. The apparent anger shaping Sontag's book can be explained by the fact that she was receiving treatment for breast cancer herself, later described in her 1988 companion volume *AIDS and its Metaphors* (Sontag 2009b).

These books did more than simply describe the fact that medicine employing martial metaphors had become a dominant discourse. Rather, Sontag argued that this discourse was negative towards patients and must be challenged. Sontag argued that metaphors circumscribing illnesses - in particular cancer – could stop patients from seeking appropriate treatments and may add to their suffering. She demanded that illnesses be stripped of their metaphorical clothing to reveal them simply as naked phenomena open to largely successful medical interventions. Using an analysis of tuberculosis as a background, Sontag argued that cancer is neither a stigma nor a curse that people bring on themselves; nor is it a punishment or an embarrassment.

Militaristic language frames cancer and its treatment as a combat zone – something that patients may not resonate with themselves, or may not feel up to engaging with. In this sense, use of martial metaphors can be counterproductive. In summary, for Sontag, diseases should be thought of without recourse to metaphor, stripped particularly of militaristic associations. But Sontag herself was a writer, and her absolute rejection of the relationship between metaphor and illness is surely too sweeping and in danger of throwing the baby out with the bathwater – a more productive argument may be to call for a shift in the focus of metaphors, away from martial language to some other form.

Metaphors are important in helping us to form meaning within, and for, illness. Switching from combative "warfare" to collaborative "welfare" metaphors may affect practices – for example, by turning attention away from a disembodied agent of illness that must be eradicated to an embodied person who needs care. Unlike Sontag, Carola Skott (2002) sees value in illness metaphors, where they create meanings and bind patients to supportive communities sharing the same metaphorical complexes. Skott, focusing on cancer narratives, also questions the uncritical acceptance of martial metaphors, where, for example, some patients see cancer as "a thing in the air" rather than being "invaded by a killer". Martial metaphors have gained a purchase in medicine and surgery, and continue to be used by doctors and surgeons, possibly because they serve a purpose in maintaining the power of such doctors and surgeons at the apex of a militaristic hierarchy as described earlier.

There is a longstanding argument in political theory that under a "state of exception" or a "state of emergency", such as a war, unusual steps may be taken to award absolute power to an individual or Government. It is then a commonly used tactic by dictators to maintain a permanent state of emergency so that they can retain their authoritarian grip on the State. Where, for example, the surgeon wishes to maintain authority, surely a good tactic is to maintain a permanent state of emergency or unrest, bolstered by reference to medicine as war? This seems to be a tactic used by some surgeons, where the permanent "enemy" in the war is not however disease or illness, but rather "management", "bureaucracy", or "protocols". The surgeon can divert attention away from internal conflict by reminding his team that the real enemies are elsewhere.

De Leonardis (2008) suggests that the widespread use of medical metaphors follows a similar logic, where:

> medical metaphors are part of the logic of dehumanization and reification of the enemy typical of war discourse … they introduce and spread the

idea that the governed must submit to the ruler with the same eagerness a
patient entrusts his/her health to a physician.

The language of war works within its own logic by eradicating its enemies,
so that it is difficult to spot alternative metaphors. Reisfield and Wilson
(2004) note that martial metaphors are inherently bullying - masculine,
power-based, paternalistic, and violent or violating. But patients may tire
of this. The authors quote a patient with colon cancer who said that seeing
his relationship with cancer as a battle "was less than palatable" because "I
had already experienced real war in Vietnam and was not anxious to repeat
anything closely resembling that".

It may then be exhausting for already exhausted patients to think that
they have a battle on their hands, and the notion of victory may be far from
the reality. Colleen Bell (2012) suggests that drawing on metaphors of war
for medicine is unethical, granting legitimacy to war itself and acts of war
such as atrocities and rape. Daniel George (2010) brings us back to
specific locations on the battlefield, noting that in care for dementia the
common and unquestioned use of bellicose terms, such as "fight", is
"metaphorically rendering the brain a seat of violence", where the
metaphor is unproductive. We might extend this critique to a range of
trials and tribulations of the elderly that do not extend to the bellicose,
such as osteoarthritis and other wear and tear diseases; or even the sorts of
infections that come at the end of life – bronchopneumonia, for example,
was once described as "the old man's friend". We are now a long way
from end of life war and violence metaphors.

Already, we can see that military metaphors in medicine are historically
transient, fraught with contradictions and conceptually weak, and fail to
capture the patient's perspective. Further, such metaphors dull the capacity
for reflection where their rhetorical style is that of the insistent bully.

Hodgkin (1985) suggests that, given the historical dominance of the
militaristic-industrial complex of metaphors in medicine, the introduction
of new metaphors may seem "precocious". Yet, medicine and illness can
readily be imagined as collaboration rather than heroic struggle, or as
exploration and a journey. Cancer, for example, has been described as a
chess match, a marathon, a drama and a dance (Reisfield and Wilson
2004). It was not always the case that medicine's interests were described
martially. For example, in early modern Europe, cancer might be
associated with impurity and rot, or with a corrosive acid, but not with an
invading enemy or a hostile presence that has to be killed. The root
meaning of cancer is "crab" or "crayfish", and the disease was so named
because the margins of some cancers send tongues of invasive tumour out
into surrounding tissue that look like the claws of a crab. A commonly

used metaphor was that of a rooting (and not even a rotting) plant that was difficult to eradicate and produced seeds, referring to metastasis (from the Greek, meaning "a change of position"). Cancer again was typified in terms of a "shifting" presence. The disease was shifty, but not aggressive.

We have already discussed issues of hospitality in Homer and in medicine. Homer, particularly in the *Odyssey,* explores the key role of domestic hospitality, and illustrates occasional breaches of this tradition that cause outcry. We see such hospitality as central to medicine ("hospitals", "house officers") in terms of keeping the stain of the tragic genre at bay, where households are disrupted. Maintaining hospitality is then a key discourse offering an alternative to "medicine as war" or as violence and conflict (Bleakley 2017).

Three other "front runner" emerging alternatives to "medicine as war" are: (i) health as balance and imbalance (homeostasis and dystasis), (ii) medicine as collaborative exploration rather than heroic struggle, and (iii) illness as a journey. People suffering in particular from chronic illnesses such as heart disease have characteristically had their identities shaped by the didactic metaphor of "illness as a journey". This metaphor offers rich cross-domain mapping drawing on speed, progress, direction, goals, and pursuit. It is not as aggressive as the martial metaphor and for this reason may be easier to accommodate for patients. Certainly it is the key didactic metaphor in self-help books about illness, now a major genre in literature, and such literature – in the key of New Age therapy-speak – is in danger of trivialising the journey metaphor, or Romanticising it as a new version of the masculine "hero's journey" with its tired dragonslaying motifs warmed over as fantasy fodder. Such metaphorical frames readily attract and absorb "alternative" therapies too.

A glaring alternative metaphor to the militaristic is the "ecologic". Concepts from the ecology movement, incorporating systems thinking, can readily be translated across to medicine, including "complexity", "dynamicism", "systems", "adaptability", "emergent properties", "holism", "integrity", "balance", "natural", "ethical use of limited resources", "quality of life", "diversity", "renewable", "sustainable", "responsibility for future generations", "community", and "conservation". Thinking with systems also challenges the hegemony of "body as machine" metaphors, replacing the linear but complicated (yet fixable) with the complex, unpredictable and ambiguous.

"Ecology" is derived from the ancient Greek *oikos,* meaning a "household". It can refer to a family, a domestic arrangement such as a family's finances, and the house within which a family lives. This returns us to metaphors of hospitality.

The use of an ecological and pacific metaphor complex may shift medicine's primary concern with aggressive treatment to co-ordinated and educated prevention, where population medicine becomes primary; also shifting values away from waste to conservation - from maintaining life at all costs to facing death more realistically. We might also temper false hope in technology-led medicine as saviour and restore "small is beautiful" values and habits of fellow feeling, mutuality, and supportive intervention to communities. Ecological, pacific and collaborative metaphors work readily together.

So, "medicine as war" is then an historically recent and problematic metaphor and should be challenged for its dominance (Segal 1997, Docherty 2001, Slobod and Fuks 2012). Let us now turn our attention to how medicine as war plays out at the level of individual psychology. What of confrontation, anger and violence within and between individuals in medicine and healthcare? Here, we will invoke Homer's guidance.

The return of the repressed

At the level of the individual, cumulative frustration can lead to anger, sometimes directed outwards and again leading, in the worse cases, to "scalpel throwing surgeons" (Scheinbaum 2012), confirming a stereotype. But more often, such anger is directed inwards and repressed, leading to chronic patterns of emotional self-hurt and an outward cynicism that is part of the well-documented phenomenon of "empathy decline" (Neumann et al 2011). This could be a modern description of Achilles' sulk after the argument with Agamemnon that opens the *Iliad*. Achilles beats himself up, loses interest in the war and becomes cynical, and has no interest in alignment with the views of others, as the Embassy scene illustrates (see chapter three).

As Freud famously argued, the repressed returns in a distorted form. But nearly three millennia before Freud, Homer had graphically depicted how repressed anger returns in patterns of both inward facing self-destructive sulk and outward facing cynicism and redoubled anger – anger as uncontrollable rage, best characterised by the trance-like furies of the Norse *berserkers*. In Book 20 of The *Iliad*, Homer describes Achilles berserker amongst the Trojans:

> Achilles lunged at Demoleon ... The lance burst through the cheek-piece of Demoleon's helmet, broke open his skull, scattered his brains. ... Achilles threw a javelin ... The point emerged from Polydorus' navel; he halted, fell groaning on one knee, pressed back the bowels as they gushed out ... . Achilles' sword swept off (Deucalion's) ... head and helmet. The

trunk fell supine, its severed backbone dripping marrow. (*Iliad* 20. 232-40).

Caroline Alexander ((2009) reminds us that: "the greater part of the *Iliad* is concerned with killing and dying ... in relentlessly inventive detail". The detail shows Homer's anatomical knowledge: a soldier is speared "in the right buttock, and the spearhead drove straight/ on and passing under the bone went into the bladder". While the battlefield needs a hospital, embracing the metaphor of medicine as war, the hospital too becomes a battlefield rather than a place of hospitality. Indeed, hospitals are relatively dangerous places to work (see chapter eleven). Hospital workers are four times more likely to be exposed to violence than those working in private sector industry (Feldmann et al 1997, National Institute for Occupational Safety and Health 2002), where patients or patients' family members in psychiatry and emergency medicine are the main sources of physical assaults on healthcare staff. More often, though, violence is enacted as verbal bullying, illustrated in this example from a scrub nurse gathered from a study of close call reports in operating theatres (internal hospital data Bleakley and Hobbs 2013):

> The surgeon was picking on me during the operation. I ignored being told off for preparing the bone donation. I ignored being told off for not having a joint replacement instrument (JRI) in hand. When I handed over the JRI, I then got a lecture 'when was I going to learn what he needed etc, etc'. (The JRI was on my trolley). The surgeon makes it clear that in his eyes I do nothing right (no mention of everything I do correctly) ... Eventually, he found another thing to moan about and I got a lecture on being useless, when would I learn, etc. It was stopped by me bursting into tears and telling him, I had had enough ... This has been going on for quite a long time, but I thought I had dealt with it, by standing up to him and being very firm: it obviously is not working, no matter how much I stand up to him.

Studies in Poland of psychiatrists (Debska et al 2012) and physiotherapists (Szczegielniak et al 2012) describe how atmospheres and cultures of aggression emerge in healthcare as a stressful triangle between individual practitioners, patients and colleagues. For example, frustrating encounters with patients may initiate clashes between colleagues. These studies define aggression as "forceful behavior, action, or attitude that is expressed physically, verbally, or symbolically".

Despite psychiatrists being the very professional group that may have most insight into such encounters, the authors suggest providing psychological support for this group. A questionnaire study of 50 physiotherapists (ibid.) showed that, on average over a month, 60% of practitioners were exposed to both patients' and colleagues' aggressive verbal abuse, 26% reported feeling discomfited by patients' self-directed aggression, and 8% suffered from actual physical aggression. Only 6% of the cohort had no report to make about aggressive encounters. The studies conclude that further research in the field is needed.

How might we address such disturbing practice issues through thinking imaginatively with Homer? This can offer an aesthetically- and morally-charged alternative to topics such as anger management in doctors without recourse to an instrumental economy, where emotions are viewed as commodities and emotional responses can be "trained" in communication skills courses, as if we were performing seals. Let us think with Homer specifically about confrontation and anger at work not to rid medicine of anger but to reinvest the emotion with meaning and purpose. Surely it is a central function of medical education, where the medical humanities are a key component (Bleakley and Marshall 2013), to articulate, help to implement, and then evaluate, strategies for turning what was previously counterproductive behaviour into something constructive?

Rageaholics and civility

Inappropriate patterns of angry behaviour in medicine can result from personality issues - such as the "acting out" typical of a Type A, impulsive personality (Ragland and Brand 1988). But they are also a product of cultural and environmental factors, as already noted. It is a fact of working life that healthcare professionals, including doctors, must become an-aesthetised to environmental issues such as inadequate or saturated lighting, and excessive background noise on busy wards. We rarely draw attention to the importance of such environmental factors, where attention and motivation may be persistently challenged by fatigue and stress (Peterkin and Bleakley 2017). Rather, we can become dulled to such perceptual overload and compensate, developing poor habits such as lack of full attention and awareness, which may subsequently bleed into poor judgement and sloppy ethical behaviour or "professionalism lapses", grounded in cynicism and using black humour as a form of displacement (Piemonte 2015).

We might work all day "on edge". In the same study of "close call" or "near miss" narrative reports from operating theatre personnel quoted above, a scrub nurse from an orthopaedic surgical team reports that the surgeon was getting by with inadequate equipment and getting increasingly frustrated and tetchy. A drill "blew up" in his hands. The surgeon then "blew up", losing his temper; and at the end of the day she reported that the team "had been skating by the seat of its pants", and had been, in various ways, "on the edge" and lucky not to have suffered an incident or accident. All who work in such stressful surroundings are open to being shaped by them, often close to blowing their tops, and in danger of compromising patient care.

The vicissitudes of anger are the central topic of the *Iliad,* which Robert Graves' (1959) free translation re-titles as *The Anger of Achilles.* Anger is also a key theme in the *Odyssey,* which culminates in one of the most gruesome accounts of insult and violence in the history of literature. Further, as Jenny Strauss Clay (1997, pp.59-60) notes, "Odysseus" may be derived from *odysasthai,* "which means 'to have hostile feelings or enmity toward someone'". This can take various forms such as "to be angry", "to hate someone", "to vex", "to trouble", and "to offend". Clay notes that the renowned classicist W.B. Stanford had said of Odysseus' name that its meanings were wide enough to include "anger" and "hatred". Dimock (1956) translates his name as "Trouble", implying "bringer of" and "sufferer from", and Shay (2002) brings the name to life by pointing out that his Vietnam veterans, on their return home, often brought trouble to their families.

In both Achilles' and Odysseus' destructive behaviours we can draw parallels with medicine's (and in particular surgery's) historical valorising of both the arrogant and the scheming hero. But Homer provides his heroes with redemptive features: in particular, Achilles' blind rage is twinned with the capacity for both moral courage and tender, homoerotic love (Achilles' passion for Patroclus).

If medicine is a battlefield, then the doctor's own body and psyche is a tent on that battlefield. Stress produces frustration and anger. These feelings are "professionally" repressed – actually, they are in danger of being chronically held under through denial. In time, the repressed, following Freud's dictum referred to earlier, returns in a distorted form – as self-directed anger, hatred or disgust, or self-loathing. Medicine, historically, has the highest rate of suicide (Shrira 2009), and alcohol and drug abuse amongst the professions (British Medical Association 1998). Stress may also be deflected and acted out rather than repressed – in violent outbursts, in behaviour such as aggressive talk or threatening body language, or, perhaps worse, in passive aggressive behaviour such as persistent cynicism, criticism, bullying and harassment. In an age in which "patient-centredness" has become both mantra and injunction, it is often forgotten that the behaviour of difficult patients is the main cause of frustration and anger amongst doctors (Halpern 2007), especially patients who refuse treatment that the doctor conscientiously believes is right or essential.

Halpern (2007) argues that it is precisely when patients are themselves deeply upset, hostile, and even aggressive, that empathy shown by doctors has its most powerful effect. However, it is at this point that doctors may either retreat into an overly "professional" relationship of cold detachment, objectifying the patient; or overstep the professional boundary by snapping - meeting hostility with hostility. Angry exchanges with clinical colleagues (Klein and Forni 2011, Debska et al 2012, Szczegielniak et al 2012) are as important to consider as angry exchanges with patients, because these exchanges can compromise patient safety. Incivility and poor care may be linked. For example, one study (Institute for Safe Medication Practices 2004) showed that 49% of nurses and pharmacists changed the way they dealt with medication orders because of a past brush with an intimidating doctor. In a USA-based survey of over 5,000 operating theatre personnel, 70% reported a range of inappropriate confronting behaviours such as berating patients and colleagues, abusive language, sarcastic and condescending remarks, and insults. This may contribute to medical error through frustrating effective team communication (O'Reilly 2011). In a further USA-based survey study of 840 doctors, over 70% said that they saw disruptive behaviour on a monthly basis (MacDonald 2011).

When George Anderson, head of a North American "anger management" consultancy was invited into the operating theatre to see at first hand the kinds of behaviour he and his colleagues might be asked to re-shape, he was horrified to find, in this day and age, "scalpel throwing surgeons" (Scheinbaum 2012). Anderson observed regular verbal abuse among the milder forms of anger, where more intense expressions of anger included a surgeon flinging an instrument (it hit the ceiling) in frustration at being handed the wrong instrument twice by a scrub nurse. A second frustrated and angry surgeon flung an instrument that hit a nurse on the shoulder.

Such behaviour is not confined to surgery. The US Joint Commission described an "epidemic" of "disruptive" doctors in a 2009 report (Advisory Board 2012). A 2005 survey of 1,500 nurses and doctors revealed that nearly 50% of the doctors said they had witnessed disruptive behaviour by nurses, where, in turn, 86% of the nurses reported doctors acting inappropriately (Rosenstein and O'Daniel 2005). Is this just the rough and tumble of medical and healthcare practice, or is this a symptom of a cultural malaise that affects the quality of that practice and places patients at risk?

In Los Angeles, after observing the surgical teams referred to above, George Anderson was asked to run "anger management" training programmes for those surgeons labelled as "rageaholics" (Scheinbaum 2012). Therapies included advice such as: when feeling a rage about to blow up, surgeons might take long, slow breaths through their noses, thinking "peace" on inhalation and "release" on exhalation. At crisis points, surgeons may use visualisation, such as imagining themselves sunbathing on a quiet beach; or replace judgemental inner dialogue such as "what an idiot!" with forgiving dialogue such as "someday we will laugh about this".

Whatever their good intentions, we are sceptical of such pious New Age therapy approaches, and of "management" gurus who turn anger into a commodity. Such chronic states of anger may be beyond "management". We suggest that the system that produces angry surgeons and doctors (the martial culture of medicine) must first change before focusing on rogue individuals. Just trying to change behaviour without understanding the historical and contextual causes of such behaviour is misguided, a legacy of shallow behaviourism. It is common knowledge that surgery in particular is grounded historically in an aggressive and competitive masculine culture. Again, however daunting the prospect, it is the culture that must be changed at root, not simply the worst-case individuals who represent the extremes of the culture. If this seems like a bridge too far, let us remind ourselves that cultures in medicine have been shaped historically through what Foucault (2001) called "conditions of possibility".

In other words, some historical events came together, perhaps serendipitously, to pave the way for an historical rupture – a major cultural change. For example, Foucault (2006) suggests that when leprosy disappeared from Europe, the leper houses were waiting to be filled. "Madness" - as a medicalised category of disease rather than a socially tolerated form of behaviour - entered the vacuum created by the disappearance of leprosy, so that a ready-made set of asylums would accommodate the newly defined "mad", once tolerated now institutionalised and treated (where the "mad" included drunks, vagrants and single mothers on the streets).

Medicine might need to cultivate more of a "culture of civility", a product of what Norbert Elias (2000) tracks historically as the "civilizing process". Elias first put forward the idea that the "civilizing" process (decency, fair exchange, manners) was intimately linked with the emergence of a political ideal – democracy. In the Middle Ages in Europe, spitting in public, for example, was acceptable. By the seventeenth and eighteenth centuries, spitting was considered a bad habit, not because it was seen as a health hazard, but because it might disgust others. Thus, the habit was democratised on the back of empathic feeling for the Other, the basis of tolerance and the democratic exchange. Elias suggested that aggressiveness underwent a similar transition to civility.

In Medieval Europe, aggression and warfare were spoken about as pleasures, and certainly there is relish in Homer's vivid, premodern descriptions of aggression. Yet we now feel uneasy at the pornographic celebration of war embodied in the character Lieutenant Colonel Bill Kilgore in Francis Ford Coppola's film *Apocalypse Now*, set in the Vietnam War. Standing on the battlefield, Kilgore says to a naïve young soldier, Lance:

> Kilgore: Smell that? You smell that?
> Lance: What?
> Kilgore: Napalm, son. Nothing else in the world smells like that. [*kneels*] I love the smell of napalm in the morning. You know, one time we had a hill bombed, for 12 hours. When it was all over, I walked up. We didn't find one of em, not one stinkin' dink body. The smell, you know that gasoline smell, the whole hill. Smelled like [*sniffing, pondering*] ... victory.

Jonathan Shay's (1994) study of posttraumatic stress after the Vietnam War is replete with accounts of soldiers who found that the more violence they engaged in during combat, the more they became inured against it. "I got very hard, cold, merciless. I lost all my mercy" says one veteran, so that violence in civilian life, such as domestic violence against women partners, was treated lightly.

Norbert Elias (2000) argues that the medieval disposition towards the love of aggression - and what we now see as its outrages such as body mutilations - was gradually civilised by the seventeenth and eighteenth centuries. Power became centralised in political institutions to either, paradoxically, aggressively control others' aggression, or to include socialising structures of civility and democracy. Eiko Ikegami's (2005) study of the relationship between manners, aesthetics and politics in Japanese society from late medieval periods also shows that as societies structure themselves, levels of civility emerge in which aggression is tightly controlled. While pre-modern Japan was a highly autocratic and structured society, where violence was institutionalised and controlled, Ikegami shows how democratic, horizontal networks of associations between people from different classes and social groups also emerged. These horizontal civilities were based around public aesthetic interests such as poetry and other arts, equivalent to our tradition of adult education evening classes.

Transformations of anger

Through the figure of Achilles, Homer shows how potential, or actual, confrontation, anger and violence can be transformed both productively and unproductively. We have already mentioned the destructive outcomes of sulking (repressed anger internalised as self-hate, or beating oneself up), and redoubling anger (berserker acting out – the uncontrollable impulse or "scalpel throwing" of "rageaholics"). Homer shows Achilles oscillating between scalpel throwing and beating himself up in the quarrel with Agamemnon early in the *Iliad*. Achilles has acquired a woman, Briseis, as war booty; Agamemnon announces that he will steal Briseis from Achilles.

Achilles' first reaction, in the heat of argument, is to reach for his sword to run Agamemnon through, but Athene interferes and Achilles sheathes his sword. However, his longer-term behaviour now swings into a sulk, a kind of emotional self-harm, a wasteland and a sapping of spirit. This drains away a powerful resource for the Greeks in the battle against the Trojans. Distaste for oneself is also projected outwards as distaste for others.

The impulse of confrontation, anger and violence can, however, be re-channelled productively. First, Homer describes *the transformation of angry impulse into reflection.* In Achilles' quarrel with Agamemnon, where, as introduced above, Achilles reaches for his sword, the goddess Athene checks his impulsive action so that his hand is forced to come away from the hilt and he in turn is forced to reconsider (figure 2-2). Cool reflection is then embedded in the hot arc of angry impulse - a model for cultivating the reflective moment in the heat of a passion. Reflection is inherent to action. This may arrive as conscience, as part of a developed moral code, or as the in-the-moment consideration of values shaping action - better termed "reflexivity". Or, reflection may be cultivated as a psychological capability of awareness – a standing back, a pause and reconsideration.

Reflection and reflexivity have large and growing literatures (Schön 1990, Bleakley 1999, Peterkin and Brett-Maclean 2017). Reflection has been anatomised as reflection-in-action (ad hoc reflection in the event) and reflection-on-action (post hoc reflection on the event). Bleakley (1999) suggests a third way – reflection-as-action – which is what Homer describes in the moment that Athene descends to check Achilles' impulse. Here, reflection is an overall performance, an embodied cognition. The body, not the mind, is doing the reflecting. Impulse is curved back upon itself so that it forms or shapes a more generous, accepting activity that is respect for the Other – the basis of democracy. This feedback curve is not a repression of impulse or desire, but a reconfiguration within the performance, an improvisation in the name of tolerance of the Other. It is a moment of recognition of difference and a transformation of impulse from tough-mindedness to tender-mindedness. It is not feedback but feedforward. It is a cultural trope of citizenship in working democracies.

Second, Homer describes *the transformation of angry impulse into moral courage*. This occurs in a remarkable and transformative scene at the heart of the *Iliad*, known as the Embassy Scene (Book 9), that is the centrepiece of chapter three. Achilles' sulk stems from having his honour smeared by Agamemnon who has stolen his spoils-of-war concubine. In an attempt to bring the estranged Achilles onside to continue the fight against the Trojans, Agamemnon sends an embassy to Achilles promising gifts, including one of Agamemnon's own daughters. Achilles stuns the embassy, which includes Odysseus, by not only refusing the proffered gifts, but also by refusing the very moral basis upon which the gifts are offered – the honour of heroism. Indeed, Achilles challenges the very basis of the genre of the hero – the epic - in an ode to the pastoral, a briefly considered return to domestic life, where greater glories and fulfilment than the battlefield may be found.

In short, Achilles considers for a moment that it may be more fulfilling to go home and live a quiet life than to stay and fight, despite the latter leading to posthumous glory. Through the pastoral alternative, you will not be immortalised in those galleries of portraits of great heroes of medicine – the reward of the heroic life (see chapters one and two). However, one can find deep satisfaction in the ordinary, the domestic, the everyday chores of work, and here achieve a different kind of heroism as the gaining of moral courage in accepting that the grind of the mundane is necessary and rewarding.

Hesiod's *Work and Days* (2008), written around 700 BC, is a poem extolling the virtues of domesticity and hard work in strong contrast to the Homeric epics. The lesson for medicine in Achilles' (temporary) turn of heart and in the themes of the pastoral genre inaugurated by Hesiod is that heroism and martial life need not be the guiding metaphors for medicine.

Again, in the UK junior doctors were once called "housemen" with the specialty unit the "house', the hospital as a whole supposedly providing the same hospitality as a home. Medicine is domestic work of care. Through the imaginative Embassy scene, Homer presents us with another way to imagine the energy of anger – not to channel it into domestic violence, but into domestic forms such as the love of the mundane and celebration of the work ethic. Further, such "house" work is shared, through what Richard Sennett (2013) praises as "the rituals, pleasures and politics of cooperation", challenging the longstanding individualistic, heroic and competitive traditions in medicine such as prize-winning.

Third, Homer describes *the transformation of angry impulse into productive pity*. We have previously argued, in chapter six, that "pity" in Homer as a form of compassion is a stronger and more telling version of what we now call technical "empathy". In the example quoted earlier, the surgeon who bullied a nurse, reduced her to tears and left her feeling powerless, may have walked away from that situation still simmering with rage, refusing reflection and rationalising his behaviour. But could that rage have been transformed into pity – deep feelings of sorrow for another's condition, now described by the technical term empathy, or being able to stand in another's shoes? This would surely have been a productive transformation of frustration and anger?

In the closing chapters of the *Iliad,* Achilles rejoins the fight against the Trojans because his close companion Patroclus has been slain by the Trojan hero Hector. Moreover, Achilles has sent Patroclus into battle on his behalf. Achilles revenges Patroclus' death by killing Hector, but then, against the code of honour, despoils Hector's body. Hector's father Priam visits Achilles under cover at night and begs that Hector's body be restored to the Trojans for proper funeral rites. In short, Achilles' anger transforms into pity for Priam and the body of Hector is restored to the enemy.

Con-frons, the Latin root of "confrontation", means "with the forehead". There are two kinds of meeting head to head – "butting" as in billy goats repeatedly hitting their heads against each other in combat. This is unproductive confrontation. Second is "but-ing", where confrontation is about talking things through, as did Achilles and Priam. Confrontation here can still be strong – the "but!" is an interruption, a challenge, but is not a head-to-head fight and carries care despite being a challenge. The evidence suggests that doctors are generally poor at such expert, reflective confrontation, preferring to simply talk over patients (Roter and Hall 2006).

Conclusion

Medicine has, historically, been more enmeshed with the love of war than the art of war. *The Art of War* is a widely studied manual of *strategy*, supposedly written by Sun Tzu in China in the 5th century BC (2008). It is a manual of paradoxical engagement with an enemy, where "the supreme art of war is to engage the enemy without fighting".

As a manual of tactics and strategy, Sun Tzu's book has been colonised by the business and management culture as a guidebook to strategic management. Medicine as war can be reframed as medicine as the art of war, where medicine is a strategy utilised not to violently crush the enemy, but to get to know the enemy intimately. This turns medicine from a directly confrontational practice into a more subtle type of confrontation as a meeting of forces rather than a clash of forces. The enemy in this case is disease.

The art of war demands engagement and dialogue with illness rather than disease, to get to know the meaning and patterns of illnesses and not to resort simply to the kind of fighting talk and practice in the wake of Thomas Sydenham, where the enemy of disease is attacked or butted head on. Thus, the martial metaphors of medicine may be mobilised in such a way as to undermine their historical meanings, just as Sun Tzu mobilised war metaphors to describe strategies of avoiding conflict. Isn't this precisely what happens at the very close of Homer's *Odyssey* as the gods call for a halt in violence, and an enantiodromia occurs where violence turns into its opposite? These energies are subsequently mobilised (within the pastoral genre) for pacific and collaborative purposes. If one prefers to think of the *Odyssey*'s natural conclusion as Penelope and Odysseus retiring to their bed to make love after the dreadful violence that precedes their reunion (after 20 years apart!), this too is a pacific scene. This mirrors the trope of the goddess of love, Aphrodite, taking Ares, the god of war, to bed to transform his martial impulse into tender care.

Homer teaches us then not to blindly *ban* anger and associated violence ("zero tolerance"), but rather to *transform* the energy of anger and possible violence into productive purposes. The very same strategy can be applied to the martial metaphors that have shaped medical practice for nearly four hundred years.

CHAPTER NINE

ERROR

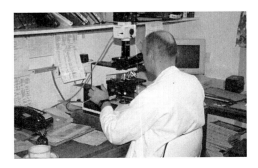

Figure 9-1: The pathologist at work

Homer and error

Error is part of the human condition. That doesn't make error right, but it does say that error will happen even when we devise sophisticated ways to reduce it. Error too can be fortunate as well as unfortunate or even disastrous. Evolution would not have proceeded as Darwin described – through natural selection – if error was not stitched in to nature. While Darwin was able to describe evolution, he could only guess at its motor. It was not until Mendel's work on genetics that chance and error were placed at the heart of biological process where it was hypothesised that gene mutations provide the means by which diversity of species occur. A gene mutation is an error of information – sometimes fortunate, but often resulting in pathology and illness.

We make sense of error through metaphors. How we make sense – the metaphors we choose (or that choose us) – is revealing. If we are driven by the "body as machine" metaphor, as medicine has been since Vesalius' influence in the 16th century, then we see inbuilt body error as something to be fixed or engineered. In industries such as airlines, nuclear and transport, a good deal of potential error has been eradicated through ever-more sophisticated feedback mechanisms in associated machinery. Anaesthetics in medicine has benefited from this engineering thinking.

However, there still remains what psychologists call "human factors". The body may be viewed as a machine with a set of feedback mechanisms that maintain homeostasis, but these are made complex through cultural-artefactual extensions such as diet, exercise, eyeglasses, pacemakers, watches, computers, and now computer offshoots such as electronic personal trainers worn like watches.

But when we suspend engineering metaphors to consider "human factors" such as emotion - sudden panic, explosive anger, passions of the heart, jealousy, envy, desire - then we are rudely shoved into the territory of the error-prone. Even gentle slippages can mount up like potential at a synapse and then burst forth as an unexpected error based on blindness caused by habit; or, error can grip in a sudden moment of irrationality that the ancient Greeks called *atē* – to be "made witless". We will discuss *atē* at length throughout this chapter.

Acting in ways incomprehensible to later analysis can then be a feature of major disasters. James Reason's analysis of the Moorgate tube disaster attempts a rational explanation of sorts (Reason and Mycielska 1982, pp.204-10.). In this event, an underground tube train in London was supposed to terminate at a temporary platform beyond which was a short overrun tunnel ending in a solid wall. The driver drove at full speed into the wall. He was seen as he drove past the platform looking quite relaxed. He and 42 passengers were killed. No satisfactory explanation was found and the official conclusion was that suicide was likeliest. Reason argues that suicide was unlikely, and that the driver mistook stations and thought he was approaching the one he had just left; numerous warning signs and lights should have alerted him of the error, but instead closed his mind down and froze him into immobility.

In our use of Homer to think otherwise about medicine and medical education, we find that while humans are error-prone, persistent error is configured as a lapse in human morality, itself a consequence of poor self-insight and reflective awareness. In a "post-truth" age, there is a danger that we mistake liberal, heartfelt human forgiveness for normalisation of habitual and malicious error. "Post truth" pundits justify and normalise their activities by contrasting them with the supposed demon of political correctness that they see as oppressive and ideological. We read Homer's figures of Agamemnon and Odysseus as characterising two kinds of serial errorists, both of whom we recognise from medicine, as this chapter explores.

The first type, illustrated by the figure of Agamemnon, persistently blames being overcome by passions beyond his control that lead him to commit errors in judgement and relationship that have hurtful consequences for others; Agamemnon meanwhile walks away unscathed, failing to show either shame or remorse.

The second type, illustrated by the figure of Odysseus as portrayed in later Greek literature, is a slippery manipulator who basically cons others into believing that he is on their side and then deceives them, again without guilt, remorse or any attempt at apology and reparation. Shame for engaging in amoral activity is again missing. Indeed, the ethics of the activity are of secondary concern to the pragmatics – getting a job done whatever the consequences for others. Pragmatism was always popular in America, but, as William James urged, must be twinned with ethical concern.

While "error" in medicine is generally seen as actions causing harm to patients or colleagues, we can extend error to include inability to embrace affirmative action and explicitly demonstrate holding values of equity, equality and diversity. This definition puts medicine in a difficult position of an error-generating culture as it continues to tacitly support, for example, authoritarianism, sexism and racism. For example, white doctors are three times more likely to be picked for senior hospital jobs than doctors from ethnic minorities (Jaques 2013b).

We might call these lingering, institutional negative habits chronic errors. Their eradication involves a long-term process of values change in medical culture, including democratising and feminising (Bleakley 2014). In medicine, acute error can be fatal for patients – a poor diagnosis, a slip-up in surgery, over- and under-medication, a mix-up in biopsy specimens. Much of this potential error can be obviated through systems, such as protocols. But the passions and personalities of doctors are another thing, often beyond the reach of instrumental safety nets. Luckily, most errors committed by doctors are one-off slips, many of which can be rectified, and most of which prompt remorse, a sense of shame and a subsequent apology and reparation. However, medicine must also deal with the serial errorist.

To understand the emotional vicissitudes of error, these days we turn to research in psychology. Homer's *Iliad* and *Odyssey* - as the primary texts on human emotion and the consequences of its expression – offer an older take on the human condition through which we can also understand error in medicine. In the Homeric world, the human is caught between nature and the gods. Nature, again, is fundamentally flawed – fault-lines of error run through nature so that the codes creating our bodies are already error-prone. Our lives can be dis-jointed at any time through genetic misinformation. Our passions are grounded in these fault-lines of nature.

The gods, on the other hand, represent fundamental forces and faces of morality. For example, while Aphrodite is the face of passion, eroticism, love, sexuality and sensuality, she represents its finest distillation as cultivated desire, rather than base desire (the goat-god Pan, the catch-all word for "nature", is the face of base desire (Hillman and Roscher 2000)). In the Homeric world-view, error is a mis-reading, ignorance, or conscious avoidance, of an ethical position that the ancient Greeks called *aidos*. *Aidos* (*Αἰδώς*) is the ancient Greek goddess who personified humility, modesty and shame.

It is this feeling of shame, as a kind of reverence for life and others, that creates an ethical choice and cultivates restraint as the forces of nature call out for direct expression. *Aidos* in modern times is, in our view, unabashed and genuine political correctness based on values of liberty and justice for all. "Post truth", by definition, is equivalent to error as it eschews shame.

Should the forces of nature burst through with no control, we are then gripped by *atē* (*ἄτη*) - literally meaning "something overtook me", or, I was gripped by a kind of madness, such as fury or jealousy. Agamemnon is often subject to *atē*, in its passive verbal form: "I was made witless", making the subject a victim of a force bigger than himself (*Iliad* 9. 115-120) – perhaps also a good excuse for bad behaviour or serial amorality. Achilles is gripped by *atē* after the death of Patroclus at the hand of Hector, when he goes on the rampage killing Trojans at will and then commits the most atrocious of errors for a hero – the ethical misconduct of not showing respect for the body of Hector after he has slain him in combat. The equivalent in medicine would be a doctor not admitting to an error that is plain to others, and then showing naked lack of remorse and shame.

Atē too is personified as a goddess. She brings a kind of madness as folly and delusion, often leading to ruin. In the gap created through an absence of shame, or as a consequence of the all-engulfing presence of *atē*, error appears. In ancient Greek myth, it is often noted that even the gods make mistakes or are error-prone. In fact, they often make mistakes, or misjudgements, sometimes through wilful and misguided interventions, often through bad peer counsel, and more often through internal squabbles on Mount Olympus. This suggests that ethical life – the playing out of our moralities – is complex and cannot be regulated by principles (personified in the Greek Olympians) such as medicine's holy quartet: respect for autonomy, nonmaleficence (above all, do no harm), beneficence (acting in the best interests of the other), and justice. Rather, ethical conduct is best seen as situational and case-based (casuistry), so that every context requires a unique, tailored judgement. In other words, every patient is an individual.

We are not contradicting ourselves in suggesting that an ethical medicine should be situational and flexible. This is not the equivalent of a "post-truth" justification for the occasion. Rather, the "what" of an ethical decision remains constant – upholding fairness and justice – while the "how" is situational (one patient's needs are different from another's). Errors occur in (i) slippage to "alternative truth", or ad hoc justifications; and (ii) attempting to apply the same moral code in the same manner to every situation (universalism).

Homer continues the discourse on error in the *Odyssey*. The Latin "error" means "wandering" (errant), and Homer's Odysseus is the personification of the error-prone wanderer who keeps on falling into trouble. Such errancy inhabits medicine, in the UK most noticeably in high profile cases such as the Bristol paediatric heart surgery scandal, and the organ retention scandal at the Alder Hay Children's hospital – both blamed on lack of transparency and medical culture protectionism, finally attracting "whistleblowing" (see the following chapter ten). The mid-Staffordshire Hospital scandal provided a case study for widespread error and neglect due to poor management, lack of resources, and habitual negligence amongst care staff where ethical concerns were sidelined by subscription to crude managerialism.

Homer reminds us again to attend to a side of error that medicine ignores: admittance to shame in the wake of habitual or persistent error. Medicine has a recent history of deflecting blame, an unreflective and unethical stance, rather than admitting to error and expressing shame and remorse as a prelude to apology – a reflective and ethical course of events.

Medicine and error: from individuals to systems

In chapter seven, we noted that medical error is a leading cause of death. Medical error has received significant management, academic and media interest only over the last 30 or so years. A major review of errors, carried out in the USA, estimated that between 44,000 and 98,000 Americans die in hospital each year as a result of medical errors (Kohn et al 2000). These figures were extrapolated from two major studies (Brennan et al 1991, Thomas et al 2000). Even the lower figure would rank these avoidable deaths eighth in mortality statistics ahead of death in road traffic events, while the higher figure is almost certainly a gross underestimate, with a mortality rate of 225,000 per annum suggested by Starfield (2000) and confirmed by Makary and Daniel (2016) as we noted in chapter seven. Medical error would then rank third in mortality after heart disease and cancer. This figure has been confirmed in a recent study by Johns Hopkins University Medical School in the USA that reports an estimate of more than 250,000 deaths per annum (McMains 2016).

In the UK, Jeremy Laurance (2014) reports that: "Doctors' basic errors are killing 1,000 patients a month". A House of Commons Select Committee inquiry into medical error suggests that this figure is almost certainly an underestimate (Barron 2009). Around a half of these errors are avoidable because they are again grounded in human factors, such as team process, open to radical improvement through both undergraduate and continuing medical and healthcare education (Bleakley et al 2011, Bleakley 2014).

For example, regular briefings and debriefings in operating theatres have been shown to dramatically improve error rates (Health, Quality and Safety Commission NZ 2016). Demonstrating the persistence of human factors, after the introduction of a Surgical Safety Checklist involving briefing, so-called "never events", such as wrong-side and wrong-site surgery, would be eradicated. However, instances of "never events" linger because of the human factor of non-compliance, often pig-headed stubbornness on the part of a certain strain of surgeons to recognise the value of protocols that are seen as part of a political correctness conspiracy (Durkin 2015). Re-educating such surgeons involves a deep re-socialisation at the sharp end of the patient safety agenda.

Currently, all hospitals should have a mechanism for reporting errors and near misses, so that these can be analysed and assessed. This is based on the fundamental principle, not recognised 30 years ago, that the mistakes of individuals are often, some would say usually or always, systemic - made in a cultural context such as a dysfunctional institution (Vincent 1997). For example McMains (2016), summarising a recent study at Johns Hopkins University Medical School, mentioned earlier, suggests that:

> ... most medical errors aren't due to inherently bad doctors, and that reporting these errors shouldn't be addressed by punishment or legal action. Rather, they say, most errors represent systemic problems, including poorly coordinated care, fragmented insurance networks, the absence or underuse of safety nets, and other protocols, in addition to unwarranted variation in physician practice patterns that lack accountability.

The system can be modelled and better understood (for example as dynamic, complex, and adaptive), and changes can then be made in the system to prevent future mistakes. Marty Makary (Makary and Daniel 2016), a surgeon from Johns Hopkins, catalogues a host of safety issues still typically left unaddressed by hospitals, exhorting all healthcare institutions to introduce safety protocols, keep records, and publish them to widen public transparency. While 30 years ago, responsibility rested with the individual doctor and particularly with senior doctors, and there was wide variation in how individuals would accept and address such responsibility morally and practically, now we frame healthcare practice differently.

Again, as we better understand the roles and responsiveness of clinical teams and their places in institutional frameworks, so we see individual actions as secondary to the complex, dynamic processes of systems. Herbert Fred (1984, 2008) reminds us that we need to distinguish between dishonesty in medicine and consequences to such dishonesty in error. Individual or organisational dishonesty does not necessarily lead to error, although dishonesty may be employed to disguise or cover up error. Fred notes, however, that dishonesty in its own right is far more common in medicine than we may think, and, in the 20 plus years since his first study, he notes with dismay that in North America, evidence shows that dishonesty amongst medical students and doctors has not decreased but increased.

Fred (2008), an ethicist as well as physician, focuses, again within a North American context, on issues such as: widespread cheating at medical school; dishonesty in giving references and letters of recommendation; making up information on ward rounds such as a physical examination having been completed when it was overlooked; not answering bleepers (bleeps in the UK) and, for example, blaming this on "dead batteries"; copycatting inpatient records; padding out or falsifying CVs in job applications; fraudulent or inappropriate billing to medical insurance companies; unprofessional conduct in supporting or favouring drug companies; misconduct in medical and medical education research and subsequent publishing; and biased peer reviewing.

These are mainly individual decisions, although they may be affected by peer pressure. We now diagnose error from the point of view of potential whole system improvement (root cause analysis) rather than moral improvement of the aberrant individual. Stangierski and colleagues (2012), however, suggest limits to such systems understanding, where:

Some medical protocols and pathways incorporated into medical practice may help in avoiding medical errors. Furthermore, it has been proven that they may act as reminders to reduce distractions in the treatment process. Unfortunately, sometimes the guidance of the protocol is not enough, and an error occurs.

Champions of protocols reply that if guidelines were more detailed, better designed, and firmly implemented then errors could be avoided. In the old model of individual responsibility, responses to mistakes and errors varied from complete disclosure to the patient to complete concealment and denial where this was possible. Institutions rarely had a role, and errors conceived as systematically formed, even if they have root causes, would be seen as a smokescreen for a faulty individual decision or action, where somebody has to "carry the can". As care became more team-based, so error recognition, management and reduction were seen as shared responses to protocols, such as a surgical safety checklist, or a central line infection protocol, where collaboration (rather than competition) is seen to reduce error.

While this shift from individual responsibility to systems functioning shows greater sophistication in our understanding of medical error, it also creates a paradox. In the "old days", errant doctors could, and would, be protected through colleagues' bonding together and turning a blind eye to "slippage" while maintaining opacity to the public gaze. Now, even in an age of transparency, the actions of a "serial offender" rogue practitioner can be masked within a dysfunctional system.

In the *Iliad*, when Agamemnon, a serial errorist, blames his errancy on the gods who have deranged him (*atē*), we quickly see through this and blame Agamemnon's *hubris*. But in the *Odyssey,* when Odysseus does not take personal responsibility for the calamity that sends his ship hurtling away from home, just as the clifftop fires from settlements in his homeland were visible, the coast almost within touching distance, we have some sympathy.

His crew seems to be a rum bunch, imagining that Odysseus is trying to trick them by hiding treasure in a bag that actually contains the four winds, that blow uncontrollably once let loose; while Odysseus himself blames his lack of vigilance on an external factor – exhaustion, thus deflecting blame:

For nine days solid we sailed night and day.
On the tenth, the fields of our homeland were already in sight,
And we were near enough to see people tending their fires.
But then sweet sleep overcame me in my exhaustion.
For I was always managing the sheets of the ship, and would not delegate
The task to my companions, that we might reach home the faster.
… They opened the sack and all the winds rushed out
And a storm seized on them and bore them back weeping
Away from the land of their fathers (*Odyssey* 10. 28-49).

We do not intend a major review of medical error. Much of the methodology for understanding and managing it has been adapted from airline industry precedents, where errors are now rare. Foremost has been a "no blame" policy to encourage individuals to report all errors and near misses without feeling that their careers are threatened. In a generic classification of types of error, James Reason (1990, pp.53-61; 2013, pp.6-12) created two broad categories: (i) slips and lapses, where the plan of action is appropriate, but the execution is at fault; and (ii) mistakes, where the actions are correct, but there is a fault in the plan itself. Reason showed that lapses, as we would expect, are associated with the absent-minded personality, and that this personality was itself affected by, and more liable to, stress (Reason 1988).

This is a mind open to what Ruth Padel (1995) calls a "tragic madness", sudden possessions by irrational forces that we might now see as impulsiveness, closed-mindedness, wilfulness, and arrogance. Homer catalogues such tragic madness through the actions in particular of Agamemnon, Achilles and Hector, who offer blueprints not just for doctors making errors, but also for the systems in which they work.

It is admirable that most doctors endure a highly stressful initial work-based learning curve as juniors without accumulating overwhelming stress and burnout, and without clocking up errors as a result of stress. Denis Campbell (2016) reports on a recent, biggest ever, survey of Britain's 54,000 junior doctors where nearly a quarter describe themselves as "sleep-deprived" and yet continuing to work intensively (43% describe their workloads as "heavy" to "very heavy"). In the UK for many years, since the "systems" view of error generation and prevention was formulated and refined, individual doctors' worlds have been seen as secondary to accounts of the National Health Service (NHS) as a system. However, because of the dominant "body as machine" instrumental engineering metaphor, "patient safety" has been reduced to mechanics and statistics rather than flesh and blood encounters.

James Reason later expanded and refined his categories of error from the duo of slips/ lapses and mistakes to the triad of: (i) skill-based errors, where the action is largely or wholly automatic; (ii) rule-based errors, where the actor is aware there is a problem and there is a solution already available; and (iii) knowledge-based errors, where the actor has to devise the solution *de novo*. There are also violations, when the actor is aware of breaking rules and may do so for different reasons. It is this last category that interests us, and where study of Homer can shed light. What makes a doctor, who subscribes to "first, do no harm", slip into multiple and compound error and show extraordinary lack of insight or will to change? But also, what of the doctor who does slip or lapse but is in no way on an error slope and shows both insight and remorse? Who cares for both kinds of doctors and how can we better understand their respective worlds?

Errancy and reparation

In his masterwork *The Normal and the Pathological* – that focuses upon the processes by which "health" and "illness" are constructed, separated and opposed in medicine – George Canguilhem (1991) says that "Man makes mistakes because he does not know where to settle". From Homer's *Odyssey* to Melville's *Moby Dick* and James Joyce's *Ulysses*, to Jack Kerouac's *On the Road,* literature has often portrayed the restless spirit as an affliction rather than a boon. The Knight Errant is either running from something – previous errors - or cannot put down roots in fear of committing error. Such wandering is portrayed as a paradoxical form of control based on a fear of commitment.

A yearning for home is a recurring theme in the *Iliad*, where, as noted in previous chapters, even the great hero Achilles is at one point tempted to cash in his destiny of a glorious and early death as a great hero, to be remembered forever, for a return home to a long and peaceful domestic life of anonymity. The pastoral is dangled as an alternative to the tragic. Achilles, of course, cannot choose the latter – every listener to the tale knows that his destiny is the tragedy of early death rather than the pastoral idyll of an easy but bland retirement. The audiences for the epics know that Fate is a bigger force than the human narrative arc.

Yearning for home is *the* theme of the *Odyssey*. Having already spent a decade fighting in the Trojan War, the last thing that Odysseus wants is a long and convoluted trip home. But of course his destiny is to suffer another decade of interrupted travel, for he is the "Man of Twists and Turns" who can never find the straight road or the simple solution. In

Canguilhem's terms, he is a person subject to serial error because he is destined, at least for the period of the *Odyssey*, to not settle.

One way of reading this is that the person who has not "settled" shows a twin psychological flaw: first, the lack of development of a moral compass; and second, an inability to form a mind that is a quiet pool for contemplation and reflection, in which actions are always thought about for their consequences. In turn, a cause of such a flawed psychological character is an inability to take the advice of others because you are never wrong, and in turn to blame others for your own poor choices.

We have already seen that, explaining why he was blown off course within sight of home, leading to wandering for years, Odysseus blames his "bad companions", and also a "wretched sleep". In other words, Odysseus is a controlling man who has lost control. We must remind ourselves again of Odysseus' style of control – that of ultimate adaptability, slipperiness, twists and turns, that can show both a positive and negative side.

In ancient Greek understanding, he too was gripped by a form of *atē* – that, according to Gregory Nagy (2013), means "aberration, derangement" and "veering off course". Odysseus has lost his compass setting, his course, and is wandering. Poseidon, Odysseus' tormentor, reinforces this through sending storms that shipwreck Odysseus and his crew. *Atē* may lead to disaster and consequences such as punishment. The disaster – the inability to settle – is the inability to live by an appropriate moral code as tether and framework (now commonly called "professionalism"); and the punishment is a mindset of irrationality that will not accept responsibility for breaching moral codes and then feeling ordinary human shame, the very emotion that re-sets a compass or drops an anchor.

Odysseus' knee-jerk reaction is not to look at his own possibly errant judgement but to complain about and blame others, or forces outside of himself, as the cause. Refusal to accept errancy and potential error is a rejection of bearing shame, that most human of feelings. We might compare this with the arrogant surgeon, a multiple errorist or wanderer who refuses advice, counsel or mentorship: I slipped up because "bad companions" damaged me (blame the surgical team), and I was at the mercy of a "wretched sleep" (fatigue) (see chapter twelve), so I did the sensible thing and went to sleep. Such errancy, like Odysseus' wanderings, can last for a decade or more without a whistle being blown, as shame is kept at bay through rationalisation or brushing under the carpet.

Taking Hector as an example, James Redfield (1994) notes how heroes make compound errors and in the process become more and more isolated from those around them who could give advice. As errors become more severe, so the hero takes greater effort to not admit to the shame that admitting to error would bring. Hector's infamous triple error occurs over a couple of days as the Trojans look as if they might rout the Greeks. First, he promises the Trojan army victory in the face of being outmanned by the Greeks; second, he refuses to withdraw the army when the Greeks rally and fight back; and third, he refuses to withdraw within the walls of Troy despite advice to do so. This is the typical trajectory of the error-prone doctor growing ever more blind to his or her failings. Not only are technical errors not recognised or rationalised away, but errors also occur through poor communication and failure to work well within teams, failure to seek second and third opinions, to work collaboratively, and both to plan ahead (briefing) and review (debriefing), again stereotyped as forms of political correctness.

But prior to these three mistakes, Hector has made an even greater error in killing Patroclus, blinding himself to the fact that Achilles will surely seek revenge; but then compounding this error by mis-treating Patroclus' body. Instead of returning the body to the Greek camp for proper burial, Hector threatens to drag the body to Troy and throw it to the dogs, seriously breaching the heroic code of honour. This is the doctor who has gone out on a limb with his or her behaviour and has now alienated colleagues as well as rupturing ethical codes. Hector's deterioration of moral character, lack of insight, increasing isolation, and overestimation of powers of survival make him a model for the failing, error-strewn doctor who refuses shame and then must be shamed through whistleblowing and subsequent inquiry.

But this is not a new tension. In the early part of the *Iliad*, Agamemnon, a serial errorist, tries a ruse that backfires. Having been sent a dream at night by Zeus, that foretells a great victory over the Trojans on the subsequent day, instead of just announcing this to his troops, Agamemnon decides to test the courage and commitment - or loyalty - of the soldiers. He says to the Privy Council of captains of the armies that when he announces to the soldiers that they should finally return to their ships, pack up on the decade-long war, and return home, the captains must protest and whip up the fervour of the men. Then he will see who has the courage to fight. But this was an error that backfired, as the Greek army took him literally and started to march towards the ships in mass evacuation. Agamemnon has to recruit Odysseus to persuade the soldiers that they must stay to fight. Agamemnon fails to apologise for his error, the misfiring ruse.

Agamemnon carries the status of "over king" – the hospital's CEO, the Chief Medical Officer, the Health Secretary – but his status as hero is flawed. Achilles is clearly the greater hero, yet he must (albeit grudgingly) recognise Agamemnon's status in the hierarchy. Agamemnon makes multiple errors in the *Iliad* as illustrated above, the first of which is to demand the woman Briseis, Achilles' prize, for his own. He admits no shame and is shown to not be up to the job. Yet he persists in error even after insulting Achilles and provoking his anger and subsequent withdrawal from the war. *Atē* here is both the cause of the quarrel with Achilles and the effect of that quarrel. It is a disaster and a punishment for disaster.

In the *Iliad* (19.76-138), Agamemnon does not take personal responsibility for the quarrel with Achilles, but blames this on the gods inflicting *atē* upon him – a derangement or aberration. Agamemnon is passive in the face of an active attack from the goddess *Atē*. But Agamemnon positions himself outside of this process – his habitual response to conflict - and then constructs an identity as flawed hero who refuses shame. In this description, we recognise the arrogant doctor who has become detached from responsibility and remains blind to error.

Doctors too are wounded by their errors

There are two aspects of medical error, one unrecognised and probably unacceptable to modern thought, the other offering insights into an area where there has been some discussion and needs to be a great deal more. Although the admission of error is more easily made today, there is still truth in Wu's (2000) statement that: "Strangely, there is no place for mistakes in modern medicine". Wu later states: "although patients are the first and obvious victims of medical mistakes, doctors are wounded by the same errors: they are the second victims". James Reason (2000) says: "It is often the best people who make the worst mistakes".

The aim of this section is to focus on how we can help those victims, first by raising awareness about doctors committing errors who are very different from the detached and arrogant kinds who consumed us in the first half of this chapter. As noted, medical errors are generally one-off lapses for which doctors are keen to make an apology and some form of reparation.

This aspect of error is illustrated by a mistake made by one of us (RM) as a pathologist. This needs a little explanation of what pathologists do. Most of the working day is spent as a diagnostician, examining biopsies and surgical specimens from the living, first with the naked eye and then down the microscope. On microscopy, one examines a very thin sample of the specimen on a glass slide. These slides are then stored for future reference (if the patient has a second specimen taken for example).

Pathology is therefore unusual in that, if a diagnostic error is made, the specimen that it was made on is preserved unchanged for future examination. If a physician misdiagnoses a patient's physical signs or a surgeon makes an error while operating, the moment is gone and the precise circumstances under which the error was made cannot be reconstructed - not so in pathology, where your errors are preserved for posterity.

About 20 years ago, RM examined a biopsy specimen from the nasal cavity and made the diagnosis of neurofibrosarcoma, a malignant tumour of cells that form part of the sheath around nerve fibres. A year or two later, one of his colleagues came to his room with a puzzled expression. She had received a subsequent biopsy of what was clearly a benign neurofibroma, had reviewed the previous biopsy and thought it was the same. RM reviewed the slide himself and agreed. It was not simply a benign tumour; it was not possible to see how any pathologist might consider the diagnosis of malignancy in the first place. Worse still, the malignant diagnosis would be rare and normal practice would be to show the case to a colleague for confirmation, which RM had not done. In practice therefore, two errors were made around the same person. Luckily, while many specialist surgeons at the time would have undertaken major, disfiguring facial surgery to attempt to eradicate the malignant tumour, the local unit at the time believed in a "watch and wait" policy and did nothing. No physical harm was then done. Nevertheless, it was a bad mistake.

Experts now would analyse such an error and look for patterns with other errors. Every aspect of departmental and personal practice that could have affected the diagnosis would be analysed in detail. Recommendations might include making it obligatory to show any diagnosis of malignancy to a colleague (as is now the case in many departments). What struck RM at the time, and still does, was that the mistake was inexplicable, made in a parallel universe where normal practice simply did not prevail. A colleague pathologist has described a similar feeling. He led a major enquiry into a series of diagnostic errors made by a pathologist in one specialty area. At the end of months of investigation, having considered all possibilities, including illegal and malicious interventions by third parties, no satisfactory explanation could be found.

This feeling is not unique to pathologists. Clinical colleagues in other specialties also express disbelief at some of their errors. They are errors made in good faith, as opposed to the doctors and surgeons we discuss in the first part of this chapter, who, through arrogance, moral blindness and lack of self-insight, continue to make errors in bad faith, which, as Jean-

Paul Sartre (2003) so brilliantly illustrates, is a refusal to confront facts or choices. Worse, it is to apportion blame to others, or to being in the grip of irrationality (*atē*), rather than recognising one's own failings.

Late in the *Iliad*, Agamemnon finally has to admit that he was at fault at the very start of the epic in taking Briseis, the prize of Achilles, away from him. Robbed of this prize, Achilles had withdrawn from combat with his troops. The Greeks had then been routed on the field of battle; Patroclus had begged Achilles to be allowed to join the battle and borrowed Achilles' armour to do so; he had been killed by Hector. This induced Achilles to see that his anger had served only the Trojans. Agamemnon then makes a speech - part explanation, part apology - that contains passages difficult to understand in modern terms. He starts with a preamble that flags it as a speech of significance, and then continues:

> Often have the Achaeans (the Greeks) spoken against me and reproached me over this matter. However, I am not to blame, but Zeus and Fate and the Fury who walks in the night. They cast a wild bewilderment (*atē*) into my mind at the assembly when I took the prize of Achilles. What was I to do? The gods bring all things to pass. The eldest daughter of Zeus, Folly (Atē), who bewilders men, the accursed. Her feet are soft, for she does not walk on the earth, but goes among the heads of men, doing them harm; and she has bound the minds of others. Even Zeus was fooled once …

There follows a story of how Zeus was fooled by Hera at the birth of Heracles, ending with him casting Atē out of heaven to live among mortals.[1] Agamemnon continues:

> So, when great Hector of the shining helmet slaughtered the Greeks on the prows of their ships, I could not forget Folly, who first blinded me. But since I was blinded and Zeus robbed me of my wits, I wish to make amends and make rich compensation (*Iliad* 19. 85-138).

This passage is examined in detail by Dodds (1951, pp.1-27) at the start of *The Greeks and the Irrational* and by Ruth Scodel (2008). The first of Agamemnon's statements – "I am not to blame" - is arresting (doubly so as he later says "I wish to make amends", which sounds like a hollow promise). His reason is that forces outside and greater than him were acting and put *atē* to work to muddy his understanding. How are we to translate and interpret this irrationality that we believe is the element missing from current accounts? The Greek lexicon translates it as: "bewilderment or infatuation caused by blindness or delusion sent by the gods, mostly as the punishment of guilty rashness" (Liddell and Scott, *atē*). A "rashness" that actually remains guilt-free and does not provoke remorse or shame; "error" says James Redfield (1994, p.128), is a "species of shame".

Nagy (2013, p.38) translates *atē* as "derangement", and describes it as "both a passive experience … and an active force". It is not a word for which a single English word translation will do. However, difficult though it may be to translate, most people will be familiar with that moment of madness or folly, which we will call "witlessness", a state that can produce actions of uncharacteristic stupidity. Our point is that such witlessness strikes us all, but, in critical contexts, perhaps only once or twice. For others, it is cultivated as a lifestyle. Even the notion that there is an active external force producing it does not always seem so unbelievable. An important aspect of this loss of wits is that, by definition, we are not aware of it at the time. Edwards (1991) sums up his view of *atē* as: "the hero's personification of the impulse which led to a foolish and disastrous act, an act which with hindsight appears inexplicable and hence is attributed to an outside, i.e. superhuman, agency".

Current analyses of errors in medicine and elsewhere consider that they are nearly always multifactorial, and occur against a background that is inevitably error prone. Reason (2013) points to several aspects that are peculiar to healthcare, for example the large variety of activities undertaken by individuals and the large and varied amount of equipment used to make a dynamic, complex environment. This complexity is usually met by linear approaches totally unsuited to a context that requires fluidity and tolerance of ambiguity. In a working environment, a doctor can be aware that her judgment is impaired by anger or grief or simple exhaustion, and awareness of that can then help her to modify her attitudes and behaviours for the better. If we are temporarily witless, however, we cannot do anything to counteract or circumvent the state.

Agamemnon's appeal to outside deities and forces sounds wrong to modern rationality but perhaps this is just semantics. The modern literature often comments that nobody makes mistakes deliberately; the corollary of this is that outside forces almost have to be involved. We now work with a complex variety of artefacts, such as computers and universal protocols, and cannot claim mastery or expertise in all areas of interface with such artefacts (for example, it is common for clinicians to experience *atē* or witlessness in the face of sheafs of protocols and record keeping!)

We are happy to accept that, if we are blocked when writing, composing or painting, inspiration can come from nowhere. Witlessness is just the negative correlate of that external force. Modern scientism will want to examine and express that in terms of psychology, the cognitive unconscious and ultimately cortical and sub-cortical functions (the limbic system fires and smudges cortical rationality). What is generally accepted, however, is that error-prone contexts generally precede individual error. Whatever the location of witlessness, certainly its consequences of shame and guilt are culturally shaped, as we discuss later.

Error precipitates more readily in ragged than in cohesive clinical teams, as the former exhibit a variety of dysfunctions; and poorly performing hospitals are usually aggregates of such ragged teams. Error analysis then would certainly include the prevailing culture within which work practices occur. The initial angry outburst of Agamemnon that precipitates the crisis of the *Iliad* is a product of context, in which hierarchy brings privilege, a context that the *Iliad* asked its audience to examine when it was performed as song, and still demands a similar engagement today as we read it from the page or screen. Still, that final individual moment of folly is needed to produce the error.

At least Agamemnon does make his apology although we ask below whether or not it is sincere. And Achilles finally agrees to release Hector's body for proper funeral rites after King Priam's plea, but with great reluctance and a warning to Priam that he could easily change his mind at any minute if Priam irritates him; and Odysseus, on his return home and disclosure of his identity, agrees to peace after slaying the suitors, but again reluctantly, having already prepared for battle with their families. Some form of reparation is made in each case but because conditions are attached, these can be seen as not genuine apologies, but guileful appeasements.

The analysis of medical errors raises the issue of whether and in what way they should be disclosed to others and what forms of reparation are necessary, even if not sufficient. National guidance would usually be that there should be disclosure to colleagues, patients and their relatives with a formal apology. The proportion of errors disclosed is often small (Berlin 2006, Wu et al 2003), but this may depend on the severity of damage done—the more severe the injury, the more likely it will be discussed with the patient and relatives (Aasland and Førd 2005).[2]

In litigious societies like the USA, there is the added problem of exactly how apologies are phrased in order to do least damage in any future lawsuit (Berlin 2006, Wu et al 2009, Bell 2012). Taft (2005) considers this a moral, not a legal or management, issue. He analyses recommendations from medical societies and business sources of what an apology comprises and how it should be delivered. He is critical of false apologies—what he calls "apologias": "a business communications model ... more than a simple justification of one's position ... it is a justification coupled with a defensive strategy." His own recommendations for a full apology are: "There should be an unequivocal admission of error", with "an admission of fault ... an expression of genuine remorse and regret for any harm caused by the violation; and an explicit offer of restitution and promise of reform" (Taft 2005).

Agamemnon's speech fulfils most or all of these criteria, so it is important to note that commentators ancient and modern have believed his apology to be graceless and insincere (Edwards 1991, pp.243-53). This is largely because their readings of the text indicate body language on the part of the king that is in contrast to his words, so offering a mixed message, a lesson for anyone making an apology. Another important feature of the apology is that, having blamed his action on the powerful external forces of Zeus, Fate and "the night-wandering Fury", he finishes his speech by appearing to take responsibility for his action, at least to the extent of offering compensation: "But since I was blinded and Zeus robbed me of my wits, I wish to make amends and make rich compensation" – again blame is laid at the door of the external force of *atē* (*Iliad* 19. 137-8).[3]

Witlessness, therefore, does not absolve him from responsibility. Remember, though, that Agamemnon had claimed at the start of his speech "I am not to blame". Here is the difference between Homer's time and modern culture. However witless we may have been, however much misled by an evil genie, modern workers in healthcare would never make the same claim. Indeed, such a cause of error would generally make us feel more culpable. Agamemnon then accepts a sort of legal culpability, but says that he accepts no blame and clearly feels no guilt for his actions. For the modern doctor, guilt and shame would usually be the main reaction, although we have suggested that suspension of any such moral attachment defines the serial errorist. Examination of medical errors is normally through a detailed forensic search of all the events that led to them and, as we have discussed, consideration has been given as to how to help affected patients and families afterwards.

Less thought, however, has been given to the damage done to the doctors involved, where 90% of doctors in one study said that they did not feel supported by their organisation (Waterman et al 2007). Although the damage done is recognised (Wu et al 2003), it is striking that, in the report of a major inquiry into medical error in the National Health Service in the UK, there is only a passing reference to the impact that these mistakes may have on those who make them (Department of Health 2000, p.16).

How does Agamemnon feel about his error? The question would not have been asked in the world of the *Iliad*. It is questionable even whether the language existed to ask it. He has not truly repented of his actions, as his language shows. There is no sincere apology to Achilles (Edwards 1991). His main concern would be with any possible loss of face through having made the initial error and through now having to make this apology, such as it is. Dodds (1951) concludes his analysis of *atē* by introducing the concept of the shame culture in which Agamemnon (and possibly Homer) operated, and the guilt culture that followed it and which prevails today. He suggests there was a move from a shame culture as described in the *Iliad* to a guilt culture in the world of Plato and Euripides.

Ruth Benedict (1946) famously compared Japanese and American cultures, where Japanese culture is described as a "shame" culture, and American culture is described as a "guilt" culture. The difference is that the Japanese look outward to social acceptability where the Americans look inward to personal, introjected morality, as differing mirrors for reflection.

We suggest that contemporary medical culture manages to contain both elements – shame and guilt simultaneously. Analysis of doctors' reactions to making mistakes shows that they are concerned both with loss of reputation among their peers (shame) and also suffer intense feelings of guilt (Swaminath and Raguram 2011). The situation is further complicated in North America by the legal implications of admission, let alone disclosure of error (MacDonald and Attaran 2009). The literature describes admission of error as being "injurious to one's pride" as well as a "threat to self-esteem" (Robbennolt 2009).

The overbearing mindset of an Agamemnon making a mistake as a doctor on the wards today would be the anxiety of being shamed among his community. There is not an internalised moral sense among Greek heroes that might produce a feeling of guilt. There are no moral implications to being affected by *atē* in Homer, apart from one possible reference to being afflicted as punishment for a forgotten sacrifice (*Iliad* 9. 535-40). It just happens. Doctors must then carry a double burden of shame and guilt in the wake of error, the shame magnified if an apology is made face to face.

Doctors are, however, expected by the public to be above error. There is an expectation of perfection: "We live in an age in which the only universally acceptable cause of death is decapitation—all else is considered reparable" (Wears and Wu 2002). And doctors are well known to set themselves punishing high standards. This may seem excellent, but, as Sutcliffe (2004) suggests:

> Medicine is often driven by the idea that perfection is the ultimate goal and
> that mistakes are a personal and professional failure. This mindset, while

praiseworthy, can blind people to the idea that mistakes are normal and can provide opportunities to learn.

This makes it particularly difficult to come to terms with mistakes. As Robbennolt (2009) says: "it is hard to have confidence in one's competence as a healer and to simultaneously accept that one has caused harm to another", while "it is most painful to people when an important element of their self-concept is threatened".

Kaldjian and colleagues (2007) talk of "a compulsive mindset among physicians which automatically views bad outcomes as failures". Swaminath and colleagues (2001) describe medical errors as "haunting the conscience of those involved". Doctors are described as reacting to their errors with shame, humiliation, agony, anguish, devastation, panic, guilt, remorse, sadness, anger, self-doubt, and self-blame – a litany of sores (Wears and Wu 2002, Taft 2005, Schwappach and Boluarte 2008). Penson et al (2001) use descriptions bordering on the sordid, such as: "anxiety about a soiled reputation". They quote one doctor as saying, in the wake of error: "I felt a sense of shame like a burning ulcer. This was not guilt: guilt is what you feel when you have done something wrong. What I felt was shame: I was what was wrong".

See how strongly the moral flame burns, so that "shame" is an inevitable consequence for the thoughtful and always competent doctor, except on this one occasion of slippage. Fischer and colleagues (Fischer et al 2006), describing the effects of making errors, bring notice to self-flagellation, quoting descriptors such as: "scared", "guilty", "embarrassed", "fear", "mad at myself", "extraordinarily awful", and "frightening and discouraging".

We are aware that our examples of error in Homer are all men. Women now form more than half the student intake to medical schools worldwide. There are adverse effects in the sphere of bullying and abuse, as we discuss in chapter eleven, but also on the reactions of women after error (Waterman et al 2007). Male students are believed by their female colleagues to be less sensitive, or more insulated from feeling, and so protected from reacting adversely to their errors (Mankaka et al 2014). The response of seniors may be felt to be sexist:

> It's true that, when you make a mistake, you're telling yourself that they [the male supervisors] think you're the featherbrain of the service. In their opinions, it was almost normal that it was a woman who had made the error. When you are a woman and have the reputation of being a bad doctor, it's hard to change it, precisely because you're a woman (Mankaka et al 2014).

There are encouraging differences too, in that women more often make constructive changes to their practice in response to error (Wu et al 2003, p.226).

Although there may be sympathy from one's colleagues, there are still not adequate mechanisms for supporting medics who have made mistakes. The medical facts are often thoroughly discussed at medical meetings, but rarely the feelings of those affected. Failure to deal with these emotions adequately leads to dysfunctional processes such as withdrawal, burnout, alcoholism and a decline in empathy (Wu 2000, West et al 2006). These are reactions to perceived failure within a guilt culture. In addition, those perceived failures can lead to responses typical of a shame culture such as breaches in integrity, changing records and covering up (Davidoff 2002, Taft 2005, Fred 2008).

Mizrahi (1984) categorised the ways in which doctors in training avoided facing the responsibilities of error: denial through redefinition of what error is, discounting (blaming others for your mistakes), and distancing. His study was from the early days of error investigation, when making mistakes was not readily recognised or discussed. It is striking, though, how well his categories describe the apology of Agamemnon.

Conclusion

In this chapter, we consider the moment of "tragic madness" (Padel 1995) that underlies some errors, and also emphasise the psychological harm that is done to the healthcare staff that commit them. In turn, we have considered the different case of the serial errorist whose behaviour, in previous generations, faithful colleagues closing ranks and the opacity of medicine concealed, but who, in an era of public transparency is now subject to whistleblowing and censure (the subject of our following chapter ten). We hope to see institutional changes that provide greater care for those staff – not only the dependable clinicians with a one-off error, but also the serial errorist, where a more therapeutic approach will be required.

It is not our intention to advocate the hard headed, thick-skinned attitude of Agamemnon, whose language - even as he offers his apology - displays his arrogance and sense of power and position. This seems to be where those advocating training for increased "resilience" and "grit" are misdirecting us (see chapter thirteen) (Peterkin and Bleakley 2017). We might look to the response of Achilles, to the offer of restitution.

Achilles has also recognised by this point that he too is at fault. His anger and intransigence have caused the deaths of many Greeks (which does not concern him), and also the death of his beloved Patroclus (which does). His response is to say that any question of recompense must wait; there is a battle to fight and an enemy to defeat. So in medicine, there is always a next task that has to be dealt with. Achilles moves on to his next task, a berserk attack on the Trojan forces, causing huge numbers of casualties and culminating in the death of Hector in front of the gates of Troy. But afterwards, he returns to his grief and organises and presides over the funeral rites of Patroclus and the subsequent games in celebration of Patroclus' death.

Doctors often, probably usually, would not revisit their error, certainly not in terms of discussing it openly with others; rather, the silt of subsequent medical events, whence it may resurface or erupt years later, covers it over gradually. Better that the cycle of error-shame is played out with full awareness, attention to moral frames, appropriate disclosure and apology, and peer and institutional support. Good doctors are hard to come by and human error is impossible to eradicate entirely. There will be slips and mistakes whatever protocols are in place, even where we are satisfied that the best possible safety climate has been set up.

Notes

1. Agamemnon thus cunningly draws an implicit parallel between himself and the king of the gods.
2. Roughly one quarter to one third of doctors stated that they would disclose errors to patients, though 70% or more thought that they should do so (Berlin 2006, Wu et al 2003). Aasland and Ford (2005) found that 68% of their doctors surveyed had discussed their error with patients but suggest this could be because they confined their definition of errors to those with severe consequences.
3. Scodel (2008, p.95) feels able to state: "In the full modern sense of the word, there are no apologies in Homeric epic". Her explanation for this view is strikingly relevant to today:

> Most Homeric quasi-apologies, however, resemble the inadequate apologies that are so familiar a feature of modern public life. Homeric characters sometimes apologise without quite admitting that an actual offence took place. Or they may acknowledge that something wrong happened, without quite acknowledging that they themselves did it: … Or if they admit wrongdoing, they still do not express actual regret.

CHAPTER TEN

WHISTLEBLOWING

WRITTEN FROM AN ORIGINAL IDEA BY, AND IN COLLABORATION WITH, VICTORIA RODULSON

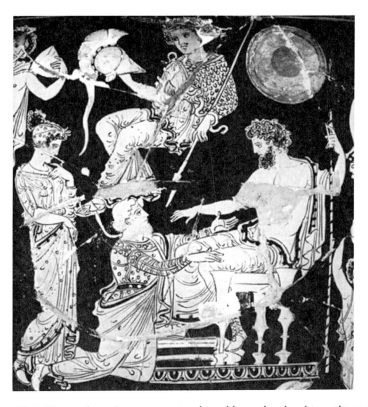

Figure 10-1: Chryses begs Agamemnon to release his captive daughter – the sequel leads to the first recorded case of "whistleblowing"

Dilemmas of "speaking out"

One current, pressing, issue in medicine and healthcare is the role of the whistleblower who recognises poor practice or ethical transgressions that compromise patient care and safety. Once, whistleblowers were ostracised as "snitches", where medical culture closed ranks. However, in a new era of public accountability in the UK after a series of scandals, medicine looks to formally embrace whistleblowing to the point that not reporting transgressions has in its own right become a transgression of professionalism.

Medical students gain an identity through an increasingly intimate identification with the history and traditions of medical culture and its specialties. Inevitably, they find themselves in situations of conflicting loyalties should they see senior clinicians behaving unprofessionally. What are the implications of facing these dilemmas for students in terms of role modelling and shaping of character as a doctor, and how might a study of Homer help with such dilemmas?

We suggest that a close reading of an opening scene in Homer's *Iliad* can help us to untangle such ethical dilemmas. We link this with the early Greek tradition of *parrhesia* or "truth telling", where frank "speaking out" against perceived injustice or inappropriate behaviour is encouraged as resistance to power and perceived abuse of authority. What we now call "speaking truth to power", or informed acts of resistance, the ancient Greeks called *parrhesia*. We encourage medical educators to openly discuss perceived ethical dilemmas with medical students; and medicine to make the transition from an historically "closed" to an "open" society (Popper 1945) where whistleblowing becomes as acceptable and necessary as good hygiene on the wards. But in an ideal medical society, whistleblowing would be unnecessary, because the offender could be approached directly.

A brief episode at the beginning of Homer's *Iliad* offers the earliest example in Western literature of what we now call "whistleblowing", and we will examine the parallels and contrasts with modern examples. The rather ugly term "whistleblowing" is modern, coined in the early 1970s by Ralph Nader (2016), an American civic activist, to replace previously negatively and loaded descriptors such as "snitching" and "informing", where "snitchers" are liable to be ostracised from a community closing ranks. These descriptors are linked to societies such as medicine and the military that are largely opaque, rather than transparent, to the public gaze. Here, closing ranks to protect one's own kind is viewed as necessary even where this offers moral contradictions.

In traditional clans, "snitches" align with despised figures - as betrayers - from Judas Iscariot to spies in the Cold War who "crossed over". Since Ralph Nader's activism, such inward-looking, self-protective, habits have been questioned, so that whistleblowing in emerging egalitarian medical and healthcare contexts is now a requirement, punishable if explicitly ignored. The term "whistleblowing" of course carries a kind of moral authority as it denotes policing. It is like flypaper, attracting bad press that sticks to it. Needham (2012) suggests it is time for re-invention, where: "Problems remain with the negative connotations of the term "whistleblowing". Perhaps it is time to whistleblow on whistleblowing? Certainly it may be time for a new word.

Whistleblowing and virtue ethics

Nader (2016) views whistleblowing as a moral responsibility or duty in both the professions and public life - a challenge to habitual practices of disguising ethical slippage. High profile public accountability incidents in medicine - such as, in the UK, the Bristol paediatric heart surgery scandal - have given whistleblowing a high profile (https://en.wikipedia.org/wiki/ Bristol_heart_scandal).

Professional guidelines, for example from the British Medical Association (https://www.bma.org.uk/404) and General Medical Council (http://www.gmc-uk.org/DC5900_Whistleblowing_guidance.pdf_57107304 .pdf), have followed, offering guidance, reassurance and support, to cancel out the historical legacy of stigma. Indeed, medical students are encouraged to raise concerns about issues or practices they perceive as unethical primarily as a "duty to report on substandard care" (Needham 2012). Whistleblowing is now seen as a healthy example of virtue ethics in action (Faunce 2004).

There has been significant development of interest in virtue ethics in healthcare, after previous widespread dismissal, where it is opposed to the dominant discourse of principles-based approaches (Statman 1997). Virtue is not formally taught in medical education – rather, it is modelled in practice by senior clinicians and is aligned with "good character" as an issue of identity construction of the "proto-professional" (medical students) and "professional" (qualified doctor). In *After Virtue* (MacIntyre 1985) - perhaps the most influential modern text on virtue ethics - Alisdair MacIntyre argued that virtue refuses reduction to universal principles because it is culture-specific. In the Homeric era, for example, the cultural model for virtue was that of the Warrior King, where in a postmodern culture, virtues might be modelled by celebrities. MacIntyre then sees virtue as plastic or contingent upon context. As cultures change, so do role models; consequently, processes of identity construction through identification with role models and cultural norms also change.

MacIntyre's *After Virtue* is over 35 years old, yet its importance has not waned. In an era of "fake news" and "post truth" public behaviour, "virtue" has become virtual, modelled by reality television. MacIntyre predicted the emergence of this ethical vacuum, suggesting that we should return to Aristotle for guidance on what virtue means. He was alarmed by the manner in which virtue had become identified with individual opinion rather than social agreement, such that fact and opinion had become hopelessly blurred. For MacIntyre, virtues are meaningful only when they are tied to the *telos,* or ultimate purpose, of a community, and not to the self-gratification of influential individuals.

In medicine, the *telos* of the culture, according to Pellegrino's (2005, 2008) rigorous philosophical analysis, is contained in the first moral precept of the Hippocratic Oath that sets out what the "good" (purpose, or end point – *telos*) of medicine is: I will do whatever is "good for the benefit of my patient, and abstain from whatever is deleterious and mischievous ...".

"Mischief", in relation to patient care, smacks of "post-virtue" values – behaving selfishly rather than for the good of the community. This may escalate into unprofessional behaviour. Pellegrino (2005, 2008) recognises that this ancient moral precept is made problematic by the often conflicting roles of the contemporary doctor, including researcher, manager, business leader, politician, educator, advocate, and so forth.

What may be considered virtuous in a medicine of the future can be read from current sea changes, such as: a shift from autocracy to democracy and egalitarianism; from masculine heroism to feminine collaboration and team process; and from paternalism (doctor-centredness) to patient-centredness. Such shifts align with Carol Gilligan's (1982) call for a situated or context-sensitive "ethics of care" (or a "relational ethics") replacing a principles-led ethics. As a feminist, Gilligan points out that the field of virtue ethics since Plato has been gender-biased, towards masculine interests and values.

Where MacIntyre suggests that virtue should align with the *telos* of the community, we see the *telos* of medical culture shifting from realising heroism (see chapters one, two and five) within an opaque community that characteristically closed ranks under adversity or challenge, to a transparent community of collaboration and shared success concerned also with social justice. Such a community is not paternalistic, but grounds itself in patients' concerns and needs, returning to the first precept of the Hippocratic Oath quoted earlier (see chapters six and seven).

In this brave new world, whistleblowers are cherished rather than ostracised, as was the case up to only a decade ago. For example, Stephen Bolsin, an anaesthetist, exposed the Bristol Royal Infirmary paediatric heart surgery scandal between 1989 and 1995, where an unusually high number of deaths were occurring but surgeons closed ranks in denial of the problem. While Bolsin's exposures led to the formation of the Kennedy inquiry and its recommendations for a framework of clinical governance in the UK, he was cast as a "troublemaker" and failed to gain work in the UK in an attempt to move away from Bristol. He eventually moved to Australia where he has pursued a successful clinical and patient safety education career, including supporting whistleblowing (Faunce and Bolsin 2004, Faunce et al 2004, Bolsin et al 2011).

Contemporary views on virtue ethics focus on the consequences of our social actions rather than on pre-ordained cultural habits. This lifts virtue out of its imprisonment as blind devotion to the main culture into which one is initiated (a kind of Freemasonry), again compromising traditional models of identity through identification with a significant tribe or clan in which personal conscience is quelled.

A significant body of research on how medical students approach (moral) "professionalism dilemmas" in the face of transgressions by senior clinicians, led by Charlotte Rees and Lynn Monrouxe, shows that identity formation amongst these medical students is no longer led solely by identification with the historical traditions of medicine (Monrouxe et al 2014, Rees et al 2013). Rather, students recognise the primacy of public accountability set against the pull of tradition as they wrestle with moral dilemmas. What most medical students aim for is authentic patient-centredness, and in the changing climate of collaborative, team-based healthcare they are necessarily caught in the inexorable drift towards a feminist ethics of care.

Whistleblowing in the flesh

Whistleblowing is widely discussed in the context of politics and national security with recent high profile cases of "leaking" sensitive political and military information to the Internet for public scrutiny. The highest profile case is Julian Assange's WikiLeaks - publishing the once imprisoned Bradley Manning's (now Chelsea Manning since a gender reassignment – itself a bold form of moral courage) leak of United States high security information; and Edward Snowden's leak of classified information from the National Security Agency.

Such bold speech has been widely discussed and historically situated as originating from Euripides (487-407 BC), who coined the term *parrhesia* or "fearless speech" to describe speech that was free from rhetoric and spoke "truth to power". *Parrhesia* literally means "to speak everything" or to speak openly and boldly, implying not just freedom of speech but speaking "truth" as a public obligation even if this means bringing risk upon oneself. Michel Foucault (2011) has almost single-handedly recovered interest in the topic of "the courage of truth", "truth-telling", or the parrhesiastical tradition and this has led to many commentaries (McGushin 2007, Bleakley 2014).

As an example, an Athenian orator Lykourgos drew public attention to the wrongdoings of Leokratis, suggesting that the law might do nothing, but the ordinary citizen can speak out publicly to denounce wrongdoing. Mansbach (2011) notes that Hellenic kings had advisors skilled in *parrhesia* who would temper the rhetoric of the monarch and this is repeated in the role of the Fool or Court Jester, who again plays a serious part in tempering royal rhetoric or bad behaviour. Whistleblowing in politics now has a major role in civic affairs and an international online network (Myers 2014). The parrhesiast often recognises and articulates a tension between corporate or professional interests and those of the public as a social injustice or abuse of privilege.

Nick Cohen (2011), writing in the UK *Observer,* suggested that the law should save whistleblowers, not silence them. Cohen notes that we still live in a climate where if you "spill the beans on your company's criminal activities" you will "not just lose your job, you could lose your career". Cohen notes Pericles' oration for the Athenian war dead, where "To be happy means to be free and to be free means to be brave", taking this as a call-to-arms for would-be parrhesiasts, who, as Foucault noted, must show moral courage without resorting to persuasion in exposing the truth. Cohen (Online, unpaginated: https://www.theguardian.com/commentisfree/2011/jul/10/whistleblowers-rupert-murdoch-nhs-nick-cohen) continues:

> On Foucault's reading, the worker who criticises his boss uses parrhesia. The boss who shouts down his worker, does not. The woman who challenges religious notions of her subordination is a parrhesiastes. The clerics who threaten her with ostracism or worse are not. In the Chinese legend, the mandarin who knows he must contradict the emperor orders carpenters to build him a coffin and takes it with him to court. Pericles would have approved.

But whistleblowing, as we suggest, goes back beyond Pericles (495-429 BCE) and Euripides (487-407 BCE) to Homer (8th century BCE) and Homer's contemporary storytellers. For example, although Homer does not include the story of the Wooden Horse and the fall of Troy in the *Iliad*, he does refer to it in the *Odyssey*. At the time of Homeric oral storytelling all members of the audience would have been familiar with the tale, later retold in Virgil's epic poem *Aeneid*. The wooden horse ruse did not fool all Trojans - Laocoon blew the whistle on the whole scheme seeing it for what it was, a trick, but was ignored by fellow Trojans. Indeed, along with his two sons he was killed by venomous and constricting sea snakes who both bit and suffocated two of the three to death (one son was said to have escaped), depicted in a famous life-size marble sculpture now in the Vatican.

Laocoon is a giant amongst whistleblowers as, in questioning the apparent gullibility of his comrades, he questioned Fate itself (or the gods' will), acting against the pre-ordained script of Troy, destined to fall. No mortal could challenge Fate, and in response Poseidon is said to have ordered Laocoon and his sons to meet the fate described above. Metaphorically, this perhaps is what whistleblowers – from high profile political WikiLeakers to local protesters – feel like when governments, corporations or even powerful seniors turn on them.

In medicine, whistleblowing is defined as:

> where an employee, former employee or member of an organisation raises concerns to people who have the power and presumed willingness to take corrective action. In most cases, the individual is unable or unwilling to raise their concerns locally either through concern for their own role or because they have raised the concern previously and no action was taken. (BMA Whistleblowing).

Despite Nader's campaign to rebrand "snitching" as the more positive "whistleblowing", the consequences of the latter remain for many stigmatising rather than liberating. Helene Donnelly, a nurse involved in the 2008 Mid-Staffordshire National Health Service (NHS) Foundation Trust scandal, exemplifies whistleblowing at its worst and best. Despite fear of reprisal and a lack of support and feedback, Donnelly was persistent in reporting her concerns over poor and fraudulent practice - falsifying waiting times - in the hospital's Emergency Department:

> The culture in the department gradually declined to the point where all of the staff were scared of the Sisters and afraid to speak out against the poor standard of care the patients were receiving in case they incurred the wrath

of the Sisters.... I was concerned about the terrible effect that our actions were having on patient care. I did raise this with Sisters [X] and [Y], however their response was extremely aggressive, basically telling me that they were in charge and accusing me and anyone else who agreed with me of not being team players. (Francis 2013).

One feels those mythical Neptunian sea snakes coiling and suffocating ready to sink their fangs and release their poison. Donnelly's concerns were not taken seriously nor formally processed by the Trust. She endured harassment and threats from colleagues so extreme that she did not feel safe walking to her car in the dark at the end of a shift. She later told the public inquiry: "I felt completely on my own" (Francis 2013).

The Iliad plunges the audience straight into the great quarrel between Achilles and Agamemnon, familiar now from previous chapters, dictating the events of the rest of the poem (*Iliad* 1. 68-113). That quarrel is precipitated by an act of whistleblowing. Agamemnon, a Greek king, has taken a woman, Chryseis, as a war prize. He refuses to release her to her father, Chryses, who is a priest of Apollo and who offers a ransom as recompense; as punishment, Apollo visits a plague on the Greek encampment. Achilles calls a meeting of the Greek leaders to determine the cause of the plague and the seer Calchas boldly steps forward saying that he can explain, as an act of *parrhesia* or fearless speech. He demands protection from Achilles because his explanation will incriminate somebody important (he is referring to Agamemnon but does not name him for fear of reprisal):

> swear to me that you will willingly help me in word and deed. For I think I shall infuriate a man who wields great power over all the Greeks and in whom they put their trust. An angry king is mightier than a lesser man. Even if he swallows his anger at the time, he will harbour resentment in his chest until he may let it forth (*Iliad* 1. 76-83).

Achilles swears to protect him: "even if you speak of Agamemnon, who claims to be by far the best of the Greeks" (*Iliad* 1. 90-1). Calchas then explains in very straightforward terms that Apollo is angry at the insult by Agamemnon to his priest in refusing to release Chryseis for the offered ransom. Calchas is right to be concerned about the reaction of Agamemnon, who rounds on him: "angry, his heart filled with a black passion and his eyes flashing like flame. 'Prophet of evil, never do you speak anything to my advantage. It is always your delight to prophesy evil'" (*Iliad* 1.103-7). Crucially however, Agamemnon has no choice but to accept Calchas' assessment. He returns Chryseis to her father but demands recompense, taking the woman who is by right Achilles' prize. It is from this final insult that the events of the *Iliad* unfold, fuelled by Achilles' quarrel with Agamemnon.

Medical students too are a good example of individuals reluctant to speak out. They regard themselves as on the bottom rung of the hierarchy, paradoxically rendered insensible and insensitive by their superiors whom they hope to emulate. Unlike their superiors, who are now specialists, as juniors they remain generalists and are present in many environments throughout the healthcare system and thus able to bear witness to a host of potential ethical transgressions; they witness examples of bad practice, some serious (Monrouxe et al 2014, Rees et al 2013); and they feel a powerful duty to do something with their knowledge, to report it somewhere (Lindstrom et al 2011). In some medical schools these issues are discussed, often in the setting of small group tutorials; however, just as often they are taken no further, despite students making formal reports to senior members of academic staff. This is akin to Calchas' request for support from Achilles. Nothing will be said without the backing of a powerful figure.

Over a quarter of a century ago, Henry Silver and Anita Glicken (1990) showed a strikingly high incidence of "medical student abuse" by seniors. Over 80% of medical students reported abuse, which is the subject of the following chapter eleven, but worse, nearly 70% reported incidents that were "very upsetting" and 16% said that such abuse had marked them for life. A study by Field (2002) showed that bullying of medical students was still common and that bullying within medicine was endemic to the culture. A later study by John Coverdale and colleagues (Coverdale et al 2009) showed unacceptably high levels of bullying even in psychiatry training, where more psychological insight, care and empathy would be expected. As noted earlier, nearly a decade of research by Rees and Monrouxe (for example, Rees et al 2013) shows that abuse and bullying can be subtle and wearing for medical students, placing patient care at risk but also numbing the potential for speaking out as students get used to the idea that "this is the way things happen around here", so that bad behaviour becomes naturalised.

Speaking out against social injustice

A comparison between an event reported in 2013 from the mid-Staffordshire UK NHS debacle and a fictional event reported some 3000 years earlier would be of passing interest only, except for the light that Homer can shed on our age. Calasso's (1994, p.103) is a memorable quotation: "Every notion of progress is refuted by the existence of the *Iliad*". This can be read in several ways – for example, is Calasso saying that the *Iliad* already contains the whole of the history of human psychology (a notion with which we can readily agree)? Or is it something to do with the unchanging nature of relationships of power between humans?

It is depressing that the weak still fear to speak out against the strong. Importantly, what we are not looking at here is an immoveable structural disposition or cultural archetype. There is no reason that medicine as a culture cannot change from restrictive hierarchy to open democracy – indeed, the introduction of governance structures after the Kennedy inquiry shows that medical culture learned much from the Bristol Royal Infirmary scandal and such lessons should be processional, progressive and far-reaching.

A groundbreaking book by the anthropological archaeologists Kent Flannery and Joyce Marcus (2012) discusses "the creation of inequality" in terms of "how our prehistoric ancestors set the stage for monarchy, slavery and empire". Following Rousseau's famous suggestion that hierarchical culture shows slippage from a more natural state of egalitarianism, Flannery and Marcus critically investigate the archaeological and anthropological evidence to show that Ice Age hunter-gatherer communities, centred on small family groups that were largely foragers, must have collaborated with other groups for survival and must have incorporated taboos against the development of hierarchy and privilege.

Egalitarianism disappears with the introduction of larger groups particularly during the transition to agriculture, as more elaborate clans develop from simpler family units. In a perceptive final chapter, Flannery and Marcus suggest that much greater egalitarianism is possible amongst contemporary societies if we look to the lessons of anthropology and archaeology, not only by restructuring distribution of wealth but through individuals learning to promote social justice. It is ironic that medical students commit themselves ethically to treat all patients as equals in terms of required medical treatment, yet are fashioned through identity formation by a culture saturated with inequality: a pincer movement of hierarchy within healthcare, and hierarchy accepted as natural between doctors and patients.

Yet, as we have said, governance is slowly re-shaping medical culture - just as Achilles encourages Calchas to "take full courage and speak out", so, as we noted earlier, the General Medical Council (GMC) promotes a culture of openness and integrity, asking doctors, and even medical students, to be brave and voice their concerns, providing several options for doing so. The British Medical Association (BMA) also recognises whistleblowing - as a "professional duty that needs to be fulfilled in a professional way" (Porter 2009).

Individuals are advised first to follow local protocol, and, while reporting to the media remains an option and is protected under the Public Interest Disclosure Act, it must only be done in exceptional circumstances (Whistleblowing Helpline 2013). In the event that local systems do not exist or fail to deal with the issue, clinicians must inform the appropriate regulatory body and discuss concerns with an impartial colleague, a defence body such as the Medical Defence Union or Medical Protection Society, their professional organisation, or the GMC (2013). For UK Foundation programme trainees, the first stop is the educational supervisor. One of the *Duties of a Doctor* listed by the GMC in their publication *Tomorrow's Doctors* (2009) is: "Act without delay if you have good reason to believe that you or a colleague may be putting patients at risk".

By incorporating this in legislation, one could say that it is easier for doctors to understand that they are duty-bound to report on substandard patient care, whereas for previous generations there may have been some ambiguity as to whether a whistleblower was doing the right thing or being an unreasonable troublemaker. Indeed, as already noted, the GMC now views doctors who do not report misconduct as accountable, even where they are not implicated. This supports the move to transparency in medicine that embraces MacIntyre's notion of virtue as the reflective or carefully thought through *telos* of a social group.

Anonymity or open confrontation?

Measures to uphold anonymity reassure health workers, as demonstrated by the GMC's confidential whistleblowing helpline that received 358 calls in its first four months of operation. One in eight of these required referral to the GMC's fitness to practise triage system (Jacques 2013). But there is a difference here between Homer and the present. Calchas is afraid precisely because his words are spoken in open assembly. Although "anonymous" is derived from Greek ("having no name"), the concept of blaming someone behind his or her back in such a context is foreign to the ancient Greek mentality. During the "Embassy scene" in Book 9 (see chapter three), when three Greek leaders are sent to persuade Achilles to return to help his comrades, there is an unexpressed need for tact in the way that they express themselves.

In a return to our theme of chapter three - speaking "bluntly" - Achilles himself feels no such need for tact: "I must speak out bluntly what I think and how it shall come to pass. Then you will not sit there muttering one after another. For I hate like the gates of Hell that man who thinks one thing and says another" (*Iliad* 9. 309-13).

These words are spoken in a group of five, but the original revelation and argument occur in open assembly of the whole army, and certainly there Achilles speaks bluntly, calling his leader "a shameless schemer" and "a drunken sot". Achilles, however, unlike Calchas, is a hero of equal status to Agamemnon. There is one other occasion when an ordinary man, this time a soldier, speaks his mind. Following the quarrel, Achilles has retired to his part of the camp vowing to take no further part in the fighting. Overnight, Zeus sends a dream to Agamemnon telling him to test the mettle of his troops by suggesting to them that they are losing the war and should return home. The plan backfires and the troops rush enthusiastically to the ships, happy to return - but Odysseus restrains them, recalling them to their duty. The troops sit quietly except for one, Thersites, who speaks out against Agamemnon. He asks him what more he wants - his huts are full of booty and he has the pick of the captured women. He urges his colleagues to return to the ships and leave Agamemnon, the man who insulted Achilles "a much better man" (*Iliad* 2. 211-77).

One might think then that ordinary men can speak out in assembly, but Odysseus reacts swiftly. He harshly warns, indeed threatens, Thersites not to speak against his king. If he does so again, Odysseus swears: "I will strip you of cloak and tunic and thrash you weeping and naked from this assembly down to the swift ships" (*Iliad* 2. 261-4). He then beats him around the head and shoulders with his staff to literally drive home the warning. We might think "so much for plain speaking, for parrhesiasts and their directness". But recall that *parrhesia* is an art and that bluff and ungainly rhetoric have no part in "truth telling".

Sluiter and Rosen (2004, p.16), warn against taking the high moral ground with parrhesia, where: "Parrhesia in Aristotle is not a virtue, it is a description of a certain type of speech, which is sometimes rightly adopted and sometimes not". *Parrhesia* is context-dependent and open to interpretation: according to van Raalte (2004, pp.279-312), *parrhesia* for Calchas, Achilles and Homer is a matter of bravery; for Socrates and Plato, it is a matter of virtue.[1] Aristotle does talk of *parrhesia* explicitly, and Mulherne (2004, 313-39) argues that *parrhesia* is a matter for both ethical and political practice.

Returning to Thersites' intervention, this is then an enigmatic passage. While Thersites has apparently only spoken the truth, we get more context from Homer. He is introduced by Homer as a braggart and given a bizarre appearance by him. He might expect some sympathy from his colleagues but they laugh at his plight and one says: "This is the best thing Odysseus has done for the Greeks to silence this loud-mouthed braggart". Thus Homer teaches us how to spot would-be parrhesiasts who are in fact common rhetoricians or troublemakers. We might spot behaviours of ambitious politicians in such tactics.

This behaviour of Thersites' colleagues is all the more enigmatic because Homer tells us they react in this way "despite being angry." Angry at what? The behaviour of Agamemnon? Being prevented from returning home? We are not told. It is suggested that Homer includes Thersites to epitomise the opposite of the heroic, represented by Achilles (Postlethwaite 1998). Certainly Thersites' speech echoes some of the words and themes that occur in the quarrel between Achilles and Agamemnon. However, if these two represent opposite ends of the spectrum of safety in whistleblowers, where does Calchas fit within such a spectrum? Perhaps we should think of another paradigm than binary opposites.

Rather, Achilles is protected by his heroic stature, Calchas by the patronage of Achilles and his stature as a soothsayer, and Thersites exemplifies the fate of those without protection or perhaps he blurts out what he sees as truth but the rest of us see as devoid of both moral courage and content. Perhaps both whistleblowing and telling the truth are particularly unacceptable if your nature is irritating and your appearance unattractive: the latter is unfortunate, where the former can be re-educated.

Speaking truth to power

Homer makes it clear that Calchas' greatest fear is that of repercussions, for he understands that: "When a king is angry at a lesser man, his is the greater power" (*Iliad* 1. 80). There are echoes of this fear of a king's wrath elsewhere in Greek literature. In Sophocles' *Oedipus Rex* (lines 300-462 and 1121-85), both Teiresias and the shepherd fear the anger of Oedipus as their stories of events following his birth unfold; and the action of Euripides' *Bacchae* revolves around the furious reaction of the king, Pentheus, to the worship of Dionysus by his people. All three kings suffer dismal fates.

Calchas and healthcare staff share a common dilemma: to blow the whistle and face possible negative consequences, or to let poor practice go unreported and, with current legislation, face later punishment for not divulging information. "Agamemnon's ability to command obedience rests on a fear of retribution" (Hammer 2002, 83), and by incurring the wrath of a king and thus jeopardising this Homeric hierarchy, Calchas knows the only person who will be able to protect him must be superior to himself in standing, and of heroic status equal to or greater than Agamemnon. To whistleblow, must one then seek at least one ally of high standing? If one does, it may only serve to threaten the "face" of that powerful person (Scodel 2008).

Unlike the other Greeks, Achilles does not fear Agamemnon, and when he refers to the king earlier in Book 1 as one "who now claims to be far the best of the Achaeans (Greeks)" (*Iliad* 1. 91), his words carry a tone of mockery. Without Achilles' promise, Calchas knows that he may lose everything at the hands of Agamemnon, and while the warrior may not be able to negate the prophet's fears, he is able to neutralise them so far that Calchas may speak the truth (Hammer 2002). Needham (2012) postulates that a medical hierarchy and intimidating senior staff members may also dissuade staff, and medical students in particular, from questioning practice - even more so where there is a perception of a "closed shop" where colleagues cover for each other leading to a lack of transparency.

As noted above, the modern UK NHS supposedly promotes approachability and mutual respect amongst all members of the multi-disciplinary team, and there are measures in place intended to protect whistleblowing doctors. In spite of this, a 2010 survey conducted by the BMA found that at some point in their careers, most hospital doctors have had concerns regarding patient care or staff behaviour, yet nearly 50% failed to report them due to fear of repercussions and lack of confidence in a resolution. And of those who did report, 10% faced reprisals (BMA 2012).

Sovereign power (exercised by authority) - its use and abuse - is a constant menace to whistleblowers ancient and modern and is reproductive of traditional hierarchies or habits. Michel Foucault's (2011) extensive study of *parrhesia* as a form of capillary power – power that runs through a system and is potentially productive of change, for example as resistance to sovereign power – offers a framework for understanding and legitimising whistleblowing in the public interest. The scene that we have described at the beginning of the *Iliad* happens in open debate in front of all the people.

It has been argued that this parallels the rise of democratic processes in the newly emerging city-states of the 8th century BCE, and has been described as "assembly democracy", a form that has given way in complex "open" societies largely to "representative democracy" (parliamentary representation) and "monitory democracy" (the rule of law or governance) (Keane 2009).

When Apollo's priest Chryses asks for the return of his daughter, offering a rich ransom: "then all the Greeks cried out that respect should be shown to the priest and the rich ransom accepted" (*Iliad* 1. 22-3). But this is not a democracy and Agamemnon refuses, bringing Apollo's plague down on the troops in punishment. To resolve the problem, Achilles calls an assembly of all the army. The revelation of where the blame lies and the subsequent quarrel happen in front of all (Barker and Christensen 2013). Events, discussions and arguments are open; decisions are not. In the argument between Achilles and Agamemnon, it is clear that Achilles is the mightier warrior but Agamemnon is the more powerful leader.

The Greek army described by Homer and the UK NHS alike both make much of teamwork and open debate, but sovereign power, in the form of potential retribution, dominates both systems. It is the mobilisation of capillary power (potency inherent in any system after one strips away sovereign power or the power of authority), or resistance (speaking truth to power) in the form of plain speaking or whistleblowing, which can counter such potential retribution through a soft revolution.

Conclusion

Whistleblowing requires "huge courage" (Porter 2009); indeed, as Foucault (2011) noted, a "moral courage" where "Free-spokenness hangs on the style of life", and organisations should, in a contemporary democracy aiming for egalitarianism, do everything they can to ensure that there are no obstacles for those who choose to voice their concerns. Yet it is those committed to a style of life that is egalitarian who will choose to whistleblow as opposed to lay low.

Examples from Homer's *Iliad* and modern medical practice demonstrate that for effective whistleblowing to take place individuals should be reassured that their personal and professional wellbeing are protected and that their worries will be heard and taken seriously, with appropriate action taken. Yet, they must also show the courage and skill of classical parrhesiasts. Recent changes to legislation in the UK are improving the situation, but staff must know to whom they can turn when in need of support and guidance. Medical students are in a particularly vulnerable position even in a rapidly changing world of medical education, and need mentorial and tutorial structures around them to find their way through the tangle of ethical mishaps and slippage of professionalism described in detail by the collaborative research of Rees and Monrouxe (Rees et al 2013, Monrouxe et al 2014).

The medical workplace – a sprawling and confusing landscape for medical students - must adopt a culture not of fear but one of openness and reflection. The Greeks learned through great loss and hardship from their mistakes in politics and warfare; the NHS needs to learn through its collective history and intelligence. Unfortunately, the signs are not good – there is much preparatory work to do on post hoc investigation of the creation of inequality in medical culture in order to develop an egalitarian, patient-centred medicine that honours whistleblowers as parrhesiasts and not as pariahs. Foucault (2011) suggested that the Church took over the ancients' parrhesiastic philosophy and invested the pastor with the role and identity of the "speaker of truth", but this role too has been traditionally ascribed to the doctor (McGushin 2007). How will doctors of the future manage such an identity heavily entwined with public trust within a politicised health service that seems to have lost moral courage?

Note

1. The "Apology" of Plato is an account of Socrates' defence at his trial for "blasphemy and corrupting the youth". Although not described as *parrhesia*, Socrates' defence is that he feels bound to try to improve the lives of his citizen-colleagues by testing their ideas and beliefs through dialectic. He keeps returning to the need to determine the truth, and is essential reading at the beginning of 2017, as we write, in an age of "post-truth" and "alternative facts". During his defence, Socrates likens himself to Achilles at the moment the latter returns to battle to avenge the death of Patroclus. The slightly ludicrous comparison has troubled commentators, but the problem is resolved by reading it as a joke. The idea of Plato making jokes can be difficult to accept.

CHAPTER ELEVEN

ABUSE

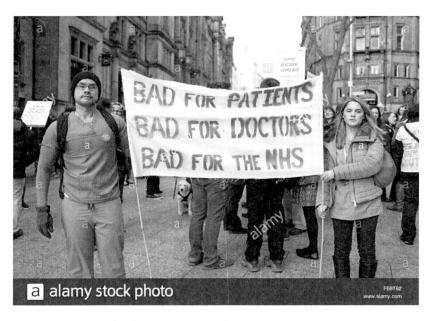

Figure 11-1: UK Junior doctors' strike 2016-17

Encounter with a surgeon

The Peninsula Medical School, UK, where both of the authors once worked, was well known for its emphasis on the medical humanities in the curriculum. Among the many Arts and Humanities Special Study Units (SSUs) offered to 4th year students was a Poetry SSU. This gave students an opportunity to capture clinical learning issues in a pithy, expressive way, bringing aesthetic and ethical dimensions to what was typically viewed instrumentally. Predictably, many students wrote poems about patients as they deepened their clinical work-based experience. Other students wrote about colleagues and senior staff who acted as their mentors and teachers. Some of these descriptions were sobering. One student wrote this poem:

Encounter with a Surgeon

His reputation precedes him,
Loud, arrogant, aggressive, manic - these are his labels.
"What's this?" he demands, offering a grey slimy tube between latex fingers
(oh no)
(what is it?)
(the pancreas lives around there I think)
(sod it)
"the pancreas"
"what?" "No!"
"the duodenum?"
His eyes shift with anger
(wrong again)
"you're a fuckwit, ok? You're a fuckwit!"
"this is the large bowel, what is it?"
"the large bowel"
"and what are you?"
"a fuckwit, sir"

Ritual humiliation in medicine

Learning through humiliation used to be standard in medical and surgical education, and still lingers as the unfortunate medical student above discovered. A pseudo-militaristic "hardening" regime was considered necessary for medical students to toughen them up as a defence against all the bad that they would meet in medicine and surgery – pain, suffering, hardship and death. As a result, medical students lost their idealism and gained cynicism (Becker et al 1961, Sinclair 1997, Narang 2014). Men, and a male mentality (and morality) of survivorship, dominated clinical education that was, pedagogically, more force-fed training than inquisitive education.

Ritual humiliation of students around the bedside, known in the USA as "pimping", was common – where the senior doctor asked the medical student impossibly hard questions and then shamed him in front of colleagues and patients. Moreover, while elders exposed students for supposed ignorance, those very students must sham competence in front of patients. This tradition continues. In a Swedish study, Lindstrom and colleagues (2011) describe a student admitting to feeling insecure in performing defibrillation, and being told by the senior: "never again, in front of a patient, admit that you are not experienced: that is unprofessional". The same study describes multiple examples of hurtful shaming of students.

The celebrated ethnographic study *Boys in White* by Howard Becker and colleagues (Becker et al 1961) captured the tenor of the late, male-dominated, 1950s culture of medicine and medical training, exposing to the wider academic community what was essentially a closed society without public accountability. The book's title reveals how things have changed – medical students in many countries no longer wear white coats and the gender intake is now only about 40% "boys". Surely, as the formal white coats disappear and medical culture's gender balance shifts from men to women, teaching by ritual humiliation must now be old news? Yet our poet student above is recent news. Perhaps the surgeon he encountered was a fossil from a previous, unreconstructed, age of "boys in white"?

Thirty years on from *Boys in White*, Baldwin and colleagues (1991) found high levels of abuse of undergraduates through a survey of ten medical schools in the USA. Over 80% of students reported being shouted at or humiliated in public, while over half reported sexual harassment. This mistreatment by senior staff must be put into the context of what medical students also encounter through patient contact. In the Baldwin study, 26% reported being "threatened with harm", where threatened or actual violence was often by patients.

Why, then, add insult to injury by humiliating students through medical education, where the same students may be exposed to dangers from patients and the public in the tender years of their apprenticeships? After Baldwin, a later (1998) USA based survey of 80% of graduating medical students, with 13,168 respondents, found that 48% reported at least one incident of mistreatment while at medical school (Mangus et al 1998).

One might imagine that such incidents can be shaken off or incorporated without serious harm, yet a 1990 study found that where 80% of the students surveyed reported incidents of abuse and two thirds of these students said that the abuses were of "major importance", one in four reported that they would have chosen a different profession had they known that such abuse was part of their training and widely tolerated (Silver and Glicken 1990). Such "hardening" of medical students merely made them more cynical, some bent on ditching medicine and turning to study of the law, perhaps to ultimately sue doctors. "My third year experience so completely soured my ideals of medicine that I am now considering becoming a malpractice consultant" (Rosenberg and Silver 1984).

In a 2006 study of 16 medical schools in the USA, 42% of students reported being harassed and 84% being belittled. In a review of similar studies, the author noted that 69% of those abused reported that at least one such episode was of major importance and very upsetting (Frank et al 2006).

Michael Greger (1999), a doctor himself, summarised over 20 studies on medical student abuse between 1982 and 1998, where medical education is described as "brutal", and physicians as highly intelligent but emotionally stunted, entering a profession where they can re-enact the abuse they themselves might have suffered within dysfunctional family contexts. The psychologist Robert Coombs (1997) echoed this view in a key study on why some doctors develop drug dependencies in the face of overwhelming work pressures.

As such probing and disconcerting literature expanded, so a counter movement of scepticism emerged. Critics pointed out that most studies were self-reports of "perceived" mistreatment, where self-reports are not valued as research evidence because of potential bias. Further, some medical students may have pre-existing psychopathology - such as depression - that would distort their judgments about medical education experiences. And, does anyone bother to study abuse of faculty by medical students (Kane 1995, Baldwin and Daugherty 1997)? Further research, however, showed that it was mainly male students who adopted this sceptical stance, some of whom reported with bravado that women medical students tended to overreact to sexual innuendo and humour (Kane 1995).

Is this history of ritual humiliation of medical students largely a North American phenomenon, where, for example, "hazing" (initiation by humiliation) is popular in Universities? The research suggests otherwise. In a 2004 study of a UK medical school, Lempp and Seale (2004) found that 19 of 36 students reported personal experiences of ritual humiliation:

> I've found my first rotation was very stressful, humiliating, I worked and read because of fear, because of being targeted - and that was just miserable ... One time, the consultant came in when I was examining the patient ... and just started asking me questions ... I just went blank and didn't know the answers to his questions - and then he got angrier... after things like that... you don't even have the confidence to take blood or anything. (Year 3 student).

In a climate in which public accountability for medicine was increasingly demanded, such research claimed public attention. A *Guardian* article reported Lempp and Seale's work under the title "Medical students humiliated by senior doctors" (*Guardian* 1st October 2004). But surely we have moved on from such abusive practices in the 21st century, confining them to the dustbin of medical education history?

When Kaji Sritharan and Muhunthan Thillai (2012) reported that: "The days of ritual humiliation are long gone", do we recognise that a corner has indeed been turned? We would like to think so, but in 2010 Jenny Firth-Cozens (Firth-Cozens and Harrison 2010) noted that ritual humiliation "used to be common practice in many medical teaching settings. That it has not disappeared entirely is a cause for concern". Drawing on the postmodern language of the new ethnographies, Claire L. Wendland (2010) reported that in an African medical school setting, ritual humiliation was still commonly practiced as "neocolonial domination" within medicine's "hegemonic moral order" and process of "enculturation". The identity construction of the medical student still appeared to be one based on traditions of the public school and military service, to educate for "backbone" and place in hierarchy, transferred to imperialistic endeavour.

While medical education has seen massive forward leaps in enlightened practices, some old traditions linger. Gágyor and colleagues (2012), in a study of a German medical school, found that 391 students surveyed reported a total of 1630 negative experiences. Only a minority (48 students) had no negative experiences. A 2013 National Training Survey by the UK General Medical Council (GMC 2013) found that 13.2% of respondents said that they had been victims of bullying and harassment in their posts, where 19.5% had also witnessed someone else being bullied in their post, and 26.5% experienced undermining behaviour from a senior colleague. A 2015 survey of final stage students from two Australian medical schools (Scott et al 2015) concluded that:

> Practices associated with humiliating medical students persist in contemporary medical education. These practices need to be eradicated, given the evidence that they affect students' learning and mental health and are dissonant with formal professionalism curricula. Interventions are needed to interrupt the transgenerational legacy and culture in which teaching by humiliation is perpetuated.

A recent large scale survey of 3,000 surgical trainees' experiences in Australia and New Zealand by an Expert Advisory Group (2015) led to that group stating that it was "shocked by what it has heard" about the reported prevalence (49%) of discrimination, bullying and sexual harrassment in surgical training. The report called for "a profound shift in the culture of surgery". Most senior surgeons were found "not equipped to provide constructive feedback". This shocking report was summarised for the public in the *Sydney Morning Herald*. Female trainees faced remarks such as: "Why don't you just go and do the grocery shopping?", and "you can join us in theatre – not to do anything, just for eye candy". One was told "I would only be considered for a job if I had my tubes tied" (Medew 2015).

A significant grey literature of online articles and blogs reveals many similar accounts of ritual humiliation in both medical and surgical training worldwide – termed, ironically, by one "insider" commentator: "the strange way we learn" (Karthikesan 2015).

Finally, the wide-ranging literature on abuse in medical culture and education, from which we have drawn illustrative examples above, was crying out for a systematic review and meta-analysis. This was conducted by Fnais and colleagues in 2011 and first published in 2014 (Fnais et al 2015). The authors used "harrassment" and "discrimination" in medical training as their key words and so were in the overall territory of ritual humiliation. They defined these terms as "a wide range of behaviors that medical trainees perceive as being humiliating, hostile, or abusive".

Their aim was "To understand the significance of such mistreatment and to explore potential preventive strategies". From the literature of 57 cross-sectional and two cohort studies, the authors report that:

> 59.4% of medical trainees had experienced at least one form of harassment or discrimination during their training. ... Verbal harassment was the most commonly cited form of harassment ... . Consultants were the most commonly cited source of harassment and discrimination, followed by patients or patients' families (34.4% and 21.9%, respectively).

They note, in summary, "the surprisingly high prevalence of harassment and discrimination among medical trainees that has not declined over time", and "recommend both drafting policies and promoting cultural change within academic institutions to prevent future abuse".

Can Homer help?

We have argued throughout this book that patient-centred and team-based collaborative practices are central to an emerging medical landscape no longer shaped by metaphors of conflict, violence, and violation, but rather those of social co-operation, respect for difference, and hospitality. In order to better understand this transition in the metaphorical landscape of medicine, as this shapes the realities of clinical education and practice, we consider Homer's move from the extreme militarism of the *Iliad* to the pacific pastoralism of the *Odyssey* – from heroic glory to homecoming. The shaping metaphor of the *Odyssey* is the "journey" – commonly used to describe patients' illness experiences. Just as the shaping of medicine is shifting from the historical influence of the didactic metaphors of "medicine as war" and "the body as machine" to a pacific metaphor of collaboration, so Homer shifts the overall metaphorical tone from conflict to collaboration at the completion of the *Odyssey*.

Moreover, the central ethical theme of the *Odyssey* is the imperative of hospitality (*xenia*): the expectations of households to provide hospitality to strangers; the expectations that guests will not abuse that hospitality; and the consequences of punishment on both sides should the rules of hospitality be broken (Reece 1993). Hospitality is then conditional, grounded in a bigger notion of reciprocity and gift exchange ("there is no such thing as a free lunch" – the National Health Service may be "free" at the point of delivery but is funded through taxation).

As discussed elsewhere, having returned home from the Trojan War after ten years of travelling, to be reunited with his wife Penelope and son Telemachus, Odysseus brutally slaughters his wife's suitors, who have assumed his death, abused the hospitality of her house, and pressured her into choosing one of them as her new husband. This fight is as gruesome as any war scene in the *Iliad*. In the final Book, the gods call a truce: "Let them be friends with one another as before, and let wealth and peace be in the land" (*Odyssey* 24. 485-6) decrees Zeus; but the fighting continues until Athene, with Zeus' approval, intervenes: "Break off – shed no more blood – make peace at once!" (*Odyssey* 24. 531-2). Odysseus "obeyed her, glad at heart" (*Odyssey* 24. 545). How will we bring such a pact to medical education to make us all "glad at heart", and not cultivators of cynicism, conflict and humiliation?

Times have changed since *Boys in White*. Yet, despite enlightened medical education, the surgeon's caustic remark that opened this article offers a reminder that humiliating abuse still lingers as ill-formed pedagogic technique - and we have shown above that this view is not anecdotal, but evidence-based. So what might study of Homer offer to better understand abuse and shame in medical education that is not already in the literature? Joel Rosenthal (2012), the President for the Carnegie Council for Ethics in International Affairs, based in New York, gave a speech at the annual Maine Humanities Council Winter Weekend Seminar in March 2012 entitled "Ethics and War in Homer's *Iliad*". Rosenthal says:

> When I was in 9th grade, confronting the *Iliad* for the first time, I had two
> questions. First, why is it so important that we read the so-called classics?

And second what is a classic anyway? It is only now, all these years later,
that I can finally answer these questions. We read the classics because they
tell us something essential about human nature. A classic text endures
because it touches on an unchanging truth of human experience.

We would like to think that while belligerence may be central to human
history, it should not be an enduring aspect of medical pedagogy. Learning
and discipline are closely tied, but the discipline of learning should not be
mistaken for learning through punishment. Whatever the teacher's
justification, ritual shaming and humiliation of learners are surely
symptoms of the teacher's personality issues or a cultural pathology than
the learners lack? Yet, despite the best efforts of medical schools to
introduce liberal pedagogies into medical education, as we have seen ritual
humiliation still lingers in clinical teaching.

Abuse in Homer

After a truce is broken early in the *Iliad*, Agamemnon rallies his troops in
a typically aggressive manner:

> What is this, Diomedes, son of Tydeus, the godlike horseman? Why do
> you cower, only watching the ranks of battle? It was not like Tydeus to
> shrink back … . But the son he bore is a worse man in battle, though better
> in debate (*Iliad* 4. 370-400).

Agamemnon's shaming of Diomedes – the commander scolding a senior
soldier - could well be a consultant surgeon berating a junior for not
showing "grit" in a tight situation. "Grit" has become a desired character
trait for surgeons, defined as "passion and perseverance for long-term
goals", and we discuss it in depth in chapter thirteen. Homeric language
would perhaps have been more blunt about those with "below-median
values" of "grit" and the need for "screening for grit", where such talk
exposes how tired martial metaphors in medicine have become.

Those with "grit" may also be those who feel free to abuse (going well
beyond "banter") - and abuse is exchanged as easily between equals as
down through the hierarchy. During a chariot race, part of the funeral
games for Patroclus, Idomeneus calls out the name of the race leader to the
rest of the kings. Then: "Swift Ajax … reproved him rudely: 'Idomeneus,
why do you brag? … . You are not the youngest of the Argives, nor are
yours the sharpest eyes. Yet always you boast. You should not brag so
much. Other, better men are to hand'". Idomeneus replies: "Ajax, you are

the most argumentative of fools. And the most lacking of the Argives in good manners ..." (*Iliad* 23. 457-84).

The argument is poised to escalate, but Achilles jumps up and intervenes. Multidisciplinary team meetings can take on the same tone, with consultants from differing specialties shaping a hierarchy based on specialty stereotyping, where no such hierarchy formally exists:

> He's a big, bold, beer swilling rugby fan, and when it comes to clinical practice he prefers to cut and run, rather than communicate with patients. She's cute and fluffy, with a permanent smile and a small koala attached to her stethoscope. He's paternalistic, kindly, with a penchant for corduroy jackets and elbow patches. These stereotypes of the surgeon, paediatrician, and general practitioner (GP) are the stuff of professional banter, along with those for doctors in all the other specialties (Oxtoby 2013).

Abuse is not always between equals. Early in the *Iliad*, as described in the previous chapter nine, Thersites, a simple foot soldier, has baited Agamemnon with greed and incompetence. Odysseus then confronts him:

> Thersites, you babbling fool, you may be a smart barrack room lawyer, but stop this. Don't argue with kings ... . If I catch you again in this sort of stupidity, I'll get hold of you, strip you of your clothes, everything that hides your nakedness, and thrash you back to the ships to go and weep.

Odysseus then hits him over the back with his staff and reduces him to tears, to the approval of the rest of the company (*Iliad* 2. 246-64). Describing conflict in the healthcare workplace, Michael Ramsay (2001) says:

> Physicians, both male and female, often have hard-driving, type A personalities and little training in interpersonal skills. They may have high IQs but lack emotional intelligence. In the past, physicians were revered as charismatic people who could do no wrong; now they are seen as one part of the health care team. Temper outbursts—with throwing of instruments and loud profanity directed at any unfortunate person who happens to be near at hand—are no longer tolerated.

The result is that:

> Communication is poor, and staff withhold information because of fear of an outburst. The information withheld may be vital for patient well-being. The physician loses staff support and may become isolated.

Such doctors are not just driven by personality profile but, again, configured by medicine's primary didactic martial metaphor, characterising themselves as fighters. As the shaping of the landscape of medicine shifts from the didactic medicine as war/ the body as a machine metaphors, it may be formed in the future by pacific metaphors drawn from ecology and feminism, resulting in the establishment of authentic patient-centred practice and inter-professional teamwork. In this climate, medical abuse will not be tolerated.

"Honour-shame" and "Guilt" cultures

Returning to Joel Rosenthal's (2012) speech about the relevance of Homer for current times, referred to earlier, Rosenthal points out that the *Iliad* is much more than a "slugging story". Rather, "The poem invites us to reflect on … the use of force as it shapes our understanding of virtues such as honor and responsibility and vices such as excessive pride, vengeance and cruelty". Here, Rosenthal is invoking a Homeric "honour-shame culture" where values are based on family - or peer - approval.

As we introduced briefly in chapter nine on "error", during WWII the anthropologist Ruth Benedict (1946) compared American and Japanese cultures. She developed a summary model that explained differences in behaviour between Japanese prisoners of war and Americans. Puzzled, for example, by the fact that Japanese POWs did not want to let their relatives know that they were alive, Benedict suggested that these POWs were ashamed of revealing their condition.

An honour-shame culture works on external (family/ peer/ public) approval or disapproval as a code of honour. American culture, noted Benedict, worked on a different logic – that of guilt based on transgressing an internalised moral code. Benedict was never able to carry out fieldwork in Japan and her work has been criticised on this basis, but her model came to strongly influence the work of an Irish Oxford-educated classicist, Eric Robertson Dodds (1951).

Dodds suggested that the study of Homeric and later Greek culture had been systematically distorted through the dominance of a twin discourse – first, the assumption that the ancient Greeks prized rationality (the Apollonic) over the irrational (the Dionysian) (Friedrich Nietzsche (1872, 2013) had pointed this out long before Dodds); and second, that we can never fully understand the early Greek world as long as we study it through the lens of a dominant Christian values framework (also a cornerstone of Nietzsche's canon). The latter framework, borrowing from Benedict, he described as a "guilt culture", where the Homeric world was shaped by a "shame culture" - where honour as peer approval is the key element.

Honour-shame cultures maintain control through rewarding honour and ostracising through shame. The most humiliating condition is to lose the approval of respected others with the threat of exclusion. Self-respect in an honour culture is gained not by reference to a moral code but by honouring what is expected by significant others. In contrast, in a guilt culture, public approval or disapproval is secondary to recognition that one has upheld or transgressed an internalised moral code, resulting in feelings of pride or guilt. Dodds saw that the distinction between shame and guilt cultures is not clear-cut, where mixed economies will always occur.

Recognition and esteem for the doctor, in particular the surgeon, operate within the tight world of peers. Such a world echoes the Homeric age of heroes. As Dodds (1951, p.17) suggests: "Homeric man's highest good is not the enjoyment of a quiet conscience, but the enjoyment of *timē*, public esteem". Losing face amongst your colleagues is unbearable, exposing you to ridicule. As the subculture protects its own kind, whistleblowers are ostracised (see previous chapter ten). But this honour/shame-based culture sits in a guilt/conscience-based wider public culture as a bad apple, presenting a paradox.

Researching and writing at the same time as Ruth Benedict, the American sociologist David Riesman and colleagues (Riesman et al 1950) described "tradition-directed" behaviour as typical of highly stratified, conservative, hierarchical and patriarchal cultures. Those at the tip of the hierarchy habitually employ techniques of ritual humiliation to shame those lower on the hierarchy. In the North American society they described, the authors note that tradition-directed behaviour had long been replaced by "inner-directed" behaviour, where the admired person was an idiosyncratic individual who had made his or her own way through singular effort (self-help).

Both tradition-directed and inner-directed persons were concerned with power – exerting heroic power or bowing to the power of heroes in tradition-directed culture, or exerting entrepreneurial power and self-control in self-directed culture. Riesman and colleagues pointed to a new, emergent, social model, that of "other-directedness". This person is not interested in power, but in relationships, looking for collaboration and social cohesion, and emotional satisfaction rather than esteem. This is the dominant social process in post-WWII liberal societies.

Contemporary medical students live in Riesman's other-directed world and Benedict's guilt culture. Yet the medical and surgical worlds into which they are being socialised have, historically, been tradition-directed, honour-shame cultures. The medical student lets him or herself down through transgression: "I didn't bother to revise for the exam"; "I didn't read up on the patient's condition", and feels consequent guilt. The reference point is not public shame and humiliation but private censure. On the wards or in the operating theatre, however, the same student is pimped and ritually humiliated – typical tactics within an honour-shame, tradition-directed climate.

The emotional response of the abused student or junior doctor may then be a mixture of shame and guilt. The process of ritual humiliation set in a tradition-directed/ honour culture framework predicts shame as a response. However, the student or junior doctor, undergoing identity construction through socialisation or enculturation, may feel guilt, as he or she is also embedded in an other-directed/ guilt culture that is the life outside of clinical medicine, such as classroom-based medical education based on contemporary pedagogical values as explained above. Lindstrom and colleagues (Lindstrom et al 2011) note that the circumstances for feeling shame can be similar for students as for patients – feeling a real or metaphoric nakedness; subordination to a greater power; and being taken by surprise.

Aidos

As discussed earlier, in chapter nine on "error", *aidos* is the ancient Greek equivalent of "shame", but has shifting meanings in the ancient world. Dodds (1951) describes *aidos* as "respect for public opinion" within an honour-shame culture. Douglas Cairns (1993) has systematically examined the meanings of *aidos* within the network of Homeric values, such as its relationship to honour (*timē*) and distinction from guilt; Cairns notes that *aidos* is rarely used as a noun - in the sense of an emotion we feel - but more usually of the effect of "bringing shame on". This fits with the honour-shame model of external approval or censure, rather than the guilt model of transgression of an internalised morality leading to a heightened emotional state.

The verb derived from *aidos, aideomai*, has two meanings: the first of feeling shame before someone, and the second of feeling respect (Cairns 1993, pp.2-3). The verb is used in the scene from the *Iliad* described earlier, where Agamemnon is urging his troops into battle and insults Diomedes (whose valour should be beyond question). We, the readers, might expect Diomedes to reply angrily, but he says nothing: "*aidestheis basileos enipeen aidoioio* - having respect for (or feeling shame before, or both) the rebuke of his respected king" (*Iliad* 4. 402).

There are, in fact, two words derived from *aidos* in this sentence – *aidestheis* and *aidoioio*, and both point to other shades of meaning of *aidos*, as respect or reverence, rather than shame. This shifts the moral right towards the person higher on the hierarchy, however distasteful the shaming.

This scene has resonances with the medical world: the abused is of lower status than the abuser; and the abuse is often unjustified or entirely disproportionate, yet the rebuke is meekly accepted. The hierarchy is crystallised where the scene goes on to have Sthenelus argue with Agamemnon only to be rebuked by Diomedes, because Agamemnon will take all the blame if the expedition to Troy fails: "great will be his misfortune if the Greeks are slaughtered" (*Iliad* 4. 415-7). This too is commonly heard in the medical context. The same excuse - that consultants take all the responsibility under great pressure in life and death situations - is an almost hackneyed justification for their bad behaviour.

It is also a commonplace for the subordinate to criticise the harshness of feedback and in the next breath to say that, in some sense, it has done them good, kept them on their toes. Watling and colleagues (Watling et al 2012), in a paper on understanding responses to feedback, also report such incidents (and their comment at the end suggests the supervisor's behaviour is acceptable, placing it squarely within the heroic tradition of "what doesn't break you makes you stronger"):

> One participant, recalling the challenging experience of working with a surgeon who routinely offered blunt criticism, admitted: "Sometimes their feedback, even though it was really harsh and cruel, did improve my technical skills". The unmistakable influence of this largely negative feedback on technical skill development suggests that negative feedback in a prevention-focused setting can be practice-shaping, even if the experience of receiving the feedback is unpleasant.

The great quarrel between Agamemnon and Achilles at the beginning of the *Iliad* relates how Agamemnon threatens to dishonour and shame Achilles by taking Briseis, Achilles' prize of war, from him. This loss of honour and public esteem (*timē*) is relevant to the medical context, especially if we see honour as analogous to status. As we have seen, "humiliation" is a word that occurs often in medical contexts. It is not just medical students and juniors who are readily shamed, but status and hierarchy so infuse medicine that a consultant from one specialty can readily shame another from a different specialty – surgeons to other doctors, consultants to senior GPs. *Timē* pervades medical culture and its loss produces a feeling of *aidos* or shame.

Cairns' treatment of *aidos* in Homer constantly resonates with the study of abuse in medicine. He discusses the subtleties of meaning in Greek and English – how shame differs from embarrassment, for example. He also deals with the difference between shame and guilt, and the extent to which the former requires an audience, while the latter needs only ourselves and introjection of morals as conscience. This echoes our discussion above concerning the differences between honour-shame/ tradition-directed and guilt/ other-directed cultures. Cairns discusses how a culture of shame requires a culture of honour; how feelings of shame and even guilt can lie outside rational analysis – we may feel both, knowing that we are not at fault; and how individuals feel shame to different degrees, leading some to underestimate the effect they have and others to feel it with undesirable strength.

Shame too has an aesthetic component – the episode that produces shame disfiguring both the abused and the abuser, resulting in ugliness in relationship. Where other-directed cultures seek to shape quality relationships, in comparison tradition-directed cultures can be seen to fall back on blunt and dull exchanges. Recall that David Riesman's (1950) other-directedness moves into a territory of mutuality that also sees beauty in care – quite different from the ugliness and brutality produced by naked humiliation of another. While the Homeric hero most keenly feels *aidos* (shame) in the presence of superiors, peers and family, this can extend to guests, strangers, beggars and supplicants. The medical equivalent is that while doctors' and surgeons' honour and shame dynamics are keenest amongst peers, such dynamics can extend to the multidisciplinary clinical team. The dynamics of guilt culture, however, also embrace the patient.

The medical abuse we have catalogued here from a variety of studies is not only heartless, or lacking compassion, but also artless – lacking style and subtlety. There is a big difference between blunt bullying and hurtful sarcasm at the expense of someone else's feeling and sharp satire, parody or lampooning - ridiculing what is ridiculous in the other. While the recipient may feel the barb, the satirist - as cartoonist, comedian or commentator - sets out to lampoon for a good reason. This may be because the target is pompous or inflated. Such shaming is then aesthetically pleasing to an audience. We might then ask, first, is the surgeon's or doctor's ritual humiliation of the medical student justified as satire? If so, then it is not abuse. Such scenarios are unlikely and point to the unreflexive bluntness or an-aesthetic nature of medical abuse where sarcasm trumps satire.

Conclusions and solutions

In the ancient context, the question whether the Trojan War could have been brought to a speedier conclusion if Agamemnon and Achilles had attended an anger management course is not productive. In the modern context, we feel that it is of the greatest importance. Having made the diagnosis that types of abuse still exist in medical culture and medical education but are often overlooked, we must now treat the symptoms. We recognise that Baldwin and colleagues' (Baldwin et al 1991) research on medical student abuse in North America had already reached an innovative conclusion over two decades ago in making an analogy with transgenerational child abuse:

> It would be difficult to see a "kinder and gentler" physician emerging from an environment in which students perceive themselves as having been mistreated or humiliated to the extent revealed in this survey. Of more serious note is the possibility that such attitudes and behaviours may be visited on younger students or even patients. If child abuse is an appropriate analogue, there may be a "transgenerational legacy" that leads to future mistreatment of others on the part of those who have been mistreated as students.

The implication in Baldwin and colleagues' conclusion is that hardened and cynical doctors and surgeons, also serial abusers, may need counselling or psychotherapy before they turn to palliative substance abuse (Coombs 1997). Well, such services have been widely available for over two decades for doctors (such as the British Medical Association's *Doctors in difficulty* and *Doctors' well-being* - http://www.bma.org.uk/support-at-work/doctors-well-being/websites-for-doctors-in-difficulty), but of course are resisted and scoffed at by those who may need them most. One often hears a justification for abuse in medicine that it is a tough profession to work in so students need to be toughened up. But this, a psychoanalyst would say, is an ego defence mechanism of rationalisation at work. Again, how can we make light of the recent report of widespread abuse in Australasian surgical training, noted earlier (Expert Advisory Group 2015) that calls for "a profound shift in the culture of surgery" in successfully addressing and preventing discrimination, sexual harassment and bullying. Again, the advisory group was "shocked by what it has heard", where "The time for action has come".

The RACS report juxtaposes comments of the abused with those of the rationalisers, elegantly demonstrating the problem of disjunction between an other-directed/ guilt culture and a tradition-directed/ honour-shame culture:

> The abused: "what really disturbed me was seeing the effect bullying had on colleagues, some who have quit, and feeling I couldn't do anything to help because my own career would end if I spoke out".

> The rationaliser: "Surgery is a stressful specialty. If you can't deal with the stress, and that includes bullying, you should choose a different profession".

The latter attempt at justification above is perhaps preferable to the hypocrisy of denying that such abuse occurs.

Abusive behaviour, such as ritual humiliation, is all the more extraordinary where it occurs in a supposedly caring profession. Perpetrators of abuse and sceptics towards its effects too will scoff at the use of the word "abuse" for what they might see as "creating backbone". Dictionary definitions of "abuse" cover enough ground to encompass our examples easily – "to take a bad advantage of", "to maltreat, injure, wrong or hurt", "to violate, defile, to wrong with words. To speak injuriously of or to" (*Shorter OED* 1971).

What then of solutions? We suggest two levels: the first is cultural, the second, pedagogical. The cultural solution has already been outlined and is certainly already in motion as an historical change. Nietzsche, and later Michel Foucault, described the historical conditions of possibility for the emergence of any major social phenomenon and gave illustrative examples. Foucault famously traces the histories of the emergence of madness, prisons, sexuality and self-care in the Western world. These do not have single, but multiple and complex, origins that cannot be predicted in advance but only accounted for retrospectively.

We suggest here that modern medicine has been shaped primarily since the 17th century by two didactic metaphors and discourses: conflict (medicine as war) and engineering (the body as machine), that naturally harmonise as an "industrial-military" complex. This twin metaphor has shaped a particular and familiar landscape of medical practice and medical education. However, we suggest that this landscape is being re-shaped through the didactic metaphor of collaboration (teamwork) within an ecological feminism (patient-centred holistic medicine) (Bleakley 2017). In Homer, we find that the theme of hospitality, especially in the *Odyssey* offers an alternative set of metaphors to those of war and engineering. The "hospital" should not simply be nominal, but exercise hospitality.

Our second - pedagogical - solution notes that the problem of abuse embedded in medicine has been recognised for at least 30 years. Pendleton and colleagues (Pendleton et al 1984) offered a corrective in possibly the single most influential book in communication in medicine, certainly for the culture of UK General Practice. The authors laid down guidelines – that later became known as "Pendleton's rules" - of how to give positive and supportive feedback rather than negative criticism. In brief, the guidelines are: to clarify matters of fact; to encourage the learner to speak first; to consider what has been done well first before what could be done differently; and to make recommendations rather than state weaknesses. Positive and constructive feedback can still be challenging, but should never be wilfully destructive. The authors offered a corrective to the ingrained habits of teaching through humiliation.

The approach was, however, strongly criticised. Kurtz and colleagues (1998) felt that "what could be done differently" was seen as a thin disguise for "what was done poorly". The learner may perceive the initial positive feedback as patronising or insincere, and be bracing herself for the hit she thinks is sure to come. Textbooks describe this as "sugar coating" – anecdotally, our medical students, less given to sugar coating, describe it as a "shit sandwich". Their "Kurtz" approach is to start with the learner's agenda, encourage self-assessment and collaborative problem solving, and use descriptive feedback to encourage a non-judgemental approach.

Claridge and Lewis (2005) criticise the language of feedback such as "trial and error" and "learning from our mistakes". Instead, they suggest we ask questions like: "what is the learning in this?"; "what is the gift here?"; and "by asking these questions, the coach acknowledges our humanness and our resourcefulness". Their emphasis is on not making general criticisms such as "you talk too much", but on dealing with specific examples, focusing on changing behaviour. Note that the authors' pedagogical inclination is towards management and leadership talk, all too common now in medical education.

We began with a poem by a medical student, let us finish with a BMA "Connecting Doctors" blog by a surgical trainee (https://www.bma.org.uk/connecting-doctors/b/work/posts/is-it-ever-right-to-tell-off-trainees-in-public) (Curtis 2014):

> "I want you to come with me," he said as he led me down the corridor to the crime scene. "I need to show you something." And then he added the ominous line: "for your education."
>
> I stood in silence as the prosecution listed my transgressions in front of the patient. The jury, composed of four medical students and two nurses, all anonymous and disguised behind theatre masks, were also silent. You

could have heard a suture needle drop. I said nothing as I walked slowly out of theatre and back to my room. But really, I was thinking: "If you're going to tell off your registrar, why do it in front of a room full of medical students, the medical students who I have to teach, who have to sit in clinic with me later today, who have to listen to what I have to say and hopefully believe what I am telling them?

"Why tell me off in front of the patient who may have to see me in clinic a few months down the line, who now must have no confidence in my opinion?"

"Go back and speak to him about it," urged the nurses, siding with the defence. "He shouldn't undermine you like that in front of the students"

A part of me wants to and I nearly go back to confront him, to ask him not to humiliate me again like that, but I don't and I fear that I have missed my chance completely.

We will leave you, the reader, to look at the many comments on this blog – all but one are supportive of the humiliated trainee. The dissenting voice echoes back to Homeric times and honour-shame culture, in which one is socialised into a potentially dysfunctional insular group that provides the source of esteem, ignoring transparency, turning its back on critics and scapegoating whistleblowers. In response to the surgical trainee's heartfelt complaints, the lone dissenting voice on the blog is from a "weary consultant" (from 4th March 2014):

Don't you think we might be going a bit over the top here? I was a houseman during the Lancelott Spratt era and it wasn't comfortable, I accept, but I don't think a telling off in public did us any harm. It happened to us all and it bred a certain camaraderie.

We rest our case.

CHAPTER TWELVE

BONE TIRED

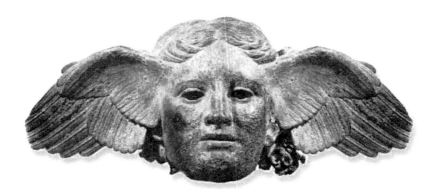

Figure 12-1: Hypnos, god of sleep

Bone tired and ready for sleep

Having spent a decade at war with the Trojans and a further decade getting home to Ithaca from Troy, Odysseus is at breaking point, storm-tossed and ragged from a series of strange and often ugly encounters. Every other action he and his crew take seems to incur the wrath of the gods, or the incumbents of the isles on which he lands. As Odysseus and his bedraggled crew ease their ship into the harbour of the isle where Circe - "the nymph with lovely braids" – resides, they must rest out of pure exhaustion: "then, disembarking, there we lay for two days and two nights, eating our hearts out, bone tired and grieving together" (*Odyssey* 10.142-3).

The ancient Greeks would have described what we call "bone tired" as a sapping of *thumos* – courage, fighting spirit, the love of competition, the desire to be the best, to show both "guts" and "heart". Bone tired kicks in when the tank of heroism runs dry. As one of Samuel Beckett's (1953) characters in *The Unnamable* says, gnomically: "You must go on. I can't go on, I'll go on".

Three times around the walls of Troy, Achilles manages to gain on Hector with a little help first from Apollo and then Athene, who spurs on the finest of the Greek warriors: "But you stand there now, and get your breath; I will go to him and persuade him to stand against you and fight" (*Iliad* 22. 222-3). The goddess then tricks Hector by appearing beside him disguised as his brother Deiphobus, persuading Hector that the two of them should stand and fight Achilles, giving Hector some hope. Achilles launches a spear at Hector but misses. Athene recovers the spear and hands it back to Hector, who decides to swoop on Achilles with sword in hand, assuming he was being aided by Deiphobus. But as he turns to look at his brother, Athene suddenly disappears, and Hector realises that he has been duped and is alone in combat with the most terrifying of warriors bent on revenge.

Despite his exhaustion, and with a last flush of adrenaline – or *thumos* - pushing around his system, Achilles charges with another bronze-tipped ash spear and thrusts it into Hector's neck, just missing the windpipe so that Hector can still speak as he dies. Homer likens the pursuit first to a hawk stalking a terrified dove and then to a dog chasing a deer's fawn. Hector's dying words to Achilles mirror back to him his lack of humanity or pity: "in your breast is a heart of iron". When *thumos* boils over the victor may show no mercy and the victim capitulates, exhausted.

Socrates warned that where unbridled and untutored *thumos* is potentially destructive, *thumos* can also be channelled into productive activity through education. Competitive games offer a culturally honed outlet for *thumos*, but Socrates suggested that philosophy too could channel such energy and be framed as competition, such as seeking the best at argument and rhetoric. The Socratic method was developed as a kind of intellectual wrestling, where you systematically expose the flaws in an opponent's argument and use the weight and tangle of the opponent's clumsy rhetoric as a means of bringing that opponent down.

Plato's *Republic* deals with the conundrum of how an educated elite of thinkers might keep a much larger population of less educated and *thumos*-heavy military under their control, lest their *thumos* explode and the soldiers turn on their superiors. Medical students are forever being reminded that they are the brightest of entrants to University at the same time as they are told that they are bottom of the medical hierarchy in a hugely competitive environment where they must cut the mustard to progress. This includes behaving impeccably, as "proto-professionals". Medical education offers a particularly gruelling education of *thumos* management.

Part of the mythology that used to be generated at medical school is that doctors, like great warriors, are not supposed to get bone tired. Long shifts, including working at night with no sleep, constitute a badge of honour. Doctors' *thumos* - courage and determination - must be inexhaustible. They must, too, develop professional hearts of iron to protect themselves from emotional entanglement with their patients' conditions. They must work through adversity including exposure to death, pain and suffering. Yet, as a raft of studies shows us, the most junior doctors in particular are overworked and suffer from stress (Peterkin and Bleakley 2017).

Around a quarter of doctors will report excessive stress and nearly a half of all healthcare workers, including doctors, report that they feel stressed at work most or all of the time (Johnson 2016), where over 70% of this group surveyed reported that stress at work had also caused them to lose sleep. Doctors are not the only ones who interpret getting by on little sleep as an heroic gesture. Margaret Thatcher famously claimed that she got by on four hours a night, and Donald Trump claims that he only needs three – 1 am to 4 am (Huffington 2016).

Thumos is not an inexhaustible reservoir and must be re-charged. Even the toughest warriors get tired and vulnerable. In the *Iliad,* Diomedes (otherwise referred to by Homer as "as tough as they come") is scolded by the goddess Athene for apparently slacking off in the fight against the Trojans:

> She found the king by his horses and chariot
> Cooling the wound, which Pandarus had inflicted with an arrow.
> For the sweat troubled him beneath the broad strap
> of his round shield. Troubled by this and weary of limb,
> He was lifting the strap and wiping away the dark blood (*Iliad* 5. 794-8).

Whereupon Athene scolded him, reminding Diomedes that although his father was slight, he was a "fighter" who never gave up:

> But you, I stand by you and protect you,
> I urge you with my favour to fight the Trojans,
> But either you are bone tired from the fight
> Or some god has robbed you of spirit (*Iliad*. 5. 809-12).

Athene fires up Diomedes in spite of his exhaustion, spurring him on to challenge the war god Ares himself, who Athene sees as a turncoat for supporting the Trojans. Diomedes spears Ares in the side causing the god of war to yell and disappear to the clouds covering Olympus like a tornado – "a darker clot of air". Ares is wounded and winded, while Diomedes gets a second wind – something that can happen deep within the fabric of exhaustion but which is dangerous, because the after-effect is so debilitating. Too many second winds offer the royal road to burnout. Too much adrenaline pumping, as athletes will tell you, can pitch you beyond extra exertion into total collapse.

A meteorological equivalent to the disappearance of Ares to the sky as a "darker clot of air", a tornado, is an annual wind of the Aegean described by the ancients as *Meltemi*. Sometimes reaching 30 knots, the wind is exhausting to sail in and can last for a week to two weeks at a time during the end of June to the beginning of September. Odysseus and his crew get caught in such a wind after the Thracian raid causing them bone tiredness:

> Zeus, cloudgatherer, sent the North Wind rushing on our ships
> in a raging storm, and covered land and sea
> alike in cloud. Night rushed down from the heavens.
> The ships were borne headlong, and their sails
> Were torn to shreds and tatters by the force of the wind.
> We lowered them to deck, fearing for our lives,
> And rowed as hard as we could for land.
> Then we lay for two days and two nights together
> Eating our hearts out with exhaustion and grief together (*Odyssey* 9. 67-75).

Translators of Homer such as Fagles and Lombardo use "bone tired" for exhaustion, as does Mitchell (2011) to describe exhausted horses in battle. The use of "bone tired" may be over-stretching the Greek *kameteen*, referring to "labouring". But we recognise from medical work this end-of-rope exhaustion for both doctors and patients, especially as the workplace is characteristically thought of as a battlefield and illness as a journey.

It is not just heroes whose *thumos* is exercised, but women, of course, get exhausted too and there are examples of that in Homer – particularly Penelope's nightly undoing of her daily weaving that would give her claim to a sleep pattern matching that of Margaret Thatcher.

Further, women can rightfully claim that the most exhausting aspects of life are pregnancy, giving birth and mothering children; and women doctors who choose to have families have, historically, had to bear this exhaustion while coping with a medical work system that demands their full-time attention, especially in surgery. This situation, thankfully, is changing, but slowly. It is not that governing bodies are slow to issue detailed guidelines for women doctors who choose to have children and then take necessary time out from work. Rather, it is lingering attitudes within an older generation of doctors and surgeons from a once wholly male-dominated profession that serve to frustrate women's ambitions.

Our point here is that exhaustion in Homer is bound up with the archetypally masculine, macho, heroic posture of "pushing through", whatever the cost. This is the badge of honour in warfare, high level and extreme sports and, historically, in medical and, in particular, surgical work.

The ancient Greeks described two dominant bodily experiences: those of *thumos* and *cholos*. Cantor and Hufnagel (2012, p.52) describe *thumos* as:

> competitiveness, the compulsion to be first in everything, aggressiveness in battle, a quick temper, sensitivity in matters of honor, a capacity for raw indignation – all linked to the basic emotion of raw anger.

Courage and senseless violence are the two faces of *thumos,* as we have seen. Like the ancient Greeks, we socially channel *thumos* into competitive sports and we educate *thumos,* following Socrates, through turning academic study into a competition replete with posturing and technical apparatus: cumbersome assessment, grades, rankings and league tables. Learning becomes combat, where a raft of metaphors distinguishes between winners and losers: distinction versus fail, Ivy League/ Oxbridge versus Red Brick Universities, high achievers versus underachievers, excellence versus mere competence. This is familiar territory for medical students, socialised into being the best. The ancient Greeks also describe *thumos* as a substance that fills the organ *phrenes* (associated with the mind, hence "phrenology", but also the lungs). Besides courage, *thumos* is then "inspiration" - also gaining a "second wind" (just what you need, too, when sailing in a *meltemi*).

Thumos, as we have seen, is usually described in Homer as the seat of rage. The prime example of this in the *Iliad* is again the killing spree that consumes Achilles as he seeks revenge for the death of Patroclus; and in the *Odyssey,* the killing spree that Odysseus embarks upon with his son Telemachus on his return to Ithaca as he mows down Penelope's suitors in an animalistic revenge.

Cholos describes quick anger, in contrast to *menis* that is the brooding rage of Achilles, a sullen anger, where *cholos* is "swallowed" and dissipated in time or digested. *Cholos* is the root of choleric – the humour that underpins a quick temper. A third kind of anger is *kotos*, one that initiates revenge, and that we now know as rancour. Thomas Walsh (2005), in a study of "anger and the Homeric poems", suggests that *kotos* is the specific kind of feuding anger that permeates the *Iliad*. The *Iliad* is, however, a song about a spectrum of wrath – opening with a sharp rage that becomes an embittered sulk and draws to it rancour. Achilles, it seems, covers the range of angers.

Thumos typically enhances activity up to a point and then over-excitation causes activity to disintegrate – this is the "inverted U" of the Yerkes-Dodson law:

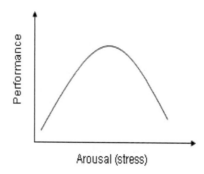

In his pursuit of Hector, Achilles' "powerful frame was bone-weary from charging Hector/ straight and hard to the walls of windswept Troy" (*Iliad* 23. 74-75, trans. Fagles 1990). In the previous line, a reference is made to Achilles' *thumos* in the context of him being exhausted not only from his dogged pursuit of Hector, but in then preparing a funeral pyre for his beloved Patroclus, where "sleep caught him ... as mists of refreshing slumber poured around him" (*ibid.*, 72-3). Later, after mourning for Patroclus, again Achilles "sank down, exhausted. Sweet sleep overwhelmed him" (*ibid.*, 266).

There is nothing we wish for more than to sink into that sweet sleep in the midst of a demanding, even overwhelming, period of over-work leading to exhaustion. Once *thumos* is exhausted, there is calm after the storm. When a disguised King Priam seeks out Achilles in the Greek camp to plead with him to return the body of his son Hector for a proper funeral rite, Achilles is reasonable with him because his *thumos* is temporarily exhausted. But Achilles warns Priam not to push him too far, in case his anger is sparked and he might then slay him on the spot.

In light of this background, it seems that medicine has followed the Homeric heroic template where work is structured to be exhausting - as a badge of honour and mark of courage. It is clear that organisational issues including chronic under-staffing promise exhaustion for many and burnout for some; but medicine's historical legacy is to shoot itself in the foot, or try to drive the car at full speed with the brakes engaged. We can admire this work ethic but also see its contradictions.

What we stereotype as the poor bedside manner of surgeons can be seen as the legacy of a dominant *thumos* – struggling to be the best, craving competition - often sublimated as the brooding rage that is *cholos*, easily giving way to a quick temper that may involve revenge (*kotos* or rancour). This complex hot temperament comes at a cost, including making mistakes of judgement through lack of impulse control, and creating cumulative stress. The oath "First, do no harm" should be extended to "First, do no self-harm". Hot, angry and spiteful outbursts in the midst of burnout can lead in time to sediments of cold ashes as self-recrimination.

In the next section, we will argue that overwork and sleep deprivation can no longer serve as badges of honour in medicine and should not be tolerated. We must make greater efforts to educate *thumos* both personally and across medical culture, so that energy is burned brightly but does not burn out, again to leave the cold ashes of despair. In parallel, structurally, health organisations such as the UK National Health Service (NHS) must find ways to support workforces without creating conditions for excessive stress and potential burnout, and without compromising patient safety through overwork. Importantly, we see this not only as an instrumental, ethical and political issue, but also as an issue of aesthetics. *Thumos*, as Socrates suggested, must be educated wilfully yet with subtlety and style.

Durational misperformance

" … it is not possible for people to be sleepless forever". Homer, *Odyssey* 19. 591-2.

"There is a time for many words, and there is also a time for sleep". Homer, *Odyssey* 11. 379.

Performances of the epics the *Iliad* and the *Odyssey*, as song cycles, were also epic - what in art circles is termed a "durational performance", where time is the frame and stamina is usually the quality required of the performer(s), originally *rhapsodes* or actor-singers, who played all the parts of the characters as they recited the epic as song.

Talking with a doctor normally sympathetic to the arts, AB discussed Marina Abramović's June to August 2014 durational performance "512 hours" at the Serpentine Gallery, London - 10 am to 6 pm six days a week over two months (Serpentine Gallery 2014). The doctor laughed:

> Eight hours a day in a confined space mixing with a group of unknown
> people and dealing with the unexpected – that's meat and potatoes to me.
> Marina Abramović should try a weekend shift on a busy emergency ward
> without sleep!

I got his point, but he missed the aesthetic purpose of durational
performance art - to bring the dark imaginary, the world of the ancient
Greek gods Hypnos (Sleep), Thanatos (Death) and Lethe (Forgetfulness)
into waking consciousness (Hillman 1979). This re-membering of the
underworld of sleep as a daytime dance with images goes with the grain of
the world of Hypnos as an honouring of sleep and its visions in waking
consciousness. Any imaginative act surely does this as it de-literalises the
everyday, inviting the world of sleep into the world of wakefulness as a
celebration.

Medicine, in contrast, does the opposite to art's celebration of Hypnos.
Traditionally heroic, medicine sets out rather to slay Hypnos - to keep
sleep at bay in the service of bright diagnostic and curative work under the
intense glare of the medical gaze, revelatory imaging technologies, harsh
hospital lighting and the operating theatre's spotlights.

This manic work of illumination - where Hypnos is enemy rather than
the bringer of gifts - goes against the naturally depressive grain of sleep
and its dark world, as doctors work caffeine-fuelled shifts. Such long
shifts, in contrast with Abramović's art, can be seen to offer durational
misperformance, frantically waving away the symptoms of sleep
deprivation as an irrational irritation and then inviting the cold ashes of
burn-out rather than the nightworld's texture and natural embrace of burnt
umber and charcoal.

What is it then to cherish - indeed, heroically nourish - the absence of
sleep? In Homer, while heroes pushed themselves to the point of utter
exhaustion, as we have seen, and sleep is seen as a sweet relief, there are
many warnings too about sleeping being dangerous, for that is when the
enemy can sneak up on you and take you by surprise. Doctors too may feel
that sleep is an abrogation of responsibility or a slippage of the mask of
professional control. They must be on watch as the enemy of disease can
attack their patients at any time of night or day.

There is a vast literature on the presence of sleep - its meanings, dream
content, cycles and phases (Wiseman 2014); and there is a growing
literature on the dangers of sleep deprivation among doctors and surgeons,
where patients' lives can be put at risk (Sanghavi 2011). However, as one
might expect, there is nothing on the heroic cultivation of wakefulness (or
intentional sleep deprivation) that mimics durational and endurance
performance art but strips it of its aesthetic and meaning - a misperformance.

Why do doctors still prize working long hours - to include sleep deprivation - in the face of the clear evidence that this leads to more risk with associated medical error, and to personal longer-term ill health? (Again, we stress that this cultural choice is different from the unacceptable timetabling of excessive work hours due to shortage of staff and resources – an organisational scandal).

Medicine serves Apollo and his son Asclepius the healer, dwelling in that harsh, persistent lighting of the hospital and the white light of the operating theatre where sleep is assigned to the bed bound or anaesthetised patient, thus making a clear division between the carers and the cared for.

In hospital medicine, the UK employs more anaesthetists - nearly 12,000 - than any other specialty: almost twice as many doctors as paediatricians, psychiatrists, or radiologists (http://www.gmc-uk.org/doctors/register/search_stats.asp). It is in the anaesthetist's caves - the anaesthetic room and the recovery room - that Hypnos lurks in the hospital, working against the grain of Apollo's presence as the patient is administered the temporary gift of painless sleep.

Despite major legislation on the recommended number of hours for professional work - such as the European Working Time Directive (EWTD) - working long hours involving significant sleep deprivation is still common practice for junior doctors. Further, and this was part of their argument with terms and conditions about to be imposed by the UK Tory Government when English junior doctors went on strike in 2016, basic pay is relatively so poor for early career doctors with large University fees loans to repay, that they must supplement this through overtime work paid at higher rates for unsociable hours – weekends and night shifts.

An argument is made by the profession that doctors, especially surgeons, will not achieve the requisite number of hours of training in technical skills and understanding if a directive such as the EWTD framework is followed. However, medical educationalists, sociologists and anthropologists point out that a significant proportion of that training time is not spent gaining the magical "10,000 hours" of practice to become an expert (Gladwell 2008), but is devoted rather to informal socialisation into subcultures of medicine and surgery by simply "hanging out" with the crew, maintaining high visibility or presence, regardless of your usefulness.

Because of the strength of resistance from within medicine itself to restricting hours at work in the face of the above rationalisations by those who study medical socialisation, there must be other reasons why doctors support the outwardly irrational practice of working long hours that include significant sleep deprivation. Sleep deprivation is indeed a key element in the socialisation of doctors and a vital element in identity production. But studies of socialisation of doctors fall short of explaining the paradox of choosing to work at risk under conditions of sleep deprivation when the invitation is now there to legitimately walk away, protected by employment law. Where sleep deprivation is historically a badge of honour in terms of legitimate entry into a community of practice - medicine or surgery - it serves a wider purpose.

From our argument above, we can see sleep deprivation - or wakefulness in the face of the call for sleep - as a durational misperformance that casts the doctor as rational and in control of the instinctual impulse to rest and dream. The doctor is heroic dragonslayer in the service of bright Asclepius, the patron of medicine, son of Apollo. Indeed, the doctor has pledged an oath to the Apollonic way and is duty bound. It is for patients to rest and dream, bruised black and blue and then yellowing in recovery from symptom, and for doctors - from surgeons through to psychiatrists - to treat the slumbering patient. These performances are virtually enacted, doubled or simulated through the genre of medical soap operas where the exhausted but willing junior doctor is a typical and celebrated figure.

However, again unlike performance art that explicitly brings a sleepworld perspective, a hypnotic trance, a suspended state into a dayworld enactment as a celebration of the imaginary and the extraordinary, sleep-deprived medical durational misperformance is rigidly instrumental and unconscious of its aesthetic potential. Indeed, these misperformances go out of their way to literalise life through medicalisation - stripping both birth and death of their trajectories, intimacies and family celebrations or mournings, passing ownership to the hospital and the clinical routine. Here, births are induced and deaths unnecessarily extended and technologised according to literal dayworld work schedules and not the natural nightworld rhythms of sleep and dream that denature the dayworld. For example, the dying patient - in prolonged terminal illness or coma - may be literally kept in the dark in paradoxical suspension in medicine's Apollonic bubble without any of the benefits of the rinse of sunlight (Gawande 2014).

The medicalisation of wakefulness has now been promoted by what is being hailed as a "wonder drug". Modafinil (street name "Daffy") is now being taken by one in five students to allow for long periods of wakefulness and concentration (Whitehouse 2016). A randomised controlled trial (RTC) on junior doctors working long hours showed conclusively that Modafinil provides chemically induced wakefulness that far outstripped the placebo effect (Harvey 2011). Modafinil is described as a "wakefulness promoting agent" - basically a stimulant - that does not appear to have side effects other than "snappiness" when concentration is interrupted (patients may recognise this as typical of some doctors in any case) and as a laxative. "Snappiness" brings to mind *cholos*, quick anger, a resting but irritable snake that is quick to strike. The side effect of Daffy as a laxative is an interesting, dark, bodily-based reply from the voice of repressed Hypnos. Shit and the underworld are old pals.

However, nobody knows what the longer-term, intensive use of the drug may lead to. The RCT concluded that: "fatigued doctors might benefit from pharmacological enhancement in situations that require efficient information processing, flexible thinking, and decision making under time pressure". Modafinil - sanitised wonderfully as "pharmacological enhancement" - then serves the heroic impulse to slay night itself and its demon of sleep, core to the dominant historical discourse of masculinised medicine.

This strenuous warding off of Sleep (Hypnos) and its associates Death (Thanatos) and Forgetfulness (Lethe) is then bought at a price. Again, the repression of sleep returns in a distorted form. Not just subsequent chronic symptoms for the doctor, but the return of repressed sleep shows in the very fabric of medicine and its organisational culture. The hospital itself - despite all efforts to bring the arts into its interior - can be seen to often deliver the wrong kind of sleep through its architecture, offering a numbing or an-aesthetic environment rather than an aesthetic experience: low ceilings, harsh lighting, over-heating, over-crowding, the smells of disinfectant and cleaning products; and - again - often over-worked, highly pressured and sleep-deprived staff. When doctors repress sleep, they do not simply hold Hypnos at bay (or rather transfer sleep to patients as a controlling gesture). In *Theogony*, Hesiod describes the brood of Night, among them Old Age, Strife, Lamentation and Doom. These forces must be kept at bay too, or medicalised.

Was the doctor right to mock Marina Abramović's project? Well, it certainly raised a point of discussion between us as to how we can best understand the work of doctors and clinical teams. At one level, their work must be understood as durational performance, especially during sleep deprivation. The work is both tightly scripted and well-rehearsed and improvised, requiring high tolerance of ambiguity or uncertainty. Yet doctors frame their work in instrumental terms and tend to deny, suspend or repress the aesthetic and performative elements. The durational performance then becomes, again, a misperformance as a militaristic and intelligence exercise, or a siege.

This martial front tends to displace the framing of work as beautiful, graceful, tender or elegant - lyrical, rather than epic or tragic, work.

Further, despite the presence of habitual and repeated aspects of the work being clearly scripted (following guidelines and protocols, filling out forms, patterns of diagnostic judgement, routine examinations, co-ordination with other teams) as junior doctors in particular learn the ropes, their performances can be stilted, they can readily forget their lines and they can fail to achieve graceful improvisation. This is only exacerbated during caffeine- or Modafinil-fuelled sleep deprivation.

The instrumental response to the dilemmas set out above is simply to restrict the number of hours that junior doctors can work, according to quasi-legislation such as the EWTD. But this misses the deeper cultural and historical reasons why junior doctors will go on committing themselves to long hours, including sleep-deprived work. Vocational calling and socialisation into medical and surgical specialties demands this as a process of identity construction. Medical culture insists that its Apollonic devotees wage war on the world of Hypnos, where Death is resident. Medicine modelled on the Homeric epics – as literal or figurative battle-hardened heroism, that the psychoanalyst Alfred Adler called "the masculine protest" and feminists call "the patriarchy" – will surely embody the paradox that exhaustion as a badge of honour is also a sure way to create an unsafe environment for your patients. Tired doctors make more mistakes and patient safety is integral to patient care.

Embracing Hypnos through a new medicine

How then can such an unproductive situation be addressed? How can the paradox of invitation and refusal of tiredness and exhaustion at the same time, that we have termed the durational misperformance of fatigue, be faced? The structural response is straightforward – first, build hospitals that do not blunt our sensibilities through poor, merely functional, design but offer authentic hospitality; and second, recruit enough staff to arrange for doctors to work reasonable hours and get enough sleep to guarantee focus on the job. In times of economic austerity these are false hopes. While fundamentally supporting this plan in the knowledge that the UK spends less on healthcare than most European nations, we have set out confounding factors beyond the structural, grounded historically in medical archetypes or relatively fixed patterns of behaviour.

Worship at the altars of father and son Apollo and Asclepius can be reframed by explicitly *performing* durational sleep deprivation without its opposition to Hypnos or Sleep. This is a conscious, reflexive performance that denatures and challenges the normal patriarchal, heroic posturing. Medicine must learn to take a deep breath and relax. This seems insulting to extremely pressured, hard-working doctors who want nothing more than to spread the workload. Our point is that medicine carries a historical burden of tension through its subscription to heroism and militaristic hierarchy. As we argue throughout the rest of this book, masculine, heroic, patriarchal, paternalistic, combative and competitive medicine must relax into the feminine and the collaborative. Where the foot is taken off the brake (a metaphor for medicine's self-inflicted symptoms - such as iatrogenesis or medically induced patient harm, and doctors' self-harm), then the accelerator need not be held down, allowing for a greater flexibility in how work is paced.

The sleepworld perspective allocated to patients - in part to guarantee their passivity - can be reclaimed for doctors too, softening the harsh, penetrating light of traditional Apollonic medicine to make it more yielding and embracing. This is a job for a fresh, innovative medical education, and not a bone tired one.

CHAPTER THIRTEEN

RESILIENCE

WRITTEN IN COLLABORATION WITH JACOB KING, ELIN BARHAM AND KIRSTEN LESLIE

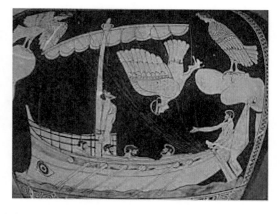

Figure 13-1: Odysseus resists the Sirens' song

Medicine's "Achilles' Heel"

Medicine is learned and performed under the most pressing of circumstances, mostly in hospital settings with chronic understaffing, excessive pressures on bed spaces and throughput, overpowering heating and harsh lighting, poor food, and, often, irritable clinical team colleagues. But, added to these organisational issues is the historical legacy of medical culture as shaped by martial metaphors embracing heroism, including a self-punishing work ethic and notorious inability for self-care.

We can describe this pincer effect of the externally imposed (dysfunctional organisational pressures) and self-imposed (medical culture's heroic legacy) as trying to drive a car with the brake engaged. Together, they form a health hazard for both patients and doctors. We have called for both organisational and cultural change throughout this book – indeed, through "thinking otherwise" with Homer we have set out a manifesto for such change, albeit complex. This composite circumstance has produced dysfunctional learning and working environments for medical education and for medical practice, that anaesthetise or numb, rather than bringing quality and sensibility to work (to formulate an ethical and aesthetic medicine).

We argue in this final chapter that there are negative, unintended consequences of this pincer effect of structural pressures and self-imposed militaristic discipline, including lack of discrimination. This can be seen in the uncritical acceptance of the current project to "train" "resilience" in order to produce healthcare workers with "grit". This involves the supposed inoculation of healthcare workers, particularly doctors, against possible exhaustion, overbearing anxiety, depression, and burnout. While acknowledging the good intentions of such schemes, we suggest that focus on the inoculation of individuals with "resilience" takes attention away from the primary issues – attending on the one hand to the dysfunctional systems within which individuals work, and on the other hand addressing the historically-conditioned habits of heroic medicine.

The 2016 annual report of the UK General Medical Council (GMC 2016) "The State of Medical Education and Practice in the UK" refers to a "challenging time" and "a state of unease within the medical profession". Doctors are experiencing higher levels of dissatisfaction and lower levels of morale than ever before, working in a system that is often described as being at breaking point. The report describes a "dangerous level of alienation" felt by doctors. A headline in the UK's *The Observer* for 12/02/2017 says: "Most young NHS doctors suffering burnout" (Campbell 2017).

This alarming headline – perhaps an extrapolation that is also an exaggeration - comes from a UK survey of 2,300 trainee anaesthetists, where "six out of seven - 85% - are at risk of becoming burned out, despite only being in their 20s and 30s". The survey offers a litany of problems. Added to hospital stress is a new factor – long commutes to work. Sixty-four per cent reported that their physical health is being affected by overwork and 61% their mental health. During a shift, 62% reported that they had gone without a meal; 75% going without adequate hydration; 95% stayed on after their shift, 68% for up to two hours longer; and 28% had done at least two hours unpaid overtime at least once within the last month. There was a lack of on-call rooms and of easy access to food and drink.

Of the top ten worst jobs for your health, paradoxically three are in healthcare, including anaesthetists and their assistants, and other surgical team members; while burnout is also on the increase in medicine (Forster 2016). That medicine is now considered a toxic profession is worrying. Yet some of the remedies that have been suggested for dealing with this are more worrying.

Where the mood of those working in the UK National Health Service (NHS) now is not good, we would like to consider a return to Homer's *Iliad* and *Odyssey* to think differently about the primary knee jerk reaction to the crisis of psychological health and balance within healthcare systems such as the NHS, where gaining "resilience" and "grit" – terms usually reserved for the military, and borrowed from studies of the forms and behaviours of physical substances - is increasingly touted as the resource we should be tapping into to help us flourish in the current working environment.

"Resilience" hardly appeared in the medical literature until about two decades ago but is now regarded as an essential personality trait for the modern clinician. There has been an exponential rise in the last 20 years of literature advocating the benefits of resilience, and educators are now considering how they may develop it in undergraduates and postgraduates (Howe et al 2012, Peterkin and Bleakley 2017).

Psychologists looking to improve the welfare of patients with post-traumatic stress disorder (PTSD), abusive childhoods, or significant relationship dysfunction initially used the word, from about 1980. From there, it emerged in the medical education literature to address the psychosocial issues of health professionals and students alike (Seoane et al 2016). Occupational health departments, faced with increasing rates of sick leave related to burnout, sought a solution in "resilience training". Like "mindfulness", a basic meditation technique, "resilience training" has become fashionable across a range of disciplines such as management, healthcare and education, and is being tailored for children. Leadership programmes - such as RobertsonCooper (https://www.robertsoncooper.com/) - advertise resilience as a "core competence".

In a post-truth age, where personal opinion is mistaken for thoughtful relativism, both instrumental and masculine heroic values maintain a strong foothold. Extreme masculinity has been normalised. Training for resilience fits perfectly with mechanical views of the human body that can be "skilled up", while resilience and grit, despite their reach into the education of children and healthcare workers, are cast as muscular.

We ask: what is wrong with education for tenderness, forgiveness and compassion, more "feminine" values? While the *Iliad* and *Odyssey* offer primary texts for courage and survival, they also reveal many lessons concerning the value of "soft", but valuable, qualities such as tenderness – qualities needed not just for sensitive patient care, but also for situations as different as apologising to families for medical error and sitting on research ethics committees. A Google search for "tenderness in medicine" directs you only to an instrumental reading: tenderness in muscles or joints, or rebound tenderness in the abdomen.

Of course, we are aware that the term "resilience" has been hi-jacked by those who wish to normalise its extreme version – of being able to cope with a high-pressure working environment (rather than working to change that environment). There is a more open reading of resilience, distinguishing it from "mental toughness":

> Emotional resilience is about adaptive coping skills, understanding and managing one's emotions and seeking social support to enable the ability to "bounce back" or even experience post-adversity growth following a stressful event. It is not only the ability to cope with stress but being able to thrive and flourish even in difficult circumstances. It is not about asking doctors to "grin and bear it" and to handle intolerable organisational pressures or excessive workloads. Neither is it about the naming and shaming of "weak" doctors for not being tough enough to cope with the pressures placed upon them. Quite the opposite, in fact.
> (https://gmcuk.wordpress.com/2015/07/15/doctors-under-pressure-need-resilience-not-mental-toughness/).

But even here, reductive instrumental language - such as "skills", and "managing one's emotions" - is used unreflectively. We examine resilience to make three points. First, there is variation in how it is defined, and it may be best to leave it as a complex, subtle strength that eludes simple definition. Second, how we develop that strength is likely to be equally elusive and complex. And third, the argument for developing resilience is that it supports healthcare workers in an environment they are finding increasingly pressing; our argument is that it is the environment that should be changed rather than those in it. Our two-pronged approach is to argue for changing the culture of medicine through metaphor framing and relaxation of the heroic impulse shown in a symptomatic work ethic; and to change the organisational setting to provide adequate resourcing. Again, it seems odd to "train" resilience to cope with a dysfunctional system rather than to address the system itself, a system obsessed with reducing complex persons to functional units.

Definitions

"Resilience" is derived from the Latin *salio*, which has meanings of jumping, leaping, or hopping. *Resilio* therefore comes to mean leaping or springing back. Pliny the Elder (1855) uses it in this literal sense of "certain fish in India (which come onto land from the rivers), and then jump back in".

However, its figurative meaning in Latin becomes one of recoiling or shrinking back from – the heat of a fire or the weight of harness for example (a definition that goes against the grain of the current image of "resilience": for most a positive spring back, rather than a reaction with negative connotations). The *Oxford English Dictionary* (1971) shows that this Latin sense was still present in the 17th and 18th centuries CE, but gradually, and particularly in the 19th century, this changed to a newer sense of returning to the original condition – the lungs in respiration or the skin following pressure, for example. This was then easily used in a metaphorical sense: "Nothing but some very transcendental claret and the resilient spirit of roving Englishmen could have induced us to sally forth" (into some foul Irish weather …) (Hole 1891, p.30); although this admirable quality could be misappropriated: "Resolute and resilient is the stout heart of the sinner, - how, like a deceitful bow, when the pressure is withdrawn, it will bound back again" (Hamilton 1876, p.150).

This negative connotation is echoed in modern times. Zolli and Healy (2013, p.21), in their examination of resilience at organisational and personal levels, point out that terrorists and criminal organisations are "highly resilient". Defining concepts like resilience can leave us scrabbling with analogy and metaphor. *Roget's Thesaurus* takes us to the heading of "Cheerfulness", subheading "Lightheartedness", where its companions are buoyancy, bounce and springiness; the adjective "resilient" is charmingly partnered with "corky".

"Corky" was a popular post-WWII name, perhaps mirroring the need to bounce back from post-war scars. Writers have come to draw analogies with saplings springing back after they are bent out of position to describe resilience. In a literature review, Jackson and colleagues (Jackson et al 2007) widen the field of the resilience metaphor to "a trajectory, a continuum, a system, a trait, a process, a cycle, and a qualitative category".

Most of the above definitions clearly refer to human resilience. Others have tried to define resilience for all circumstances:

> … the capacity of a system, be it an individual, a forest, a city or an economy, to deal with change and continue to develop. It is about how humans and nature can use shocks and disturbances like a financial crisis

or climate change to spur renewal and innovative thinking (Stockholm Resilience Centre).

Zolli and Healy (2013, p.8) examine resilience across a spectrum of professions and in ecology and business. They find that "each of these definitions rests on one of two essential aspects of resilience: continuity and recovery in the face of change", and suggest a common definition: "the capacity of a system, enterprise, or a person to maintain its core purpose and integrity in the face of dramatically changed circumstances".

The UK Government's report *No Health Without Mental Health* (DOH 2011) places resilience at the centre of a mental health strategy focused on supportive communities and ready access to services. What, however, does it mean by "resilience"? For Howe and colleagues (Howe et al 2012): "resilience is a dynamic capability which can allow people to thrive on challenges given appropriate social and personal contexts". They complicate matters by saying that several qualities ("dimensions") are subsumed within this definition: "self-efficacy, self-control, ability to engage support and help, learning from difficulties, and persistence despite blocks to progress".

Other apparent synonyms, such as "buoyancy" above (personified as "corky"), are clearly regarded as a different entity from resilience in some studies (Martin and Marsh 2009, Martin et al 2013). Southwick and Charney (2014, p.7) link resilience with metaphors of returning from deformation to normality (springing back), while Bonanno (2004) and others suggest or specify growth through adversity: "a dynamic process encompassing positive adaptation within the context of significant adversity" (Luthar et al 2000); and "the ability of an individual to adjust to adversity, maintain equilibrium, retain some sense of control over their environment. And continue to move on in a positive manner" (Jackson et al 2007).

Inevitably there are now measures of resilience (Howe et al 2012), part of the entrapment of resilience within encompassing instrumental and engineering metaphors. Windle et al (2011) reviewed these and found no gold standard against which they could be tested, nor other adequate validation. Smith et al (2008) are critical of the proxy qualities that some measures use - equanimity, perseverance, and patience, for example - feeling these lack the essential qualities of bouncing back and thriving in adversity. Windle et al (2011) also point out that most resilience scales were developed for specific age groups and fail to allow for lability. Different measures are needed for an adult and child, or for a young child and an adolescent. The authors start by recognising the difficulty of measuring an entity for which there is no agreed definition. Thus, they include measures of "psychological hardiness", "ego-resilience", "stress coping ability", and "ability to bounce back". The definition that they suggest is: "Resilience is the process of negotiating, managing and adapting to significant sources of stress or trauma". It is always dangerous to develop measures for a notion that lacks proof of concept – "measure" implies fixity, where notions of "resilience" are elastic at best and liquid at worst.

Through measure, resilience is again subject to a larger, dominant metaphorical frame of objectifying, reducing and instrumentalising, within an economic frame of "management". While we like the idea that resilience is a process rather than an object, "negotiating" and "managing" in the definition above smack of instrumentality and paradoxically turn resilience itself into an object, even a commodity.

We recognise the difficulty of measuring an entity that is so culturally dependent, while we are familiar with this in a related area - assessing entrants to medical school. In selection for our medical school, applicants are given various scenarios and asked how they would react. To us, without any wish to stereotype, it seemed that certain groups of males felt the need to appear tough ("gritty"?), and were not able to express feelings of being out of their depth, or the need to ask for help. McCann et al (2013) found variations in the concept of resilience across five different healthcare professions, so the definition of resilience depends on social context as well as historical meaning and cultural context.

What quality do we need?

We are not going to find a straightforward dictionary definition of resilience. It is best to accept its conceptual complexity, refuse its reduction to instrumental forms that can be measured, seeing it perhaps as a rich stew open to taste. We need to identify its ingredients, but also recognise the subtleties of the cooking, and that a goulash is different from a hotpot. Two ingredients bubble up from the literature (Jackson et al 2007, Luthar et al 2000): first, that there must be some exposure to adversity (how, otherwise, can you know how tough, bouncy, or gritty you are?); and second, that there must be a positive response to that adversity. This is a helpful starting point because at once it raises problems: how severe must the adversity be? One student can be greatly stressed by an exam that another will breeze through, and neither, in the UK, has to worry about his mother starving to death, like one of our students in an Ethiopian medical school with whom we have formed a partnership.

Second, what criterion does one use to judge the response? Is a lack of response a good or bad thing? Hunter and Chandler (1999) found that traumatised adolescents described resilience as being disconnected, isolated and insulated from emotional pain. This is the exact opposite of current views of resilience as an educated form of sensibility: almost painfully acute awareness and sensitivity. Such disconnection and defensive reaction as described in Hunter and Chandler's study is not hard to see in medicine, but there is a paradox at work: "without such disconnection and emotional insulation", say many doctors "I could not do my job". It is getting too close to the emotional lives of patients and their families that is potentially overwhelming. "Resilience" then becomes an elastic notion that refuses concretisation.

Other questions arise. Over what period is the response measured? What is the significance of mental health problems after a decade of apparently good recovery? What if there is a good response academically and a poor one socially? These issues cause resilience to be described as "multidimensional" and "dynamic" (Luthar et al 2000, Southwick and Charney 2014). Again, resilience can be thought of as a dynamic, complex, adaptive process rather than a chunk of emotional capital or a personality trait.

The distinction between "resilience" and "recovery" matters because the latter implies an initial loss of normal function, whereas resilience implies standing firm from the time of the initial assault. This is not a distinction that all would make. The metaphor of the sapling springing back to its normal position means there is an initial deformation. Nevertheless, the apparently impassive clinician is familiar in medicine and a figure to which many would aspire. Returning to the sapling metaphor, we might be cautious of those gaining "over-resilience", who, fresh from their resilience training, showing true grit, spring back so hard as to smack their colleagues. Such "whiplash resilience" can also create irritating zealots for training programmes, as resilience missionaries or evangelists.

The complexity behind resilience becomes evident from the literature. There, families coping well with a child with learning difficulties may "become resilient through finding positive meaning in the event, gaining a sense of control and continuity, and maintaining valued identities across the family network" (Howe et al 2012). Much of the literature is concerned with children and adolescents. Bonanno (2004) suggests that resilience in adults may present a simpler problem. At least we need to be aware of the effects of age on resilience.

It will be clear to the reader by now that we have an interest in how metaphors shape medical performance. Recently, the quality recommended to survive at work has moved from notions of springiness and bounce to notions of hardiness, with the introduction of "sturdy" and "tough" as synonyms (Judkins et al 2005, Southwick and Charney 2014, p.7):

> Hardiness consists of three dimensions: being committed to finding meaningful purpose in life, the belief that one can influence one's surroundings and the outcome of events, and the belief that one can learn and grow from both positive and negative life experiences (Bonanno 2004).

A wall is resilient, not if it rebounds to force, but if it endures assault. An elastic band might be described as resilient not for doing its job in recoiling to its original form, but if it fails to break when stretched to the limit. These are not just linguistic games but have significant implications for the psychological state that is being recommended. Again, the metaphors are of prime importance. Are we to be unflinching in the face of adversity, or able to recover from a setback? If we take the former, then techniques regarding mental toughness, crisis management, and staying cool under pressure should be nurtured; if the second, then the processes of assessment, reflection and analysis - that have been co-opted by the business term "self-management" - become relevant. ("Manage" has its origin in the "hands on" process – Latin *manus* – of training horses).

These are two very different goals for a teaching programme to develop. "Unflinching" is not a newly recommended virtue. One of William Osler's most celebrated addresses was entitled "Aequanimitas" (1946, pp.3-11). In it, he advocates to newly graduated medical students two qualities, one that he considers a bodily virtue: imperturbability; the other mental: equanimity. He adds flesh to the bones of the former:

> coolness and presence of mind under all circumstances, calmness amid storm, clearness of judgement in moments of great peril, immobility, impassiveness, or, to use an old and expressive word, phlegm.

Many admirers of Osler have been puzzled by this address, as it seems as if the great man is throwing out empathy and compassion as key to medical practice. Osler was aware of possible misinterpretation: " … the general accusation of hardness, so often brought against the profession, has here its foundation". He then recommends "callousness" over "sensibility".

Grit

Resilience has recently been translated, in surgical contexts, as "grit", and seen as a desired character trait. Grit is defined as "passion and perseverance for long-term goals" (Burkhart et al, 2014), where:

> grit appears to be a promising marker and risk factor for attrition from surgical residency. In an effort to retain residents, programs should consider screening for grit … and directing support to those residents with below-median values.

Passion and perseverance are the two critical ingredients of grit for Angela Lee Duckworth (2016), who finds them better predictors of success (at an American military academy) than natural talent. She has an unusual take on passion too seeing it as a quality of enduring commitment rather than one of intensity. This is a frightening scenario to those with a more tender-minded rather than tough-minded approach to medical education. "Directing support" to those with less "grit" seems to chime with modern medical education values. But the very notion of classifying ("below-median values") grit levels seems archaic and merely an old staple - masculine heroism - in new guise.

The popular surgical "skeptical scalpel" weblog (http://www.kevinmd.com/blog/2014/08/selecting-grittier-surgeons-harder-think.html) for August 19 2014 has a discussion point: "Selecting grittier surgeons is harder than you think", where:

> In case you haven't noticed, a hot new topic in education is "grit." In order to reduce the long-standing 20% attrition rate of surgical residents, some say we should select applicants who have more grit or conscientiousness.

This blogger misinterprets the findings of a Harvard symposium (https://hms.harvard.edu/resiliency-and-learning-implications-teaching-medical-students-and-residents) as advocating US Navy Seal training for medical education. This is corrected by another writer on the blog, who states that the recommendation actually was:

> First, let people experience success: Assign them to a successful group. Second, create a surveillance system and safety net, and provide encouragement, mentoring and training. Finally, mitigate the impact of stress by promoting "self-efficacy"—the belief that we are agents of change.

The original blog recasts resilience as grit and as a macho trait, but resilience can also be thought of as the forming of inventive strategies that turn apparent difficulty into opportunity. Resilience is not necessarily a "hardening up". Indeed, it may be a softening towards others and particular events. Its core is not just "bouncing back" from difficulties, but adaptability in general. Here, of course, we speak with the voice of the hero Odysseus rather than Achilles. The latter would plump for "true grit". For Odysseus, grit would be whatever makes the pearl.

Finally, more attention should be given to how resilience changes with age. This is only mentioned in passing in most of the literature - for example: "Across the life course, the experience of resilience will vary" (Windle et al 2011). The issue deserves more careful consideration. We assume that medical students are tender shoots that need protection, but do they mature into gnarled oaks, stubbornly resisting the elements but with the loss of a limb or two; or into yews, of famous longevity, whose means of survival are mysterious but may involve loss of their heartwood along the way?

"Thinking otherwise" about resilience and grit through Homer

Day-to-day existence for the combatants in the Trojan War was hard and Homer's description of the battles gives us an idea of what the aftermath must have been like in terms of the dead and wounded. Individual scenes are analysed in detail by Wolf-Hartmut (2003), mainly with a stylistic eye, but he gives a clear idea of the endurance needed to survive. Homer's descriptions are so vivid they have led to the (tongue-in-cheek) suggestion that he was "Agamemnon's aide-de-camp or else his secretary" (Wolf-Hartmut 2003, p.104).

It is tempting, therefore, to suppose that the need for resilience, however defined, would not have occurred to a Greek hero, because it was such an integral part of his heroism and manhood. This is to ignore the many occasions when Homer shows us heroes expressing doubt and fear to themselves, such as the moment when Hector challenges the Greek heroes to a duel and there is a reluctance to take up the challenge (*Iliad* 7. 67-102); or when Hector comes face-to-face with Achilles, trapped under the wall of Troy, and realises that he cannot begin to match the latter's leonine presence; or when, in a rather ludicrous misunderstanding early in the epic, the Greek army runs for their ships believing the war is being abandoned and they can return home (*Iliad* 2.1-210) thanks to a ruse by Agamemnon that backfires – scenes we have amplified elsewhere with appropriate commentaries.

We have described already the moving scene when Hector says farewell to his wife and baby son as he leaves Troy for battle (*Iliad* 6. 369-502). Andromache tries to dissuade him from fighting; his reply shows that a mix of shame and duty compel him to go out (*Iliad* 6. 440-6). Many doctors must have stood outside a patient's room, deliberating whether to go in or to avoid them because there was nothing they could do for their pain or disability or because they were dying. Shame is a driving force for Hector (he says so), but probably less so for our doctor. We have described duty as part of the motive force behind Hector's return to battle but that is a liberal interpretation of Homer's words. Hector actually says:

> and my spirit (*thumos*) urges me not to (avoid battle), since I learned always to be noble (*esthlos*), and to fight in the front rank of Trojans, defending the honour of my father and myself (*Iliad* 6. 444-6).

The two Greek words are deceptively simple to translate. *Thumos* – as discussed in previous chapters - occurs very often in Homer and is usually translated as "spirit/ breath" or "heart/ blood". It resides in the chest cavity, urging heroes to some intensive course of action, stirring them into action with a passion that may form into kinds of anger or resentment. What guides that impulse is not stated. *Esthlos*, translated above as "noble", develops the meaning of "good" in a moral sense in the later, classical Greek world.

For Achilles, what is good is what brings him honour and glory, and lacks moral overtones. For Hector, in the very domestic scene described, his motives are partly overt – shame – and partly obscure. "My spirit urges me to write" says no more than "I want to write", "I write", or even "writing". The motivating force has not been revealed. The forces motivating doctors when they are unobserved, in the middle of the night, to enter a room or stay longer with a patient at home can also be unexamined. They may spring from a sense of duty rather than shame, certainly an internalised ethic, when their actions are unobserved, and also from an identity that is constructed during their education and training.

We have come to call this "professionalism" but this is a modern obfuscation of an ancient honour code that refers to moral duty. One problem with couching resilience as a thing to be trained is that it shifts the locus of interest from a complex moral stance (values) into a staged performance. This shifts a metaphor into a literalism and drains the power of the former. The equivalent would be to take the purposefully metaphorical phrase "s/he shows true heart" and translate this into a training programme in which "heart" becomes protocol or five-stage process. We look forward to *thumos* training workshops!

Odysseus was clearly regarded in the ancient world as the epitome of fortitude and endurance. One sign of this is the epithet often assigned to him throughout the Odyssey *polutlas* – "much enduring". *Polu* is a common prefix, meaning "many", and becomes "poly" in English, from which we have polygamous and polysyllabic, for example. The verb *tlao* means "endure". One must be careful in the interpretation of epithets in Homer because of their formulaic use, which we discuss in chapter four. There is a very large literature on this issue and some have argued that such epithets are essentially meaningless – either used so often that they lose significance ("godlike Achilles"), or inappropriate ("noble Aegisthus", of one of the great villains of Greek myth). *Polutlas* is different in that it is only used in the *Iliad* and *Odyssey* to refer to Odysseus. It is odd in the *Iliad*, where he is no more "enduring" than any other, and exhibits his other main quality *polumetis* – "of many counsels, cunning, or crafty", which is used of him much more often. Adam Nicolson (2015, p.228) describes him as a "multiple of multiples" – much enduring, of many counsels, and also *polumechanos* - of many stratagems. These descriptors already make us think that the resilience shown by Odysseus is not "toughness" or "grit" but different – perhaps "elasticity" and "adaptability".

"Training" for this would surely follow a different pedagogical line than "training" for toughening up. A postgraduate medical education "Odysseus workshop" might spend time on how to be "wily" at work, in sharp contrast to an "Achilles workshop" in how to face down tough opposition. Imagine a time in medical education when we might offer, under the heading of "resilience education", workshops in "patience" modelled on the narrative of Penelope; or on "using eroticism wisely" based on the narrative of Helen.

To return to epithets linked to Odysseus (with the root "poly" or "many") - in the *Iliad*, these are used in a formulaic way to fill the metrical requirements of the end of a line, often where Odysseus is replying in a conversation. In the *Odyssey*, however, where *polutlas* appears frequently - 37 times – (Dunbar 1858, p.316), it can be formulaic, but is also used where the context gives it significance – when he is fearful that he is being tricked by the nymph Calypso (*Odyssey* 5. 159-180); when he is shipwrecked yet again and fears drowning (5. 313-64); or when he collapses exhausted having finally swum to shore (5. 464-66).

In relation to "resilience", Odysseus makes two telling statements. He appears in person late in the *Odyssey*, in book 5. On this first meeting, we find him in tears longing for his home. The nymph Calypso warns him that if he knew the hardships awaiting him he would not leave her. He replies:

"I shall endure, with a spirit (*thumon*) inured to suffering. Already I have born many evils and suffered much at sea and in war. Let the hardships come" (*Odyssey* 5. 222-4).

Almost as soon as he leaves her, the malice of Poseidon shipwrecks him (retribution for Odysseus blinding Poseidon's son the Cyclops Polyphemus, even though Polyphemus has broken the hospitality rule by eating his guests one by one rather than entertaining them). Later, he ventures to the underworld to consult the prophet Teiresias. There he sees his mother and this is the first knowledge he has of her death. Here, surely, is a lesson for education of resilience in doctors. The doctor often knows before the family of the death of a loved one, and then has to "break bad news". The resilient moment is moral, not technical or professional.

We teach medical students how to break bad news in a formulaic way as a communication skill, but it is actually a moral dilemma. Holding knowledge of the death of a person prior to those who are close to and love or care for that person is both a moral privilege (to not be abused) and a burden (I have what I do not own). Doctors must become as "many sided" or adaptable as Odysseus to know how to best proceed in each singular case of breaking bad news. They are meeting their own dead mothers without knowing that she has died. Carrying the simultaneous moral gift and burden requires a resilience and grit that cannot be simply translated from the complex moral sphere into the instrumental act of communicating information.

The doctor is the "fortunate unfortunate" in this context. Odysseus' mother refers to him as "unfortunate above all mortals". For when he finally arrives home, he finds his palace taken over by arrogant princelings vying for the hand of his wife, whom they presume is a widow. (We only find out later in the narrative that some of the suitors had also taken some of the women servants in the household to their beds).

The doctor too, in breaking bad news to family or friends, is a visitor to his or her own home. The doctor must be true to the meaning of "hospital" by providing authentic hospitality: you are a guest in my house who takes precedence over me (unless you abuse the privilege, for example by engaging in abuse, violence or perverse non-compliance with, for example, a necessary prescription). This sacrifice of indwelling one's workplace is again an ethical gesture, and not a skill, that requires resilience or grit as moral courage.

After Odysseus' return, he makes a statement regarding endurance to one of the more sympathetic suitors: "Of all the things that breathe and crawl about earth, she bears nothing weaker than man .... . When the blessed gods bring misery upon him, then he must bear it with an enduring spirit" (*Odyssey* 18. 130-35). This seems like a straightforward lesson for doctors, who literally spend much of their career in odyssey as they gain expertise in generalism and then specialism, moving geographically as opportunities appear; but also have a parallel odyssey in moving around such a variety of patients and presenting conditions; and circumstances of relative wellness and illness, encompassing deaths.

Further, Odysseus conceals his identity even from those he most loves until a final bloody denouement, when he and his son slaughter all the suitors and the women servants. We suggest a radical reading of this scene that can be taken as a metaphor for challenging the increasingly difficult work contexts under which doctors have to maintain exacting levels of performance and ethical behaviour. We suggested early in this chapter that focus upon increasing resilience and grit in individual doctors is missing the main issue – that of changing the systems in which they work, and the cultural tropes that have, historically, shaped their activities. Youngson and Blennerhassett (2016, p.355), in a recent impassioned article, argue that we have to build a more compassionate society: "Although health professionals care deeply about patients, the values of the wider system are competition, rationalism, productivity, efficiency and profit".

Bouncing up, not bouncing back

However resilient we think ourselves, trauma may undo us physically and mentally. Jonathan Shay (2002) draws parallels between veterans returning from the Vietnam War (whom he treated, largely for Post Traumatic Stress Disorder) and the tribulations of Odysseus and his men, where homecoming equates to illness. Shay's is the best study we know of making sense of a contemporary psychological phenomenon through "thinking otherwise" using Homer. Among the veterans, he noticed that those most liable to extremes of violence were those who had suffered trauma before going to war. He draws parallels between this and the wounding of Odysseus in a wild boar hunt as a young man, as some explanation of the violence he unleashes at the end of the *Odyssey*, which requires the intervention of the gods to stop.

Odysseus was already marked as a person who lived at tipping point after this initiatory encounter. The story repeats the mytheme of the vulnerability of the hero (such as Achilles' heel), reminding us that one of the problems with resilience training approaches (bouncing back to normality) is that it can perpetuate the myth, or ideal, of the perfect doctor who toughs it out whatever the circumstances. Yet flaws are precisely what make doctors human and open to compassion for their patients.

The "boar gore" wound (a classic symbol of vulnerability) is a way in to character, not a character flaw – we should learn from our mythemes. In particular, Odysseus' wound in the "thigh" (a euphemism for genitalia) has been read as a symbol of castration of the male and an opening of a symbolic vagina – in other words, a feminising of the heroic (Shuttle and Redgrove 2005).

The pressure of working in many areas of medicine is continuous, but there can be episodes of trauma out of the ordinary. These may occur to young undergraduate students, and inevitably some arrive having experienced previous childhood trauma. If they are then exposed to trauma later in their career and abreact, we should worry that the lesson of Shay and Homer is that their reaction is likely to be extreme and may involve harm to themselves or others; and this is compounded by the well-known profile of medical students as high achievers with high anxiety levels and a competitive spirit.

Second, the above parallels are with Achilles, Odysseus, and a few other Greek heroes. We have said nothing about resilient women in Homer. This stems from the original definition of resilience as having connotations of bounciness and springiness. We describe above the power of endurance of Odysseus. Women in Homer are models of endurance: Helen's willingness to test the fruits of abduction; the captive women at the start of the *Iliad*; Andromache begging Hector to stay within the walls of Troy and mourning his death at the end; Penelope yearning for the return of her husband and having to tolerate the loutish behaviour of her suitors. In current theatres of war, women rarely have agency - things are done to them, rather than by them - and they must endure. Throughout this book we have commented insistently on the implications and importance of the current shift in the gender balance in medicine, and resilience is yet another area where this must have an effect. It is as if medicine is suffering its thigh wound.

Julie Ann Freischlag (Freischlag and Silva 2016) throws some light on this issue of resilience and the changing role of women in medicine and surgery. She describes her career trajectory - to become one of the top women surgeons and medical academics in North America - as a constant challenge to a uniform "sea of black suited men". The secret to her success, she claims, is "resilience" – the ability to "bounce back" from setbacks, usually engineered through blatant gender discrimination within surgical and surgical education circles.

But Freischlag extends "bouncing back" to the metaphor of "bouncing up". She says that the point about resilience is not to recover your original position, but to discover a new and more interesting position further down the line or higher on the ladder of opportunity. This beautifully illustrates the combination of resilience with endurance, described by Freischlag as "rising with adversity". She also says: "it is not the strong, but the responsive who survive", a saying that Freischlag found, to her surprise, on a Fortune Cookie.

What is Freischlag's key to a new, feminine kind of resilience? She calls it "a culture of meaningful support" – a shift from (potentially narcissistic) individualism to productive collectivism. This is precisely what is called for at the end of Homer's *Odyssey* after Odysseus' rout of Penelope's suitors and his terrible mass slaying of the women associated with them. Athene demands that Odysseus and the families of the slayed suitors seeking revenge together put down their weapons and make peace across the warring factions. As Dorothea Wender (1978, p.14) suggests: "Homer likes to move in a crowd". The close of the *Odyssey* places the reader in the midst of a congregation who are collectively bouncing up and forward to a new chapter of collective living and working after a period of dire stagnation and self-interest.

Moving forward

The situation is not hopeless. We must be clear about the qualities that we want to instil, resist the siren calls for gritty doctors and nurses, and above all pay constant attention to the environments in which we expect to work. We would argue that those working in healthcare are exemplars of how to flourish in difficult circumstances, and others should be learning from them. For some it is a question of survival rather than flourishing and it is those that we seek to help, but the starting point must be the quality of the system in which they work. Quality of a system such as the NHS cannot be reduced to functionality - it includes sensibility or awareness of workers' emotional needs and provision of an environment in which potential can flourish, rather than working at a level of mere "competence".

Several studies examine coping mechanisms which are effective, and distinguish two potential resources, those present within the individual and those present within their environment (Tusaie and Dyer 2004, Jackson et al 2007, McCann et al 2013). Although we reject the adoption of a military mindset in healthcare (again, the hegemony of the "medicine as war" metaphor must be challenged), the military too do not put the onus entirely on the individual, but see resilience or "psychological fitness" in terms of a balance between personal and environmental resources (Bates et al 2010).

Much can be learned about resilience from survivors of trauma such as natural disasters, accidents, political conflicts, and wars. Gonzales (2012) describes how forms of resilience developed in the aftermath of trauma may themselves become additional symptoms, where the effort to seek help is minimal. After the 9/11 attack on the World Trade Centre, the Federal Emergency Management Agency made $155 million dollars available for post-trauma counselling, expecting up to a quarter of a million to apply. As Gonzales says "Just 300 people turned up". The mindset, that many, probably most, people need psychological help after trauma is prevalent in many western societies now and is challenged by Bonanno (2004). His take on resilience is both "that it is more common than often believed" but also that "it represents a distinct trajectory from that of recovery".

Stephen Joseph (2011) argues for what he calls "posttraumatic growth" in the wake of trauma, ranging from losses such as separation, divorce, illness and bereavement, to more intense events such as assault, accidents and natural disasters. Joseph catalogues powers of deep recovery - supposedly upholding the maxim that what doesn't kill us makes us stronger - where trauma can facilitate "new meaning, purpose and direction in life". Sennett (2013) challenges such models of stoic self-reliance, pointing to the value of the "rituals, pleasures and politics of cooperation" rather than autonomous self-recuperation. For Sennett, collaboration is the best antidote to pervasive adversarial competition that brings communities into conflict and isolates individuals. This collaboration should be not only across medical specialties but also across the disciplines. McCann et al (2013), in their cross-disciplinary review of resilience, found a distinct shortage of studies of doctors' resilience and, in general, different strategies were described for "coping" within each healthcare profession.

There is no shortage of suggestions for strategies to enhance resilience (Tusaie and Dyer 2004, Jackson et al 2007, Seoane et al 2016): building positive relationships at work, staying positive, developing emotional insight, achieving a good work-life balance, and being reflective, for example (Jackson et al 2007). These suggestions at first sight seem facile.

Other factors associated with resilience include having caring and supportive relationships, being able to make realistic plans and taking steps to carry them out, having a positive view of oneself, being able to communicate and problem solve, and the capacity to manage strong feelings and impulses. Seoane et al (2016) recommend keeping a "daily gratitude journal", suggesting, almost incidentally to the rest of their paper, that this will "promote reflection and resilience". McCann et al

(2013) found that there were some coping mechanisms shared between professions in medicine – laughter and humour, self-reflection, beliefs and spirituality, and professional identity. We have referred to the pervasiveness of black humour in medicine in previous chapters, and it is recognised as a feature of resilience in both doctors and nurses (Tusaie and Dyer 2004), and a coping feature in Vietnam POWs and American military personnel (Southwick and Charney 2014).

The *American Psychological Association* (http://www.apa.org/help center/road-resilience.aspx) identifies the following ten ways to build resilience:

1. Make connections.
2. Avoid seeing crises as insurmountable problems.
3. Accept that change is a part of living.
4. Move towards realistic goals.
5. Take decisive actions.
6. Look for opportunities for self-discovery.
7. Nurture a positive view of yourself.
8. Keep things in perspective.
9. Maintain a hopeful outlook.
10. Take care of yourself.

It is easy to see this list as facile or stating the obvious. We need more sophisticated analyses and suggestions for change. Peterkin and Bleakley (2017) note that for doctors, the following elements are highly predictive of professional resilience:

1. A strong sense of identity and agency.
2. Possessing clear values and beliefs.
2. Not forcing values on others.
3. Self-awareness.
4. A healthy temperament and a good sense of humour.
5. Not taking things personally.
6. Valuing your work - feeling that it does make a difference.
7. An ability to learn from past challenges and stressful situations.

Again, reduction to a list easily trivialises a complex issue. Bates et al (2010) give a comprehensive and detailed list of possible resources, based on five domains: awareness, beliefs and appraisals, coping, decision making, and engagement. It is based too on a belief that "psychological fitness can be developed using the same training principles as physical fitness", again reducing resilience to a machinic equivalent. Howe et al (2012), reviewing this and other military strategies, highlight only one of their resources: "challenging scenarios" to help develop coping skills. This method resembles the, again highly reductive, "stress inoculation" of Bates et al (2010), that:

> attempts to immunize an individual from reacting negatively to stress exposure. This process takes place before experiencing the stressful conditions of concern. One critical hallmark of stress inoculation is the requirement for increasingly realistic pre-exposure through training simulation.

This is increasingly used in medical education in clinical skills training for medical students and postgraduates, which may start with simulated settings in medical school but progresses to more realistic and challenging scenarios.

Doctoring is tough and those working in healthcare know that they will have difficult times in their careers. Many of those who work in tough jobs and professions must feel frustration at the lack of understanding of those who stand outside, particularly those offering to toughen them up. It is like Nietzsche's (1872) comment on our lack of understanding of the brutality displayed in the *Iliad*: "Why did the whole Greek word exult in the fighting scenes of the *Iliad*? I am afraid, we do not understand them enough in 'Greek fashion', and that we should even shudder, if for once we did understand them thus".

We have analysed resilience, hardiness, grit and other mechanisms suggested to help individual doctors through challenging times. We are suspicious of the examples of human resilience suggested by Southwick and Charney (2014, pp.8-9, p.62) – former prisoners of war in Vietnam, and instructors in the American special forces – as models for the rest of humanity; and suspicious of their calls for "toughening up" courses, as found in the military, particularly for "intensive educational programmes" such as medicine.

At worst, this strikes us as heroic posturing and simply reproduces everything that needs to change within the systems that support medical practice, such as heroic individualism over collaboration, conflict over co-operation, hierarchy over democracy, masculine forms over feminine, managerialism over professional style, and reductive protocol-based instrumentalism over innovative practice. What is striking now in the UK is that there is so little suggestion that what needs changing is the environment of the NHS, before we toughen the workers within it. The importance of the environment is, however, not ignored in the resilience literature. Howe and colleagues (Howe et al 2012) quote "a lower ... vulnerability to adversity" as driving the need for resilience and recognise that "The environment in which an individual must survive may support or undermine his or her personal resilience".

The importance of the environment is, as one would expect, generic, so that for parents of disabled children: "factors such as neighbourhood stress, deprivation and inequality have all been found to reduce social coherence and resilience" (Zautra et al 2008).

We saw earlier the suggestion that surgeons should be selected on the basis of grittiness. It is only a step from there to suggest that these sorts of criteria should be used in the initial selection for medical school. Howe and colleagues (Howe et al 2012) advocate selecting for interpersonal skills, though the qualities they suggest as forming this are an odd group: "autonomy, resilience, team orientation and self-questioning". To revert to our examination of definitions at the beginning, some lent naturally to interpretation of resilience as a personal attribute, others as an operational spectrum of responses. The danger with the former is that: "Any scientific representation of resilience as a personal attribute can inadvertently pave the way for perceptions that some individuals simply do not 'have what it takes' to overcome adversity" (Luthar et al 2000).

We have a concern that these lists are oriented towards self-help and autonomy, in the traditional narrative of heroism and instrumentalism within the Protestant-Capitalist framework brought to a head by Samuel Smiles' (1859) *Self Help*. Smiles' second edition of 1866 extended the subtitle to include "perseverance", sister to "resilience". We would like to see greater emphasis on collective responsibility, support and development in team contexts, and "shared" or "distributed" heroism (see chapters one and two). We also note the big gap between these instrumental, checklist, self-help competences, so characteristic of our era in which doctors are hungry for an educational quick fix; and the literary, complex, disturbing and nourishing poetry of Homer that invites contemplation, exegesis including multiple readings, and, above all, appreciation as song, poetry and theatre. In Homer, the principles of resilience are illustrated through character and plot, especially in contexts of uncertainty, rendering them as aesthetic rather than functional or economic.

Homer does not prescribe through lists of required attributes, but presents optional scenarios and shows the consequences of each. Medical education, in our opinion, does not benefit from being reduced to lists. We are serious when we say that doctors can learn more about character and ethics from reading Homer than from tick-box lists.

APPENDIX

SYNOPSES OF THE *ILIAD* AND THE *ODYSSEY*

There are many summaries of the stories of the *Iliad* and the *Odyssey* in journals, books and online. We give them here for the convenience of the reader, particularly if you are new to the texts. We make no connections to medicine here – that path begins with our Introduction.

The *Iliad*

"Iliad" translates literally as "the song of Ilium (Troy)". The Trojan War was fought between the Greeks (called the Achaeans or Argives or Danaans by Homer) and the Trojans. The Greek force was assembled from the local rulers of mainland Greece and its surrounding islands under the overall command of Agamemnon, King of Mycenae. They sailed to Troy, which sits at the opening of the Hellespont, the Greek name for the Dardanelles. The reason for war was the abduction of the Greek Helen by the Trojan Paris. Helen was the wife of Menelaus, Agamemnon's brother; Paris was the son of Priam, the King of Troy. Helen was considered the most beautiful woman in the world.

The war was fought over ten years, with the Trojans mainly sheltered behind the walls of Troy. It is essential to an understanding of the *Iliad* that most of the stories of the Trojan War that have been passed down through the ages – the judgement of Paris, the abduction of Helen, the wooden horse, the death of Achilles, the destruction of Troy - are not part of the *Iliad*. Some of these events appear in the *Odyssey*, such as the wooden horse and Odysseus' meeting with the dead Achilles in Hades. The *Iliad* relates events that take place over a period of only 40 or so days towards the end of the war. The central theme of the *Iliad* is the anger of Achilles.

Books One and Two

The epic begins with an invocation to the Muse: "Sing, Muse, of the wrath of Achilles, the son of Peleus". At once there is a difficulty for the translator - that the first word in the Greek is *menin* (wrath), which you want to hit the listener between the eyes. It is grammatically natural there in the Greek but looks forced if placed there in English, though some translations try. Robert Graves' controversial translation cuts to the chase in entitling the book *The Anger of Achilles* rather than the *Iliad*.

The epic song cycle, and later the written text, focus on the seething and brooding angers of one man – Achilles – first, the cause of an eruption of anger; second, its repression in resentment; and third, its expression in an outburst of extreme violence. Every event in the *Iliad* is coloured by these three phases of Achilles' anger: cause or trigger, repression or sulk, and expression in revenge (for the slaughter in battle of his companion Patroclus by the Trojan Hector). Woven into Achilles' story is that of the leader of the Greeks, Agamemnon, whose series of blunders creates a counterpoise to Achilles' story. Agamemnon is the formal leader but proceeds by blunders, where Achilles is the recognised champion. The narrative tension in the *Iliad* is created by Achilles' stutter (his sulk) that is temporary, and the death of Patroclus that releases the valve previously containing Achilles' pent-up anger.

Homer maps the brutal Trojan War spatially in such a way that the reader cannot help but feel the tensions felt by the opposing camps. The Trojans are compressed into a besieged space behind the walls of Troy; and the war has already been grinding away for ten years on a battlefield set on the pinched plain between the walls of Troy and the gathered ships of the Greeks. Beyond the Greek ships is open "wine dark" sea and the promise of freedom and escape – but this theme is saved for the *Odyssey*. These pinched spaces set an atmosphere for the song that is the *Iliad*. This atmosphere is captured in the poet Christopher Logue's free rendering of parts of the epic as "All Day Permanent Red" – the ground soaked in blood, the air a fine red mist between bouts of slaughter. Out of this atmosphere, populated by the minor figures of the epic, mainly described in the throes of terrible deaths, the larger figures come in and out of focus and play out the main scenes.

The first pleasure of the *Iliad* is how we are plunged immediately into the action: "Which of the gods was it", the poet asks, "that caused to fight in strife Agamemnon, king of men, and godlike Achilles" The audience knows it was Apollo, who, aggrieved by Agamemnon's treatment of his priest, Chryses, brings a plague on the Greek camp. Chryses had come to ask for the return of his daughter Chryseis, a captive of war, and had offered a large ransom. All the Greeks thought the offer fair except Agamemnon, who refuses, insults the priest, and throws him out of the camp. The plague continues for nine days, and on the tenth, Achilles calls a meeting of the Greek leaders. He asks if anyone present can explain why this affliction has come on them. The seer Calchas says that he can, but that his explanation will annoy one of the leaders and he wants his safety guaranteed. Achilles agrees to do this and Calchas explains Agamemnon's offence and that Chryseis must be returned and Apollo propitiated.

Agamemnon is indeed annoyed but has to agree. However, he demands recompense because it is not suitable that he, the overall leader, should be deficient in prizes. Homer sets up one of many moral dilemmas explored in the *Iliad*. Achilles replies reasonably that all the prizes have been shared out and there is no store from which to replenish Agamemnon's loss. At this point, Agamemnon precipitates the argument from which the rest of the *Iliad* unfolds - either the Greeks find him a new prize or he will take one from Achilles or one of the other leaders. Achilles then makes a speech that makes clear his contempt for Agamemnon's greed and states that he intends to sail back to his home in Greece. Agamemnon personalises the argument even further by saying that he will take the captive woman of Achilles "so that you may learn how my power exceeds yours" (*Iliad* Book 1.187).

Achilles is then on the point of drawing his sword to kill the king but the goddess Athene pulls him back by his hair and prevents the retaliatory action. A contemporary psychological reading might invoke a moment of "reflection" within impulse. Nestor, an old warrior and counsellor, attempts to calm the situation and offers advice to both men, but Achilles launches a withering attack on the character of the king and withdraws from any further part in the fighting in a deep sulk.

Direct speech launches the action of the *Iliad* and the speeches portray vividly the passion of the quarrel and the characters of the protagonists. There is then an interlude for us to draw breath, while Chryseis is returned to her father, and offerings are made to Apollo to assuage his anger. Agamemnon carries out his threat to take Briseis, the prize of Achilles, who offers no resistance to the two nervous heralds who are sent to convey her. However, Achilles then goes to the seashore to talk to his mother Thetis. She is a sea nymph, therefore of divine origin, and is persuaded to ask Zeus, king of the gods, to intervene in the war and see the Achaeans defeated and beaten back to their ships, so that Agamemnon may learn how greatly they depend on the prowess of Achilles.

With some reluctance, Zeus agrees and sends a dream to Agamemnon, misleading him into thinking that Troy is his for the taking if he attacks immediately. Agamemnon takes the dream seriously, but decides to test the mettle of his troops with a perverse plan. He summons all his troops and suggests that they abandon the war and sail home as he thinks the war is now fruitless. The ruse backfires. Rather than challenging Agamemnon and bravely declaring that they will fight on, the troops rush for the ships. Agamemnon now has to bring the troops back. Thersites, a buffoonish character unique in the *Iliad*, criticises the leadership of Agamemnon and urges his companions to abandon the war and return home. Odysseus beats him for his insolence, and delivers a rousing speech to the troops, supported by Nestor, and they are persuaded back to their duties.

The Greeks muster for battle. Their leaders and the number of ships that they brought to Troy are described in a list of over 200 lines. This may well be a list dating back to the early days of the creation of the *Iliad* and has puzzled many commentators as inappropriate. It is hard to imagine a poem or novel of the modern era giving such a list of personnel, but this constitutes the important atmosphere, rather than the action, of the war. What is unique to Homer is the pairing of a main narrative (the story of Achilles) with this parallel atmosphere or mesh of events including the intimate details of minor soldiers' deaths. It is as if we are watching events unfold from the front and back of a mirror simultaneously. Principal characters (heroes) constitute a foreground, acting out a tragedy against a background of the atmosphere and stench of battle as a composite of minor figures.

Iris, a messenger of the gods, goes to the Trojans to spur them to action. She speaks to the leading Trojan warrior Hector, in the guise of another of Priam's sons, to warn him that the Greeks are advancing. Hector leads the Trojans out onto the plain sandwiched between the walls of Troy and the ships of the Greeks.

Books Three to Six

Paris offers to fight Menelaus in single combat on the understanding that the victor wins Helen and all her possessions, and that the war is ended. The duel is a brief affair because, when Paris comes close to defeat and death, he is concealed in a mist by his protector, Aphrodite, and smuggled away to his bedroom in Troy. This puts the mortals in a quandary as to the winner of the duel. The quandary is echoed on Olympus, where Zeus (apparently forgetting his promise to Thetis which demands battle and defeat for the Achaeans) is considering bringing the war to an end. His wife, Hera, has an inveterate hatred for Troy and its people and persuades him to continue the war. There is a bloodthirsty conversation between them. He is reluctant to allow the destruction of a city for which he has great regard and insists that when the time comes for him to destroy a city beloved of Hera, she will not object. Such is her hatred of Troy, she agrees. Given the gods' agreement. Athene races to Troy and inspires the Trojan Pandarus to shoot an arrow at Menelaus, which wounds him superficially. This is more than sufficient to break the truce and the two armies rejoin battle.

The *Iliad* is about war and much of it is given over to fighting, wounding and killing. The deaths of the many warriors could become another catalogue, but Homer embroiders each with details pertaining only to that warrior to give him an identity and make him an individual standing out from the crowd. Many deaths are associated with similes, for which Homer was famous, now acting as memorials. Readers fresh to Homer might be surprised at how the epic and tragic are meshed with the lyrical so effectively.

After the truce is broken, the fighting largely concerns Diomedes and his *aristeia*. This word describes a passage of fighting that concentrates on one particular hero and his successful rampage through the enemy ranks. During this episode of fighting, Hector is persuaded to return to the city and instruct his mother Hecuba to offer sacrifices to Athene asking that she take pity on Troy and its people. After doing this, he again urges Paris to return to battle and then goes to find his wife Andromache and baby son. They finally meet in a scene that was famous in the ancient world and justly remains so, as she tries to persuade him to remain in the city and organise its defence from there, and he remains implacable that his duty is to return to the battle outside the city walls, where we know he will die. This is one of a catalogue of errors committed by Hector that lead ultimately to his death at the hand of Achilles.

Books Seven to Eleven

The success of Diomedes and the other Achaeans does not conform with the plan of Zeus following his promise to Thetis. He forbids the other gods to assist either side and the Trojans gradually win success. As night falls, the Greeks are facing defeat and an assembly is called, at which Nestor recommends sending a small group of leaders to beg Achilles to return to the battle. This again is a famous scene of the *Iliad* and occupies much of one book (Book 9). Odysseus, Ajax and Phoenix are the chosen leaders. They go to the tent of Achilles and use argument and the promise of rich gifts to try to persuade him; but to no avail. Each, in his own way, blunders in argument employing poor rhetoric, where Achilles shows elegant and insightful thinking.

The three ambassadors return to the Achaean leaders and report that Achilles has refused any compromise and intends to return to his home the next morning. The leaders prepare for the following day's fighting. There is an interlude when Diomedes and Odysseus go to spy on the enemy. Agamemnon arms for battle and conducts his own *aristeia*, driving the Trojans back to their city gates. Finally, he is wounded and forced to leave the battle. Hector then rallies his troops and the fighting becomes general and evenly balanced for a while. Gradually, many of the Greek leaders are wounded and have to leave the battle in their turn. It is then the turn of the Greeks to be driven back.

One of the wounded is Machaon, of whom Achilles catches a glimpse as he is driven past to receive aid. Achilles sends Patroclus to find out who the wounded man is ("and so the beginning of his evil end drew near him" (11. 604)). Patroclus meets Nestor who suggests that, if Achilles will not fight himself, he might lend his armour to Patroclus. Sight of Achilles' armour alone may be sufficient to panic the Trojans.

Books Twelve to Seventeen

The action returns to the battle. The Greeks are beaten back, and hemmed in behind a wooden barricade and trench that they built around their ships. The gods have been forbidden from taking part, but Hera seduces Zeus, and the gods join battle as he enjoys a post-coital sleep.

Patroclus returns to Achilles and asks to join the battle wearing Achilles' armour. Achilles gives permission on the understanding that Patroclus only beats back the Trojans from the Greek ships and does not advance towards Troy itself. Patroclus, with the soldiers of Achilles, the Myrmidons, joins battle and beats back the Trojans. For a while it is Patroclus' turn for success and fame in battle. But he forgets, or ignores, Achilles' instruction not to advance on Troy and tries to assault the walls. Finally, the god Apollo, the main defender of Troy, strikes him on the back and renders him senseless; a Trojan puts an arrow in his back and Hector finishes him off with a spear in the belly. A long struggle takes place over the body to seize the armour of Achilles.

Books Eighteen to Twenty-One

News of Patroclus' death is brought to Achilles. He is poised to go back to battle but is prevented by his mother who begs him to wait until morning. In the meantime, she will go to Olympus and beg the craftsman god Hephaestus to make him a new set of armour. Achilles agrees, but at the urging of Athene, appears in the front line and utters a cry, reinforced by Athene, that turns back the Trojans in terror. It is an animal howl, a mix of a keening for Patroclus and a warning call to the Trojan army and Hector in particular.

As night falls, the Trojans encamp outside the city. Achilles receives the body of Patroclus and prepares it for burial. The pathos of this scene is given context by his promise that: "I will behead twelve glorious children of Troy before your pyre".

The creation of Achilles' new armour is described in great detail. Description of armour was a familiar motif in ancient poetry (Agamemnon's armour has already been detailed before his earlier *aristeia*). Achilles' armour, however, is described obsessively, particularly his new shield. Much learned commentary has been devoted to this. One striking aspect is that it is illustrated not with warlike themes (as is Agamemnon's), but rather with pastoral and domestic ones. Perhaps this is to emphasise what Achilles is about to lose by choosing war abroad over peace at home, a choice that he briefly considers, but his Fate is to reject the domestic option for a glorious death on the battlefield and immortality amongst the halls of heroes. The pastoral and domestic option is delayed until the story of Odysseus' homecoming (*nostos*) in the *Odyssey*. The *Iliad's* concern is *kleos*, the glory of the hero.

Achilles' mother presents him with the armour. Achilles calls a general assembly, renounces his anger and calls for an assault on the Trojans. Agamemnon replies with the speech of a weak man, explaining how he came to make such a wrong decision in the first place.

The Greeks now rush enthusiastically back to battle. On Olympus, Zeus is worried that they may be so victorious that Troy is destroyed before its time. Fate was considered a higher force than the gods, who themselves were subject to destiny, and so the gods acted on behalf of the spinners of Fate. Zeus had, earlier in the epic, forbidden the gods from taking any part in the war (a command circumvented several times by various ruses, one described above). He now gives permission for the gods to become involved again. The gods face each other in an amateurish and slightly buffoonish way. The audience knows that the gods are also subject to Fate. And the advance of Achilles is, at first, an anticlimax: he comes up against Aeneas, starts to fight but is robbed of victory because Poseidon whisks Aeneas away from the action. The same thing occurs when he faces Hector. The audience might expect this to be the climactic moment of the epic, but Hector too is taken away, this time by Apollo.

The above scenes are by way of introduction to the savagery to come. Achilles becomes uncontrollable physically and morally as he slaughters every enemy before him. He slips into an animal state, or that of the berserker. He refuses all pleas for clemency and even tries to battle with a river god who complains that Achilles is clogging his stream with corpses. The Trojans fly back behind the walls into Troy leaving the field to the Greeks and Achilles - all except one Trojan who makes a series of tragic blunders.

Books Twenty-Two to Twenty-Four

Hector knows that the reasonable action is for him to go back within the city's walls, but his pride and sense of duty will not permit it. We reach the climax of the epic, and one book, 22, is given over to describing the death of Hector.

Despite his resolve, as soon as Hector sets eyes on the all-conquering Achilles, his heart fails him and he runs away. Achilles pursues. Three times they circle the walls of Troy. The gods have by now withdrawn from the battle and are watching from Olympus. The heart of Zeus goes out to Hector, but he sends Athene to settle his fate. She takes on the guise of Deiphobus, one of Hector's brothers, and offers to fight with him against Achilles. Hector rallies. Before they fight, Hector tries to persuade Achilles that whoever wins should not spoil the body of their opponent but only take his armour. Achilles refuses. Achilles casts his mighty spear at Hector but misses. This should put him at a disadvantage, but Athene returns the spear to him. Hector now realises that he has been deceived but draws his sword and advances on Achilles, who drives the spear through his neck, the one weak point in his armour.

Achilles strips the armour from the body and does defile it, cutting in front of the ankle tendon (the Achilles tendon) to insert leather thongs to drag the body behind his chariot around the walls of Troy - this in front of Hector's father, mother and wife watching, distraught, from the walls above.

This could be the ending of the *Iliad*. Achilles has achieved his aim of making Agamemnon and the Greeks realise how much they depend on him, but he has lost his dearest companion through his actions. The quarrel is resolved and he is revenged on Hector. It is not difficult to imagine a Hollywood revenge movie feeling complete at this point. Homer, however, lifts the *Iliad* to a different level by returning us to the two most important dead heroes.

Achilles returns to the Greek camp and orders the building of a great pyre for the body of Patroclus. He makes sacrifices around the pyre, including twelve noble Trojan youths, and finally sets fire to it. The following morning, the bones of Patroclus are collected, put into a funeral urn and sealed, until the remains of Achilles himself can be added to them.

These funeral rites then move without pause into games held to honour Patroclus.

These games occupy much of the twenty-third book. They probably seemed a more natural sequel to a funeral in ancient times. They also mirror some of the greater events of the *Iliad* – the gods cannot resist interfering in the chariot race to support their favourites, for example, and Achilles shows himself a master of tact and diplomacy in contrast to his actions through the rest of the epic.

The last book of the *Iliad* starts with Achilles unable to overcome the grief for his lost comrade. Each day he drags the body of Hector around the site of the funeral pyre. The body remains unblemished because Apollo protects it. Finally, the gods decide that the body must be returned to his father for burial. Zeus summons Thetis, Achilles' mother, and orders her to tell Achilles to accept a ransom from Priam and return the body. Iris, a messenger of the gods is sent to Priam to instruct him what to do. He prepares a rich ransom and sets off for the Greek encampment. He is guided to the tent of Achilles by the god Hermes, who keeps him invisible to the other Greeks.

Having reached Achilles' tent, Hermes returns to Olympus. Priam enters and grasps the knees of Achilles, the traditional approach of a suppliant. Priam knows that he is risking his life by entering the camp. He asks Achilles to think of his own father beset by problems but at least with the hope of seeing his son again, whereas he, Priam, has lost most of his 50 sons, including the best of them, Hector. He ends this opening speech:

Respect the gods, Achilles, and pity me,/ Remembering your father. I am more pitiable,/ For I have born what no other mortal man has born,/ To bring to my lips the hand of the man who killed my child (*Iliad* 24. 504-6).

The two men weep and Achilles considers the sad state of his father Peleus, for Achilles knows his own fate is to die at Troy. And he thinks too of the decline in fortune of Priam, once rich in wealth and sons. Hector's body is restored and Achilles insists that the two of them share a meal. Achilles generously grants a truce of ten days so that the funeral rites of Hector can be completed. In the morning, Hermes rouses Priam from his bed so that the Trojan King can pass back through the Greek camp before dawn. Hector's body is brought back to Troy and to the three women for whom his death has most resonance. Andromache his wife, Hecuba his mother and Helen, to whom he is one of the few in Troy to have shown kindness, make speeches over his body.

A funeral pyre is built; the body is burned and the remains buried. The people of Troy return to a funeral feast. And we come to the quiet last line of the 15,000 of the *Iliad*: "Thus they tended the grave of Hector, tamer of horses" (24. 804).

The *Odyssey*

Introduction

Where the *Iliad* deals with individuality, or the idiosyncratic personality of the loner in the wild, the *Odyssey* is a meditation on the collective – family and community values. Where the *Iliad's* focus is *kleos* (glory), the *Odyssey's* is *nostos* (homecoming). The hero of the *Iliad*, Achilles, burns out young in battle, where Odysseus lives to a ripe old age in domestic retirement after returning home from the Trojan War.

This tension between the hero who dies young, in a blaze of glory, and the one who returns home to settle in to domestic routine and dies in old age, mirrors the timeless conversation between the virtues of independence and collectivity. The other Ur-text of the West, the *Old Testament,* contains two, apparently contradictory, origin myths: the Garden of Eden and the Seven Days of Creation. The first is an older myth and tells of an idyllic readymade world, expulsion from which is promised through any brazen act of independence such as temptation. The fabric of this world is woven through interdependence and resistance to hierarchy. This creation myth is anti-heroic. The Seven Days of Creation tells an entirely different story – one of building hierarchy and independence, an evolution of dominion with the human at the apex of Creation. This creation myth praises the heroic.

The poet Wallace Stevens describes two conflicting energies at play in the world: "presence" and "force". The Eden myth illustrates "presence" (interdependence), where the Seven Days of Creation myth describes the emergence of "force" (authority). Homer too can be read in this way: the *Odyssey* as a celebration of Presence; the *Iliad* as an eulogy for Force. Longinus, the 1st century AD Graeco-Roman author of *On the Sublime*, compared the *Iliad* and the *Odyssey* as, respectively, the blazing sun and the setting sun, where with the setting sun: " … the size remained, without the force".

In other words, Homer was still an important "presence" with the *Odyssey*, but was wholly magnificent in the *Iliad*. We think Longinus' judgement - that the Homer of the *Odyssey* shows "a mind in decline" - is however unfair. Odysseus is a more complex character study than Achilles. While the *Iliad* hits you between the eyes, the *Odyssey* is a more psychologically astute narrative. For example, where the *Iliad* deals almost exclusively with the masculine psyche in the theatre of war, the *Odyssey* grapples with gender relations. Women play central roles in the unfolding narrative, but more, domesticity of an embracing, feminine kind, is ultimately the prize for Odysseus at the close of his odyssey.

An odyssey is a long, exacting journey. Odysseus' journey home, as recounted by Homer, is for one particular purpose – to restore order to his disrupted household. Hospitality is a primary ethical concern in Homer, and this must be restored in Penelope's household after its disruption. During Odysseus' 20 years' absence Penelope, Odysseus' wife, has become increasingly the object of admiration of a number of suitors who have rudely camped out in her home and seek her hand in marriage, assuming that Odysseus will never return home, breaking hospitality rules. They brazenly live off and deplete the household's resources. Odysseus has been ten years fighting at Troy, seven trapped on Calypso's island, and three travelling on, by turns, "wine dark" and "loud-roaring", seas. Odysseus is the person who has been tossed and turned as well as the "man of many twists and turns" - master of disguise and guile.

Aristotle, in the *Poetics (55b)*, written in the 4th century BC, offers a summary of the *Odyssey* in 63 words:

> A certain man has been abroad many years; he is alone, and the god Poseidon keeps a hostile eye on him. At home the situation is that suitors for his wife's hand are draining his resources and plotting to kill his son. Then, after suffering storm and shipwreck, he comes home, makes himself known, attacks the suitors: he survives and they are destroyed.

We hope to flesh out Aristotle's skeleton key. The German psychologist Eduard Spranger (1882-1963) identified six value orientations that can provide a framework for discussion of any topic or event: the theoretical, social, economic, aesthetic, religious, and political. Aristotle's plain outline tells us nothing of the dramatic influence of Homer, referring only to the story's plot. In both the *Iliad* and *Odyssey*, Homer asks: how shall we understand our lives (theoretical values); live with others communally (social values); what value shall we ascribe to objects that circulate across a community (economic values); what do we mean by "quality", "form", "beauty" and "sublimity" in our lives (aesthetic values); how do we give life meaning (religious values); and what are the relationships of power between people (political values)?

The *Odyssey*, written down probably two centuries before the Old Testament, is a primary source text for addressing these value questions through "thinking otherwise", where, through the character of Odysseus, Homer asks us to address such values issues not head-on in brash

Achillean mode (absolute values), but through "many twists and turns" in Odyssean mode (values as relative and context-bound). Odysseus' framework is contemporary.

Books One to Three

So, to the text - Homer first surprises us with a series of brilliant narrative devices that again make the *Odyssey* look contemporary. Odysseus does not appear until Book Five, a fifth of the way into the text. And there he is introduced by way of flashback to his entrapment on the island of Calypso, described later. The first four books are concerned with Telemachus, son of Odysseus and Penelope, who recognises the gravity of the situation that is developing under his roof with the suitors, sensing danger. Telemachus decides that he must try to seek the whereabouts of his father, if he is alive at all. Homer also uses the literary device of flashback elsewhere – it is in the *Odyssey* that we discover how Troy eventually fell (the story of the wooden horse), and how Achilles died.

The singer of the epic that has come down to us as the *Odyssey* invokes the Muse to allow him to sing of "the man of many twists and turns/ who wandered much….". This introduces the reflective character who excels at plotting a way through life by cunning, tact and deft behaviour, in sharp contrast to the impulsive Achilles. In Book One, the goddess Athene visits Penelope's house in disguise, to let Telemachus know that Odysseus is still alive and will return. Telemachus must tell the suitors to vacate the house. Amongst them, Antinous plots to kill Odysseus' son.

Telemachus calls a meeting of the suitors and rebukes them for their style of courtship of Penelope and their unthinking rape of the household's resources (this includes women servants). Antinous responds by reminding the suitors that Penelope has tricked them – she had promised to choose a new husband as soon as she had finished weaving a coffin shroud for Laertes, Odysseus' ailing, elderly father. However, every night she has been unpicking what was woven the day before, tricking the suitors.

A pair of eagles is spotted overhead, locked in combat, and is taken as an omen that the suitors will be killed by a returning Odysseus if they do not leave the house. Telemachus prepares for a trip to Pylos and Sparta to learn the whereabouts of his father. Athene appears in the disguise of Mentor, Odysseus' friend and advisor. The subplot of Books One and Two is the coming of age of Odysseus' son Telemachus, who must abandon the nest and go on his own journey of discovery.

Telemachus arrives in Pylos, to ask King Nestor if he knows of Odysseus' whereabouts. Nestor has no information, but is able to inform

Telemachus that, upon his return from Troy, Aegisthus had killed Agamemnon with the help of Agamemnon's queen, Clytemnestra, who had been seduced by Aegisthus. This is a warning that the hero's return home may not be a comfortable one! An enduring subplot emerges: absence and heroism in war does not guarantee a hero's welcome home, but may create conditions for a problematic homecoming as life goes on during the hero's absence. The *Odyssey* grapples with this conundrum and presents a scenario of resolution of the "return of the warrior".

Books Four to Six

Telemachus arrives in Sparta, where Queen Helen and King Menelaus recognise him and reminisce about his father's exploits during the siege of Troy. It is a masterful literary ploy, as the character of Odysseus is introduced in layers before we meet the flesh and blood person. The story of the fall of Troy, including the wooden horse, is told. Menelaus has also learned that on his return voyage, Calypso had trapped Odysseus on her island, against his will.

Penelope learns that the suitors are planning to ambush and kill Telemachus on his return, but Athene, in the form of Penelope's sister, reassures her that her son will be protected. The family unit must be kept strong, for this is the magnetic archetype that draws Odysseus home to restore justice (and to a house that has become a viper's nest). We learn from these early chapters of the central role that hospitality (*xenia*) plays in the *Odyssey*. Indeed, the grand theme of the epic song is the play of currents between the magnetic hospitality of a household and the many upsets that can occur, through fate, as one circles an "attractor" of hospitality. We can read the *Odyssey* through a contemporary lens, as a dynamic, complex adaptive system, in which various natural forces (the gods' interventions, mythical beings) and psychological presences (the major characters) are emergent properties of that system, pulled to the main attractor of Penelope's and Odysseus' household that strives for stability.

In the absence of the sea god Poseidon, Odysseus' sworn enemy (Odysseus had blinded the Cyclops Polyphemus, the son of Poseidon), the gods persuade Calypso to release Odysseus, after eight years of entrapment. His crew has long since perished. He builds a boat and leaves. Eighteen days later, he sees an island, but just before landing, Poseidon spots him and sends a storm that nearly drowns Odysseus. Athene saves him and he is cast ashore, taken safely up a river and into a forest. Book Five segues into Book Six, where we find the naked Odysseus recovering from his near death by drowning to encounter the Phaeacian princess Nausicaa and her handmaidens, washing their clothes.

Nausicaa falls in love with the handsome Odysseus and gives him directions to the palace of her mother Arete, Queen of the Phaeacians, with advice on how he might best benefit from the latter's hospitality. Within these scenes – the shipwreck and the open encounter – Homer introduces many subtle issues about manners and what we now call "reflexive" social behaviour. Much of what happens with Odysseus is heavily coded, and nuances of behaviour are often ascribed to the appearance of a goddess who shapes that behaviour. In contrast to Achilles, who is characteristically blunt and direct, Odysseus is a master of performance, guise and guile. A comedy of manners runs in parallel with the epic that is Odysseus' homecoming. The audience is presented with the moral dilemma that the man of many twists and turns also falls in and out of sexual encounters in his long journey home, where Penelope is cast as faithful, warding off her suitors.

Books Seven to Nine

Book Seven sees Odysseus welcomed by Phaeacian royalty, but for the "man of many twists and turns" nothing is ever direct or to the point. Odysseus is smuggled into the court in a shroud of mist, as if a god, to prevent xenophobic comments, and declares himself a mortal to the king and queen who promise him a ship to continue his journey. But the queen recognises that Odysseus is wearing clothes borrowed from her daughter Nausicaa. Odysseus explains the earlier encounter at the river, with such eloquence that King Alcinous offers him his daughter in marriage. The audience knows that Odysseus' eloquence is also part of his slipperiness. He had introduced himself as a master of "craft" – in other words, he is "crafty", a schemer. The Greek *dolos* ("craft") is what Jacques Derrida describes as a "pharmakon" or "healing poison", a word carrying two encapsulated, contradictory, meanings – *dolos* can be used as praise or abuse, compliment or accusation.

In Book Eight, Alcinous calls an assembly to discuss the presence of Odysseus, where it is decided that he shall receive a ship to continue his voyage, while a feast and games celebration is planned in his honour. A blind bard Demodocus sings of the quarrel between Achilles and Odysseus during the Trojan War, upsetting Odysseus.

The duplicity of Odysseus (literally a "doublefold" nature) is again anathema to the direct, in-your-face style of Achilles. Reluctant to participate in the games, when forced to by goading from his young hosts,

Odysseus wipes the floor with the other contestants. The audience is reminded that Odysseus is already expert and the young men who goad him, suspecting frailty, are novices, interested only in physical prowess and not in the wisdom that shapes the appropriate expression of the physical.

At the post-games celebrations, Demodocus sings of the wooden horse and the sack of Troy and Odysseus breaks down, crying, forcing Alcinous to ask Odysseus to come clean – who is he really and where is he bound for? Odysseus is forced to reveal his identity and history, but Homer continues to create an ever more complex knot for Odysseus' character, refusing transparency.

Book Nine recounts Odysseus' adventures: swept by winds to the land of the Cicones, Odysseus' men are consumed by greed and plunder the land, only to be forced out by the Cicones, who kill many of Odysseus' crew. Swept by a storm to the land of the Lotus Eaters, Odysseus' crew become intoxicated, having eaten the local fruits that cause them to lose their memories or any desire for change. Odysseus has to drag his crew back to the ship and lock them up. What Homer begins to do is to describe a side to Odysseus that the audience has not yet fully appreciated – he can be a caring leader.

The crew sails to the land of the Cyclopes where they aim to refresh their stocks from a hoard of milk and cheese discovered by chance in the cave of Polyphemus, son of Poseidon. Despite the crew urging him to snatch what they can and get out of Polyphemus' cave while the going is good, Odysseus makes the mistake of lingering, and they are trapped in the cave by the Cyclops who eats two of the men and promises the same tomorrow. While Odysseus can care, he can also be careless.

Unable to roll back the stone covering the cave's entrance and exit, Odysseus must come up with a plan for escape. He gets Polyphemus drunk on wine brought from his ship and drives a sharpened stake into his eye, blinding him. Previously asked by the Cyclops "what is your name?", Odysseus had replied "Nobody". The blind Polyphemus staggers out of the cave, screaming that "Nobody's killing me", so no help comes. Odysseus and his crew escape from the cave by clinging to the bellies of sheep as they move out to graze.

They manage to return safely to the ships despite Polyphemus hurling rocks, where Odysseus, in an act of hubris, stupidly calls out his name to Polyphemus as a taunt, attaching the little used epithet "raider of cities". For a moment, Odysseus is overtaken by the desire for *kleos* or glory, forgetting the trajectory of his destiny that is *nostos*, homecoming. The Cyclops, in response, calls on his father Poseidon to punish Odysseus and his crew. It is Odysseus' almost fatal error to incur the wrath of the sea god Poseidon – for he must return home by storm-tossed sea.

This chapter is told as flashbacks, a narrative technique that collapses time in the epic to provide a hugely concentrated account. The story is not spun out, but gathers intensity around the strengths and weaknesses of Odysseus' duplicity. The mythological genre provides scope for allegory. While the audience admires his cunning and bravery in the plan to outwit the Cyclops, this is sandwiched by two pieces of outright stupidity on the part of Odysseus: lingering in the Cyclops' cave and calling out his name as the ships set sail. It is Homer's reminder that all heroes, of whatever stamp, are flawed. Indeed, the audience may show more sympathy with Polyphemus, who shows tenderness towards his animals, a child-like innocence, and some regard for Odysseus and his crew before he is irked.

Books Ten to Twelve

Odysseus can practically touch the shores of Ithaca in Book Ten as he sails so close to home that he can see fires burning on the cliff. But again, he makes a silly mistake. From the land of the Cyclopes, Odysseus and his crew reach the land of Aeolus who rules the wind. Here, the winds are put in a bag apart from a westerly wind, stirred up to send Odysseus safely back to Ithaca. The journey takes ten days. In sight of home, Odysseus falls asleep at the wheel. His crew, curious to see what is in the bag and imagining that Odysseus may be hiding treasure from them, opens the bag to release the winds. The audience sees that a scheming person may never be able to obtain the full trust of others, no matter how much he cares for them. A storm drives the ships back to Aeolia, where further help is angrily refused.

The crews row the ships to the land of the Laestrygonians, giants who eat Odysseus' scout patrol who have gone ahead of the main party. The giants throw boulders at the ships as Odysseus and his men try to escape, with only Odysseus' ship surviving. The crew arrives at Aeaea, home of Circe, in one of the most famous incidents in the epic. Circe enchants the crew, turning them into swine, but Odysseus is met by Hermes disguised as a young man, who tells him to eat the plant Moly to protect himself from the drug used by Circe to transform the crew into pigs.

Thom Gunn's poem "Moly" describes human consciousness embedded in the pig-body, knowing that the flesh is "streaked" like ham, with "jostling mobs" of unknown germs, the pig rooting for moly so that transformation back to human form can take place. Of human form, the pig retains only "pale-lashed eyes". Otherwise human flesh is "buried in swine". Odysseus will not taste this unwelcome transformation and entrapment as he ingests the moly plant. Hermes too had told Odysseus to lunge at Circe if she should try to strike him with her sword. He does this successfully, but in the ensuing glance and embrace, something clicks.

Odysseus becomes Circe's lover. He persuades her to turn the pigs' flesh back into his crew's human forms. Odysseus and his crew stay a year, but boredom sets in and the crew gets itchy feet, persuading Odysseus that they should resume their journey to Ithaca. Circe tells Odysseus that he must however first visit Hades, the place of the dead, to talk with the blind prophet Tiresias who will tell him how to get home.

Elpenor, the youngest of Odysseus' crew, had fallen drunk from a roof, broken his neck and died on the morning of departure, and it is Elpenor that Odysseus first meets as he carries out a ceremony given to him by Circe to attract the souls of the dead. Elpenor pleads to be given a proper burial. This is a wonderful human touch amongst the fantastic geographies and mental states that Books Nine and Ten have conjured. We might see these Books as dreams, and Book Eleven continues this exploration of a dark psychogeography with the visit to Hades, that inspired both Virgil and Dante.

Odysseus then had travelled to the land of the Cimmerians and visited the River of Oceans that is the gateway to Hades, as instructed by Circe. After Elpenor's ghost, Tiresias' shade appears to tell Odysseus that Poseidon is punishing him, trying to drown him, but that Odysseus fate is to return home and confront the suitors in his palace, and that Penelope will be his prize. He must, however, travel once more to a distant place in order to appease Poseidon. Further, he will travel to the land of Thrinacia on the way to Ithaca, but there, he must not interfere with the cattle of the sun god, otherwise he and his crew will suffer greatly.

Odysseus meets the shade of his mother Anticleia, who explains how she died of grief when he did not return immediately from the war; and, in particular, he talks with the ghosts of Agamemnon, and then Achilles, who has taken on the psychological tone of the underworld and is deeply depressed at his fate, wishing that he could return to the world of the living to carve out a different fate. Hades is misery. The audience is able to fill in the blanks from the *Iliad*, to gain some continuity of story between that and the *Odyssey*. The treatment of Achilles as fed up with his lot says much – it signals a favouring of *nostos*, homecoming, domesticity and longevity, over *kleos,* glory in battle and an early death; presence over force; the hero's absorption into the collective rather than the autonomous act.

Elpenor is indeed given a proper burial as Odysseus and his crew say goodbye to Circe who advises him on how to navigate dangers ahead. Odysseus remembers her advice as they sail past the island of the Sirens, who would seduce them, as he plugs his men's ears with beeswax to dampen the Sirens' calls, and ties himself to the mast. Only he can hear the call of the Sirens and it drives him to desperately plead with his crew to release him from his bindings – but they have been instructed to only bind him tighter. They then navigate between Scylla, a six-headed monster, and Charybdis, a fatal whirpool. They have been advised to stick close to Scylla, whatever the consequences, and indeed the sea monster eats six members of the crew.

At Thrinacia, the island of the sun, despite misgivings, the crew beach there and stay for a month as a storm passes. Eurylochus, a member of the crew, persuades others to slaughter the cattle of the sun god, against Odysseus' advice. It is a fatal mistake. Odysseus again has slept on his watch. The sun god informs Zeus of the transgression and Zeus sends a storm that destroys the ship and the entire crew except for Odysseus, who clings, barely alive, to a timber from the stricken ship. He is swept past Charybdis, barely surviving the ordeal, and is beached at Calypso's island, Ogygia.

Homer reveals the logic of the *Odyssey* as the myth of Eternal Return. Similar things happen to humans on cycles through a life course, but they must deal with them differently, according to inflections and contexts. Importantly, humanity as a whole must learn from the past. Odysseus breaks from telling his tale to the Phaeacians. They now have heard his misadventures in the round. It is a kind of confession, but one beyond belief, as would be expected of the trickster.

Books Thirteen to Sixteen

Book Thirteen sees Odysseus preparing for his final voyage, from Scheria to Ithaca, brought by a Phaeacian crew. Odysseus sleeps the whole way and is deposited on the shore of Ithaca still asleep. Poseidon is so angry at seeing how the Phaeacians helped Odysseus that he turns their ship to stone as it enters its home harbour, drowning the whole crew. The Phaeacians think twice about the reach of their hospitality and this questioning of the moral authority of the hospitality rule presents a conundrum to the audience. It is best addressed by an even higher principle than *xenia* or hospitality – harmony amongst the gods. Zeus does not wish to fall out with Poseidon.

True to the trickster theme that runs through the epic, Odysseus finds himself at home in a land he now does not recognise, for Athene has shrouded it in mist. Disguised as a shepherd, Athene assures Odysseus that he is indeed in Ithaca. But, instead of simply making his way to his home and presenting himself as a returning hero, Odysseus slips into the habit of guile, disguising himself even in his meeting with Athene, which delights her as the mistress of disguise. She further disguises Odysseus as an old good-for-nothing beggar and tells him to stay in the hut of the swineherd Eumaeus. Further, she lets him know that his son Telemachus is looking for him.

Eumaeus, in Book Fourteen, fails to recognise his old master Odysseus, but Odysseus decides not to blow his cover, pretending that he was a foot soldier who fought with Odysseus at Troy and had now returned home via Egypt, where, he heard, Odysseus was indeed still alive.

Telemachus is still in Sparta. Athene urges him to hurry on home, avoiding the ambush set by the suitors. As he leaves Sparta, an eagle swoops down by him with a goose taken from a pen in his claws. This is seen as an omen that Odysseus will swoop mercilessly to take revenge upon the suitors. Meanwhile, Odysseus, still in disguise, swaps stories with Eumaeus. Book Fifteen closes with Telemachus arriving on the shore of Ithaca to see a hawk carrying a dove in its talons – another sign that Odysseus is about to swoop on the suitors.

Book Sixteen opens with Telemachus arriving at Eumaeus' hut, unaware that the stranger is his father. Eumaeus suggests that the stranger go back with Telemachus to the palace, but Telemachus resists this in fear of what the suitors might do. Eumaeus goes to the palace on his own. Athene appears at the hut and calls Odysseus outside, stripping him of his disguise. He stands before Telemachus and there is joyful recognition, embrace and tears. They hatch a plan to surprise and overthrow the suitors who, meanwhile, are now in confusion about killing Telemachus. The audience also learns that while Antinous remains a villain, other suitors such as Amphinomus are reasonable and do not wish to harm Telemachus. Homer then introduces a dilemma – if Odysseus and Telemachus are to slaughter the suitors en masse, will they, wrongly, be tarring them all with the same brush?

Books Seventeen to Twenty Four

Books Seventeen and Eighteen prepare us for the climax of the epic, the showdown between the suitors and the returning hero and its political consequences. Telemachus returns home but does not reveal that he has met with his father. Rumours abound that Odysseus is in Ithaca. Odysseus appears at the palace in disguise and is roundly abused by Antinous, such that Penelope asks to see him. In Book Eighteen a beggar appears at the palace and insults Odysseus. A boxing match ensues in which the beggar is roundly thrashed and the audience senses that Odysseus' disguise is wearing thin. He takes the moderate suitor Amphinomus aside and warns him to leave – a warning that is not heeded, for Amphinomus is fated to die at the hands of Telemachus.

Penelope appears in full glory and beauty before the suitors and demands that if one is to take her hand in marriage, he must shower her with presents rather than depleting her household's resources. The suitors respond with a display of gifts. Odysseus' anger is coming to a boil. Still in disguise as the beggar, he tells the servants to go to Penelope, scaring them with threats. Athene is pleased to see that Odysseus is spoiling for the showdown with the suitors. She provokes Eurymachus into insulting Odysseus. He throws a stool at the beggar, but it misses, hitting a servant instead. Telemachus steps in to cool the situation down.

The kettle is coming to a boil. Books Nineteen to Twenty One maintain the high tension. In Book Twenty Two, the violent finale erupts.

The beauty of the *Odyssey*, reflecting the theme of duplicity in its various disguises - both good and bad, useful and useless - is that high drama is interspersed with tender revelations. Characters are developed in both contexts. In Book Nineteen, Odysseus and Telemachus remove the arms from the palace (so that the suitors cannot use them), and Penelope, curious, talks to Odysseus without recognition. He assures her that her husband will return within the month.

Odysseus' old wet nurse, Eurycleia, comes to wash his feet after Odysseus refuses the offer of a bed from Penelope, saying that he will sleep on the floor. Eurycleia sees a wound on Odysseus' thigh and recognises it as a scar he got from being gored while boar hunting. He is finally unmasked. He swears the old nurse to secrecy.

Penelope returns and informs Odysseus that she had a dream in which an eagle swooped down on 20 geese, killing them all. The eagle then spoke to her saying that he is her husband and has killed her lovers. Odysseus attempts to explain the meaning of the dream, but Penelope brushes this aside, saying that she has finally decided to marry one of the suitors who can pass a test – firing an arrow cleanly through the holes of 12 axe heads set in a line. This seems an impossible task and is difficult to conceive.[1]

In Book Twenty, the suitors are still tormenting Odysseus in his beggar disguise. There is a scene in which a vision grips the entire hall – the suitors appear as deathly ghosts and the walls are covered in blood. Prior to this there is an ominous thunderclap. Homer builds the tension. Odysseus is at breaking point, ready to drop his disguise. In Book Twenty One, Odysseus' bow is brought out for the archery test, but the suitors fail to even string it. Odysseus easily strings the bow to send an arrow straight through the aligned holes of the 12 axe heads. This is the prelude to the slaughter.

Book Twenty Two is an account of an incident as bloody as any in the *Iliad*, indeed, any in literature. With bow in hand, having just shot through the axe heads and before anyone can draw a breath, Odysseus wheels and shoots an arrow straight through the throat of Antinous. At first, the suitors imagine that this is an accident, but Odysseus reveals himself and the suitors panic. They are trapped and brutally slaughtered by Odysseus, Telemachus, Eumaeus and Philoetius. It is another "All Day Permanent Red" (Logue 2003), but Homer too includes slapstick violence of the kind we are used to in the modern era from Quentin Tarantino, including a brutal castration. Eurycleia is asked to round up the disloyal women servants who clear the hall of corpses and blood, and are then led outside to be slaughtered in the most terrible fashion, hung and strangled by a wire. The house is then fumigated.

Penelope has slept through the slaughter and still does not know that the beggar is Odysseus. Eurycleia wakes her and brings her downstairs, where Odysseus is now recognised. There is no instant reunion, but a stunned moment as Odysseus works out how he will now handle the situation that he has just killed all the eligible young noblemen of Ithaca. Penelope tests Odysseus by asking Eurycleia to move their marriage bed. Odysseus knows that it cannot be moved as it was carved out of the trunk of an olive tree around which the house was built. Penelope now knows that this is indeed her husband, and they go to bed, where he tells her of his travels and of the trip he must make to appease Poseidon.

The *Odyssey* could finish here, at Book Twenty Three on a moment of tension, the audience left wondering what the outcome of this slaughter will mean for the people of Ithaca; and on the moment of erotic reunion of Penelope and Odysseus. But Odysseus is yet to be reunited with his father, and peace must be made across the land.

In Book Twenty Four, the dead suitors enter Hades, surely an aberration as the bodies have received no proper burial. Odysseus visits his elderly father Laertes at the latter's farm, and after a period where the father doesn't recognise the son, Odysseus shows his scar and recalls the fruit trees Laertes gave him as a boy. They embrace. Odysseus recounts the slaughter in the hall. The scene seems stiff and forced after the songs that precede it.

Meanwhile, news of the slaughter has spread through Ithaca. The response is mixed. Antinous' father however suggests seeking revenge and organises a kind of lynch party whose members bear down on Laertes' farm. Everybody readies himself for a new fight, and there is brief violence, where Antinous' father is killed by one of Laertes' spears. But Athene interrupts and demands that the violence end and that a new era of peace should prevail. This is just as Odysseus is about to swoop on his enemies, halted by a thunderbolt from Zeus.

Finishing the *Odyssey* with Penelope's and Odysseus' tender and erotic reunion in book 23 would make sense to us romantics, but also leaves a lot of unfinished business. Most commentators see the final book as an unsatisfactory patchwork of tales from elsewhere and some doubt its authenticity. It is difficult to see quite what "authenticity" means in this context. The scene of the dead suitors conversing with the dead Greek heroes in Hades is certainly bizarre. However, the book has survived from antiquity; and Odysseus' acknowledgement that his son is now a mature warrior, his reunion with his father and the restoration of the latter to his "heroic splendour" fit both theme and narrative.[2] But it does have a strange and abrupt end. It is as if a new story wants to be told, but is not yet ripe.

There is, however, a certain logic in this poorly constructed ending – it fits the transition from the martial to the pastoral, from heroic individualism to a more feminine collective endeavour, The pacific ending allows the two stories of the *Iliad* and *Odyssey* to fit together as a whole, as two sides of life: Force and Presence.

Notes

1. Several possible arrangements are suggested by Jones (2002, p.185).
2. See Jones (2002, pp.216-17).

BIBLIOGRAPHY

Aasland, O.G., and Førde, R. "Impact of Feeling Responsible for Adverse Events on Doctors' Personal and Professional Lives: The Importance of Being Open to Criticism from Colleagues." *Quality and Safety in Health Care* 14 (2005): 13–17.

Advisory Board. 2012. "When surgeons throw scalpels, anger-management experts get the call." Accessed April 10, 2013.
http://www.advisory.com/Daily-Briefing/2012/08/06/When-surgeons-throw-scalpels-anger-management-experts-get-the-call

Agency for Healthcare Research and Quality (AHRQ). *National Healthcare Quality Report*. Rockville, MD: US Department of Health and Human Services. HealthGrades Quality Study. *The Eleventh Annual Health Grades Hospital Quality in America Study October 2008*. Health Grades, Inc., 2008. Accessed July 2, 2011.
http://www.healthgrades.com/media/DMS/pdf/HealthGradesEleventhAnnualHospitalQualityStudy2008.pdf

Agerholm, H. 2016. "One in Five CEOs are Psychopaths, New Study Finds." Accessed December 30, 2016.
http://www.independent.co.uk/news/world/australasia/psychopaths-ceos-study-statistics-one-in-five-psychopathic-traits-a7251251.html

Alexander C. *The War that Killed Achilles: The True Story of the* Iliad. London: Faber and Faber, 2009.

Allard, J., Wyatt, J., Bleakley, A., and Graham, B. "Do you really need to ask me that now?": a self-audit of interruptions to the 'shop floor' practice of a UK consultant emergency physician." *Emergency Medicine Journal* 29 (2012): 872-6.

Allums, L. (ed.) *The Epic Cosmos*. Dallas, TX: The Dallas Institute, 1992.

Antonaccio, C.M. *An Archaeology of Ancestors. Tomb Cult and Hero Cult in Early Greece*. Rowman & Littlefield Publishers Inc, Lanham, Maryland, 1995.

Arbery, G.C. 1992. "Soul and Image: The Single Honor of Achilles." In *The Epic Cosmos,* edited by L. Allums, 27-58. Dallas, TX: The Dallas Institute, 1992.

Arnheim, R. *Visual Thinking*. Berkeley, CA: University of California Press, 2004.

Arnold, M. *On Translating Homer*. New York, NY: Routledge and Sons, 1905.

Arnold, L., and Stern, D.T. "What is Medical Professionalism?" In *Measuring Medical Professionalism*, edited by Stern, D.T. 15-38. Oxford: Oxford University Press, 2006.

Arrigo, B.A. "Martial Metaphors and Medical Justice: Implications for Law, Crime, and Deviance." *Journal of Political and Military Sociology* 27 (1999): 307-22.

Asadpour, M., Sabzevari, L., Ekramifar, A., and Bidaki, R. "The Attitude of Medical Students Towards Death: A Cross-sectional Study in Rafsanjan." *Indian Journal of Palliative Care* 22 (2016): 354-61.

Baggini, J. "Compassion Fatigue." *Financial Times Weekend*. 21/ 22 Jan, 2017, 9.

Bakker, E.J. *Poetry in Speech*. Ithaca: Cornell University Press, 1997.

Bakker, E. "The Study of Homeric Discourse." In *A New Companion to Homer*, edited by Morris, I., and Powell, B. 284-304. Leiden: Brill, 2011.

Baldwin, D. C., Daugherty, S. R., and Eckenfels, E.J. "Student Perceptions of Mistreatment and Harassment During Medical School - A Survey of Ten United States Schools." *Western Journal of Medicine* 155 (1991): 140-5.

Baldwin, D. C., and Daugherty, S. R. "Do Residents Also Feel 'Abused'?" *Academic Medicine* 72 (1997): S51-53.

Barfield, O. *Poetic Diction: A Study in Meaning*. Middletown, CT: Wesleyan University Press, 1973.

Barker, E., and Christensen, J. *Homer. A Beginner's Guide*. London: Oneworld Publications, 2013.

Barron, K., Atkins, C., Bone, P., Dowd, J., Gidley, S., Hesford, S., Naysmith, D., Scott, L., Stoate, H., Syms, R., and Taylor, R. 2009. *House of Commons Health Committee Patient Safety: Sixth Report of Session, 2008-9*. Accessed January 10, 2017. http://www.publications.parliament.uk/pa/cm200809/cmselect/cmhealth/151/151i.pdf

Bates, M.J., Bowles, S., Hammermeister, J., Stokes, C., Pinder, E., Moore, M., Fritts, M., Vythilingam, M., Yosick, T., Rhodes, J., Myatt, C., Westphal, R., Fautua,D., Hammer, P., and Burbelo, G. 2010. "Psychological Fitness." *Military Medicine* 175 (2010): 21-38.

Bauman, R. *Verbal Art as Performance*. Long Grove, Illinois: Waveland Press Inc., 1977.

Bazalgette, P. *The Empathy Instinct: How to Create a More Civil Society*. London: John Murray, 2017.

Becker, H. S., Geer, B., Hughes, E. C., and Strauss, A. L. *Boys in White: Student Culture in Medical School.* Chicago, Ill.: University of Chicago Press, 1961.

Beckett, S. *The Unnamable.* New York, NY: Grove/ Atlantic, 1953/ 1978.

Bell C. "War and the Allegory of Medical Intervention: Why Metaphors Matter." *International Political Sociology* 6 (2012): 325-8.

Bell, S.K., Smulowitz, P.B., Woodward, A.C., Mello, M.M., Duva, A.M., Boothman, R.C., and Sands, K. "Disclosure, Apology, and Offer Programs: Stakeholders' Views of Barriers to and Strategies for Broad Implementation." *The Milbank Quarterly* 90 (2012): 682–705.

Benedict, R. *The Chrysanthemum and the Sword.* London: Houghton Mifflin, 1946.

Bergonzi, B. *A Study in Greene.* Oxford: Oxford University Press, 2006.

Berlin, L. "Will Saying 'I'm Sorry' Prevent a Malpractice Lawsuit?" *American Journal of Roentgenology* 187 (2006): 10-15.

—. "When Things Go Wrong. Responding to Adverse Events". 2006. Massachusetts Coalition for the Prevention of Medical Errors. Accessed on February 12, 2017. http://www.macoalition.org/documents/respondingToAdverseEvents.pdf

Bleakley, A. "Sublime Moments in the Body of the Double Pelican." In *On the Sublime in Psychoanalysis and Analytic Psychotherapy*, edited by Clarkson, P., 46–68. London: Whurr Publications, 1977.

—. "From Reflective Practice to Holistic Reflexivity." *Studies in Higher Education* 24 (1999): 315-30.

—. "You Are Who I Say You Are: The Rhetorical Construction of Identity in the Operating Theatre." *Journal of Workplace Learning* 18 (2006a): 414-25.

—. "A Common Body of Care: The Ethics and Politics of Trust in the Operating Theatre are Inseparable." *Journal of Medicine and Philosophy* 31 (2006b): 305-22.

—. "The Proof is in the Pudding: Putting Actor-Network Theory to Work in Medical Education." *Medical Teacher* 34 (2012): 462-7.

—. "Gender Matters in Medical Education." *Medical Education* 47 (2013a): 59-70.

—. "Working in 'Teams' in an Era of 'Liquid' Healthcare: What is the Use of Theory?" *Journal of Interprofessional Care* 27 (2013b): 18-26.

—. *Patient-Centred Medicine in Transition. The Heart of the Matter.* Dordrecht: Springer, 2014.

—. *Thinking With Metaphors in Medicine: The State of the Art*. London: Routledge, 2017.

Bleakley, A., Bligh, J., and Browne, J. *Medical Education for the Future: Identity, Power and Location*. Dordrecht: Springer, 2011.

Bleakley, A., Farrow, R., Gould, D., and Marshall, R. "Making sense of clinical reasoning: judgement and the evidence of the senses." *Medical Education* 37 (2003): 544-52.

Bleakley, A., and Marshall, R.J. "The Embodiment of Lyricism in Medicine and Homer." *Medical Humanities* 38 (2012): 50-4.

Bleakley, A., and Marshall, R.J. "Can the Science of Communication Inform the Art of the Medical Humanities?" *Medical Education* 47 (2013): 126-33.

Bleakley, A., Marshall, R.J., and Levine, D. "He Drove Forward with a Yell: Anger in Medicine and Homer." *Medical Humanities* 40 (2014): 22-30.

Bloom, P. "Empathy's Perilous Pull." *New Scientist* 3111 (2017): 24-25.

—. *Against Empathy: The Case for Rational Compassion*. London: The Bodley Head, 2017.

Bolsin, S., Pal, R., Wilmshurst, P., and Pena, M. "Whistleblowing and Patient Safety: The Patient's or the Profession's Interests at Stake?" *Journal of the Royal Society of Medicine* 104 (2011): 78-282.

Bonanno, G.A. "Loss, Trauma, and Human Resilience. Have We Underestimated the Human Capacity to Thrive After Extremely Aversive Events?" *American Psychologist* 59 (2004): 20-28.

Bonner, T.N. Iconoclast: Abraham Flexner and a Life in Learning. Baltimore, MD: Johns Hopkins University Press, 2002.

Boodman SG. "Doctors' Diagnostic Errors Are Often Not Mentioned But Can Take A Serious Toll", May 6, 2013 *Kaiser Health News*. Accessed on February 12 2017. http://khn.org/news/doctor-errors-misdiagnosis-more-common-than-known-serious-impact/

Bowra, C.M. *Heroic Poetry*. London: Macmillan Press, 1978.

Brecht, B. *The Life of Galileo*. Scene 13. London: Methuen, 1995.

Brennan, T.A., Leape, L.L., Laird, N.M., Hebert, L., Localio, A.R., Lawthers, A.G., Newhouse, J.P., Weiler, P.C., and Hiatt, H.H. "Incidence of Adverse Events and Negligence in Hospitalized Patients. Results of the Harvard Medical Practice Study I." *New England Journal of Medicine* 324 (1991): 370-376.

British Medical Association (BMA). "Doctors in difficulty/ Doctors' well-being." Accessed January 15, 2016.

http://www.bma.org.uk/support-at-work/doctors-well-being/websites-for-doctors-in-difficulty

British Medical Association. *Misuse of alcohol and other drugs by doctors*. London: BMA, 1998.

—. 2012. *Whistleblowing.* Accessed October 18, 2016.
https://www.bma.org.uk/advice/employment/raising-concerns/guide-to-raising-concerns.

Brixey, J., Johnson, T.R., and Zhang, J. "Evaluating a Medical Error Taxonomy." *Proceedings of the AMIA Symposium. American Medical Informatics Association* (2002): 71-5.

Brooks, S.K., Gerada, C., and Chalder, T. "Review of Literature on the Mental Health of Doctors: Are Specialist Services Needed?" *Journal of Mental Health* 20 (2011): 146-56. Accessed December 28, 2016
http://www.tandfonline.com/doi/full/10.3109/09638237.2010.541300

Burke, K. *Language as Symbolic Action: Essays on Life, Literature and Method*. Berkeley, CA: University of California Press, 1966.

Burkert, W. "The Song of Ares and Aphrodite: On the Relationship between the *Odyssey* and the *Iliad*." In *Homer's Odyssey. Oxford Readings in Classical Studies,* edited by L.E. Doherty. Oxford: OUP, 2009

Burkhart, R. A., Tholey, R., Guinto, D., Yeo, C. J., and Chojnacki, K. A. "Grit: A Marker of Residents at Risk for Attrition?" *Surgery* 155 (2014): 1014–22.

Burston, D. *The Wing of Madness: The Life and Work of R. D. Laing*. Cambridge, Mass: Harvard University Press, 2nd ed., 1998.

Cairns, D.L. *Aidos: The Psychology and Ethics of Honour and Shame in Ancient Greek Literature*. Oxford: Clarendon Press, 1993.

Calasso, R. *The Marriage of Cadmus and Harmony*. New York, NY: Vintage, 1994.

Campbell, D. "Junior doctors' sleep deprivation poses threat to patients, says GMC." *The Guardian*, Thursday 1 December 2016. Accessed on February 12 2017.
https://www.theguardian.com/society/2016/dec/01/junior-doctors-sleep-deprivation-poses-threat-to-patients-says-gmc

Campbell, J. *The Hero with a Thousand Faces*. New York, NY: Pantheon Books, 1949.

—. *Historical Atlas of World Mythology 1: The Way of the Animal Powers*. New York, NY: Times Books, 1984.

—. *Historical Atlas of World Mythology 2: The Way of the Seeded Earth*. New York, NY: Times Books, 1988.

Canguilhem, G. *The Normal and the Pathological.* New York: Zone Books, 1991.

Cantor, P.A., Hufnagel, P. "The Olympics of the Mind: Philosophy and Athletics in the Ancient Greek World." In *The Olympics and Philosophy* edited by Reid, H.L. and Austin, M.W., 49-67. Lexington: University Press of Kentucky, 2012.

Carpenter, L. *Why Doctors Hide Their Own Illnesses. The Guardian* Friday May 16, 2014. Accessed December 25, 2016. https://www.theguardian.com/society/2014/may/16/why-doctors-hide-their-own-illnesses

Cartledge, P. *The Greeks. A Portrait of Self and Others.* Oxford: Oxford University Press, 2002.

Chapman, G., trans. *The* Iliad *and The* Odyssey *of Homer.* Ware: Wordsworth Editions Limited, 2000.

Charon, R. "The Novelization of the Body, or, How Medicine and Stories Need One Another." *Narrative* 19 (2011): 33-50.

Chen, P. "When the Patient Gets Lost in Translation." April 23 2009. Accessed 19 February 2017-02-19 http://www.nytimes.com/2009/04/23/health/23chen.html

Chesterton, G.K. *The Man Who Was Thursday: A Nightmare.* New York, NY: Bartleby, 1908/ 1999.

Cicero, Marcus Tullius. "*De optimo genere oratorum.*" In M Tulli Ciceronis. *Rhetorica*, edited by Wilkins AS. Oxford: Oxford University Press 5:14, 1903, translated by RJM.

Claridge, M-T., and Lewis, T. *Coaching for effective learning.* Oxford: Radcliffe Publishing, 2005.

Clark, A. *Being there: putting brain, body and world together again.* London: MIT Press, 1999.

Clarke, M. "Manhood and Heroism." In *The Cambridge Companion to Homer*, edited by Fowler R, 74-90. Cambridge: Cambridge University Press, 2004.

Clay, J.S. *The Wrath of Athena: Gods and Men in the* Odyssey. London: Rowman & Littlefield, 1997.

Cohen, N. Let the law save whistleblowers, not silence them. *The Observer,* Sunday 10 July 2011. Accessed October 11, 2016. https://www.theguardian.com/commentisfree/2011/jul/10/whistleblowers-rupert-murdoch-nhs-nick-cohen

Coid, J. 1991. "Interviewing the Aggressive Patient." In *Developing communication and counselling skills in medicine,* edited by Corney R, 96-112. London: Routledge.

Coleman, M., and Ganong, L. "Resilience and Families." *Family Relations* 51 (2002): 101.

Cooke, M., Irby, D.M., and O'Brien, M. *Educating Physicians: A Call for Reform of Medical School and Residency.* San Francisco, CA: Jossey-Bass, 2011

Coombs, R.H. *Drug-impaired Professionals.* Cambridge, Mass.: Harvard University Press, 1997.

Coulter, A. *The Autonomous Patient: Ending paternalism in medical care.* London: The Stationery Office, 2002.

Coverdale, J.H., Balon, R., and Roberts, L.W. "Mistreatment of Trainees: Verbal Abuse and Other Bullying Behaviors." *Academic Psychiatry* 33 (2009): 269-73.

Cowan, B. (ed.) *The Prospect of Lyric.* Dallas, TX: Dallas Institute Publications.

Curtis, A-M. 2014. "Is It Ever Right to Tell Off Trainees in Public?". British Medical Association (BMA). 20th Feb 2014. Accessed January 15, 2016. http://www.bma.org.uk/news-views-analysis/work/2014/february/is-it-ever-right-to-tell-off-trainees-in-public

Dalby, A. *Rediscovering Homer: inside the origins of the epic.* New York, NY: W.W. Norton, 2006.

Davidoff, F. "Shame: The Elephant in the Room." *British Medical Journal* 7338 (2002):623–4.

Dębska E, Szczegielniak A, Skowronek A, Wydra K, Frey P, Skowronek R, and Krysta K. "Different dimensions of aggression occurring in the work environment of psychiatrists." *Psychiatr Danub* 24 Suppl 1 (2012): S165-8.

De Leonardis, F. "War as a Medicine: The Medical Metaphor in Contemporary Italian Political Language." *Social Semiotics* 18 (2008): 33-45.

Department of Health and Social Security. *Prevention of harm to patients resulting from physical or mental disability of hospital or community medical or dental staff.* London: DHSS, 1986.

——. *An Organisation with a Memory. Report of an Expert Group on Learning from Adverse Events in the NHS Chaired by the Chief Medical Officer.* HMSO. Crown Copyright, 2000.

——. *"No Health Without Mental Health."* 2 February 2011. Accessed 19 February 2017. www.gov.uk/government/publications/no-health-without-mental-health-a-cross-government-mental-health-outcomes-strategy-for-people-of-all-ages-a-call-to-action

Derrida, J. *Of grammatology*. Baltimore and London: The John Hopkins University Press, 1997.

Dimock, G.E. "The Name of Odysseus." *Hudson Review* 9 (1956): 52-70.

Docherty J.S. "Four Reasons to Use the War Metaphor with Caution." September 16, 2001. Eastern Mennonite University, Center for Justice & Peacebuilding. Accessed February 12, 2017. www.emu.edu/cjp/publications/beyond-september-11th/2001/use-the-war-metaphor-with-caution/

Dodds, E.R. *The Greeks and the Irrational*. Berkeley, California: University of California Press, 1951.

Doherty, L.E. (ed.) *Homer's Odyssey*. Oxford: OUP, 2009.

Donnelly, W.J. "Righting the Medical Record; Transforming Chronicle into Record." *Journal of the American Medical Association* 260 (1988): 823-5.

Dougherty, C. *The Raft of Odysseus: The Ethnographic Imagination of Homer's Odyssey*. New York, NY: Oxford University Press, 2001.

Dovey, S.M., Meyers, D.S., Phillips, R.L., Green, L.A., Fryer, G.E., Galliher, J.M., Kappus, J., and Grob, P. "A Preliminary Taxonomy of Medical Errors in Family Practice." *Quality & Safety in Health Care* 11 (2002): 233-8.

Dryden, J. "Dedication to the Aeneid". Preface to his translation of "The Works of Vergil". Bartleby.com. Accessed October 2, 2016. http://www.bartleby.com/13/1002.html.

Duckworth, A. *Grit. The Power of Passion and Perseverance*. London: Vermilion, 2016.

Dunbar, H. *A Complete concordance to the* Odyssey *and Hymns of Homer*. Oxford: Clarendon Press, 1858.

Durkin, M. "Revised Never Events Policy and Framework". NHS England, 2015. Accessed February 12, 2017. https://www.england.nhs.uk/wp-content/uploads/2015/04/never-evnts-pol-framwrk-apr.pdf

Edwards, M.W. *The Iliad: A Commentary, Volume 5: books 17-20*. Edited by Kirk, G.S. Cambridge, Cambridge University Press, 1991.

Elias, N. *The Civilizing Process*. Oxford: Wiley-Blackwell, 2000, 2nd ed.

Eliot, T.S. *Little Gidding*. London: Faber & Faber, 1942.

Elmer, D.F. *The Poetics of Consent: Collective Decision-Making and the Iliad*. Baltimore, MD: The Johns Hopkins University Press, 2012.

Embrey, D. "Understanding Human Behaviour and Error." Accessed 16 December 2016. http://www.humanreliability.com/articles/Understanding%20Human%20Behaviour%20and%20Error.pdf

Euripides. *Bacchae*. Edited by Dodds, E.R. Oxford: Oxford University Press, 1963.

Eva, K. "What Every Teacher Needs to Know About Clinical Reasoning." *Medical Education* 39 (2005): 98-106.

Expert Advisory Group (EAG) Report to the Royal Australasian College of Surgeons on Discrimination, Bullying and Sexual Harassment. 28th Sept 2015. Accessed January 14, 2016. http://www.surgeons.org/media/22086656/EAG-Report-to-RACS-FINAL-28-September-2015-.pdf

Fagles, R. trans. *The Iliad of Homer*. London: The Folio Society, 1999.

Faunce, T. "Developing and Teaching the Virtue-Ethics Foundations of Healthcare Whistle Blowing." *Monash Bioethics Review* 23 (2004): 41-55.

Faunce, T.A., and Bolsin, S.N.C. "Three Australian Whistleblowing Sagas: Lessons For Internal and External Regulation." *Medical Journal of Australia* 181 (2004): 44-7.

Faunce, T.A., Bolsin, S., and Chan, W-P. "Supporting Whistleblowers in Academic Medicine: Training and Respecting the Courage of Professional Conscience." *Journal of Medical Ethics* 30 (2004): 40-43.

Feldmann, T.B., Holt, J., and Hellard, S. "Violence in Medical Facilities: A Review of 40 Incidents. *Journal of the Kentucky Medical Association* 95 (1997): 183-9.

Field, T. "Bullying in Medicine." *British Medical Journal* 324 (2002): 786.

Finlay, I.H. *The Blue Sail.* Glasgow: WAX366, 2002.

Firth-Cozens, J., and Harrison, J. *How to survive in medicine personally and professionally.* Oxford: Wiley-Blackwell, 2010.

Fischer, M.A., Mazor, K.M., Baril, J., Alper, E., DeMarco, D., and Pugnaire, M. "Learning from Mistakes: Factors that Influence How Students and Residents Learn from Medical Errors." *Journal of General Internal Medicine* 21 (2006): 419–23.

Flannery, K., and Marcus, J. *The Creation of Inequality: How Our Prehistoric Ancestors Set the Stage for Monarchy, Slavery, and Empire.* Cambridge, MA.: Harvard University Press, 2012.

Flexner, A. *Medical Education in the United States and Canada: A Report to the Carnegie Foundation for the Advancement of Teaching.* Forgotten Books (reprint), 1910/ 2016.

Flexner, A., and Pritchett, H.S. *Medical Education in Europe. A Report to the Carnegie Foundation for the Advancement of Teaching. Bulletin Number Six.* BiblioLife, LLC. Leopold Classic Library, 1923/ 2016.

Fnais, N., Soobiah, C., Chen, M. H., Lillie, E., Perrier, L., Tashkhandi, M., Straus, S.E., Mamdani, M., Al-Omran, M., and Tricco, A.C. "Harassment and Discrimination in Medical Training: A Systematic Review and Meta-Analysis." *Academic Medicine* 89 (2014): 817–27.

Foley, J.M. *The Theory of Oral Composition: History and Methodology.* Bloomington and Indianapolis, IN.: Indiana University Press, 1988.

Forster, K. "Morale Crisis Among NHS Doctors 'Puts Patients at Risk'." *The Independent.* 27 October 2016. Accessed January 10, 2017. http://www.independent.co.uk/life-style/health-and-families/health-news/nhs-doctors-morale-gmc-report-specialising-state-of-medicine-general-medical-council-working-a7382606.html

Foucault, M. *The Birth of the Clinic: An archaeology of medical perception.* London: Routledge, 1973.

—. "Technologies of the Self". In *Ethics: Subjectivity and Truth,* edited by Rabinow, P. New York, NY.: The New Press, 1997.

—. *The Order of Things: Archaeology of the Human Sciences, 2nd ed.* London: Routledge, 2001.

—. *The hermeneutics of the subject: lectures at the Collège de France 1981-1982.* New York: Picador, 2005.

—. *Madness and Civilization.* London: Vintage Books, 2006.

—. *The Courage of Truth: The Government of Self and Others II.* Basingstoke: Palgrave Macmillan, 2011.

Francis, R. *Report of the Mid Staffordshire NHS Foundation Trust Public Inquiry.* London: The Stationery Office. Vol. 1, 2013.

Frank, E., Carrera, J. S., Stratton, T., Bickel, J. and Nora, L. M. "Experiences of Belittlement and Harassment and Their Correlates Among Medical Students in the United States: Longitudinal Survey". *British Medical Journal* 333 (2006): 682-4.

Frankel, H. *Early Greek Poetry and Philosophy.* New York: Harcourt Brace Jovanovich, 1975.

Fred, H.L. "Dishonesty in Medicine." *Southern Medical Journal* 77 (1984): 1221–2.

—. "Dishonesty in Medicine Revisited." *Texas Heart Institute Journal* 35 (2008): 6–15.

Fredrick, D. "Introduction: Invisible Rome." In *The Roman Gaze: Vision, Power, and the Body*, edited by D. Fredrick, 1-30. Baltimore, MD: The Johns Hopkins University Press, 2002.

Freischlag, J.A., and Silva, M.M. "Bouncing Up: Resilience and Women in Academic Medicine." *Journal of the American College of Surgeons.* Accessed on December 18, 2016:

https://www.ucdmc.ucdavis.edu/leadership/speeches-writings/PDFs/
JACS_Resilience%20Article_April2016.pdf.

Freud, S. "Humour." *International Journal of Psycho-Analysis* 9 (1928):
1-6.

Friedrich, W-H. *Wounding and Death in the* Iliad: *Homeric Techniques of
Description*. London: Gerald Duckworth and Co Ltd., 2003.

Fuks, A. 2009. The Military Metaphors in Modern Medicine. Freeland,
Oxfordshire Inter-disciplinary.net. Accessed April 7, 2015.
http://www.inter-disciplinary.net/wp-content/uploads/2009
/06/hid_fuks.pdf

Furbank, P.N. "On Reading Homer without Knowing any Greek." In
Homer. Readings and Images, edited by Emlyn-Jones, C., Hardwick,
L., and Purkis, J., 49-62. London: Gerald Duckworth and Co Ltd.,
1992.

Furness, J.B., Callaghan, B.P., Rivera, L.R. and Cho, H.J. "The enteric
nervous system and gastrointestinal innervation: integrated local and
central control." *Advances in Experimental Medicine and Biology* 817
(2014): 39-71.

Gágyor, I., Hilbert, N., Chenot, J-F., Marx, G., Ortner, T., Simmenroth-Nayda,
A., Scherer, M., Wedeken, S., and Himmel, W. 2012. "Frequency and
Perceived Severity of Negative Experiences During Medical Education
in Germany – Results of an Online-Survey of Medical Students". *GMS
Zeitschrift für Medizinische Ausbildung* 29: Doc55.

Garrouste-Orgeas, M., Philippart, F., Bruel, C, Max, A., Lau, N., and
Misset, B. "Overview of Medical Errors and Adverse Events. *Annals
of Intensive Care* 2 (2012): 2.

Gawande, A. *The Checklist Manifesto: How to Get Things Right*. London:
Profile Books, 2010.

—. *Being Mortal: Illness, Medicine and What Matters in the End*. London:
Profile Books, 2014.

General Medical Council, UK. *Good Medical Practice*. GMC, 2006.

—. *The New Doctor*. GMC, 2007.

—. 2009. *Tomorrow's Doctors.* Accessed January 7, 2015.
http://www.gmc-uk.org/TomorrowsDoctors_2009.pdf_39260971.pdf

—. 2013. *Good Medical Practice.* Accessed January 7, 2015.
www.http://www.gmcuk.org/static/documents/content/GMP_2013.pdf
_51447599.pdf

—. 2013. *National Training Survey 2013*: *Undermining.* Accessed January
15, 2016.
http://www.gmc-uk.org/NTS_2013_autumn_report_undermining.pdf_
54275779.pdf

—. *GMC Policy on Whistleblowing*. Accessed January 11, 2017. http://www.gmc-uk.org/DC5900_Whistleblowing_guidance.pdf_ 57107304.pdf

—. *The State of Medical Education and Practice in the UK.* Accessed December 17, 2016. http://www.gmc-uk.org/SOMEP_2016_Full_Report_Lo_Res.pdf _68139324.pdf

George, D.R. "Overcoming the Social Death of Dementia through Language". *The Lancet* 376 (2010): 586-7.

Gilligan, C. *In a Different Voice.* Cambridge, Mass.: Harvard University Press, 1982.

Gladwell, M. *Outliers: The Story of Success*, New York: Little, Brown and Co., 2008.

Goethe, J.W. "Zum bruderlichen andenken wielands." In *Translation – Theory and Practice. A Historical Reader*, edited by Weissbort, D., and Eysteinsson, A., 198-204. Oxford: Oxford University Press, 2006.

Goffman, E. *The Presentation of Self in Everyday Life.* New York, NY: Random House, 1959.

Gonzales, L. *Surviving Survival: The Art and Science of Resilience.* New York, NY: W.W. Norton, 2012.

Graban, M. 2011. *Statistics on Healthcare Quality and Patient Safety Problems – Errors & Harm.* Updated May 26, 2011. Accessed July 2, 2011. http://www.leanblog.org/author/admin/

Grandinetti, D. 2000. "Sex and the Satisfied Doctor." *Medical Economics.* Accessed February 12, 2017. http://medicaleconomics.modernmedicine.com/medical-economics/content/sex-and-satisfied-doctor

Graves, R. *The Anger of Achilles – Homer's Iliad.* London: Cassells, 1960.

Green, A. "Remembering Health Workers Who Died from Ebola in 2014." *Lancet* 384 (2014): 2201-6.

Greene, G. *The Woman Who Knew Too Much.* Ann Arbor, University of Michigan Press, 2001.

Greger, M. 1999. Appendix 16 – Medical Student Abuse. Accessed February 12, 2017. http://upalumni.org/medschool/appendices/appendix-16.html

Griffin, J., ed. *The Iliad.* Oxford: Oxford University Press, 1959.

Griffin, J. "The Speeches." In *The Cambridge Companion to Homer,* edited by Fowler, R., 156-167. Cambridge: Cambridge University Press, 2004.

Grober, E.D., and Bohnen, J.M.A. "Defining Medical Error." *Canadian Journal of Surgery* 48 (2005): 39-44.

Hackett, D., and Martin, C.L. *Facilitation skills for team leaders.* Boston: Thomson Course Technology, 1993.

Hainsworth, B. *The Iliad – A Commentary. Volume III: Books 9-12,* General editor Kirk, G.S. Cambridge: Cambridge University Press, 1993.

Hall, C. "Influx of women doctors 'will harm medicine'", *The Telegraph*, 03 August 2004. Accessed December 30, 2016. http://www.telegraph.co.uk/news/uknews/1468508/Influx-of-women-doctors-will-harm-medicine.html

Hall, E. *Greek Tragedy: Suffering under the Sun.* Oxford: Oxford University Press, 2010.

Hall J. "David Bowie dead: German government thanks late singer for helping to bring down the Berlin Wall." *The Independent*, Monday 11 January 2016. Accessed January 3, 2017. http://www.independent.co.uk/news/people/david-bowie-death-german-government-thanks-late-singer-for-helping-to-bring-down-the-berlin-wall-a6805931.html

Halpern, J. *From Detached Concern to Empathy: Humanizing Medical Practice.* Oxford: Oxford University Press, 2001.

—. "Empathy and Patient–Physician Conflicts." *Journal of General Internal Medicine* 22 (2007): 696–700.

Hamilton, J. *Moses, The Man of God.* London: James Nisbet and Co., 1876. Accessed October 27, 2016. https://archive.org/stream/mosesmanofgod00hami#page/150/mode/2up

Hammer, D. *The Iliad as Politics: The Performance of Political Thought.* Norman, OK.: University of Oklahoma Press, 2002.

Hanson, P.G. *Learning through groups.* San Diego: University Associates Inc., 1981.

Harris, W.V. *Restraining Rage. The Ideology of Anger Control in Classical Antiquity.* Cambridge, MA: Harvard University Press, 2001.

Harvey, C. "Anti-Fatigue Drug Helps Tired Doctors -- Good Idea?" *New Scientist* blog 24 October 2011. Accessed June 3, 2015. http://www.newscientist.com/article/dn21084-antifatigue-drug-helps-tired-doctors--good-idea.html#.VW7do17zCTM

Havelock, E.A. *The Muse Learns to Write.* New Haven, CT.: Yale University Press, 1986.

Hawhee, D. *Bodily Arts: Rhetoric and Athletics in Ancient Greece.* Austin, TX: University of Texas Press, 2004.

Hawton, K., Clements, A., Sakarovitch, C., Simkin, S., and Deeks, J.J. "Suicide in Doctors: A Study of Risk According to Gender, Seniority and Specialty in Medical Practitioners in England and Wales, 1979– 1995." *Journal of Epidemiology and Community Health* 55 (2001): 296–300.

Hayashino, Y., Utsugi-Ozaki, M., Feldman, M.D., and Fukuhara, S. "Hope Modified the Association Between Distress and Incidence of Self-Perceived Medical Errors among Practicing Physicians: Prospective Cohort Study." *PLoS One* 7 (2012): e35585.

Haywood, L. "Translation Emergency Toolkit", University of Cambridge, Faculty of Modern and Medieval Languages, 2012. Accessed December 30, 2016.
    http://www.mml.cam.ac.uk/call/translation/toolkit/

HealthGrades Quality Study. 2004. *Patient Safety in American Hospitals.* Health Grades, Inc. Accessed 06 Jan 2015.
    http://www.healthgrades.com/media/english/pdf/HG_Patient_Safety_S tudy_Final.pdf

—. *The Eleventh Annual HealthGrades Hospital Quality in America Study October 2008.* Health Grades, Inc., 2008. Accessed July 2, 2015.
    http://www.healthgrades.com/media/DMS/pdf/HealthGradesEleventh AnnualHospitalQualityStudy2008.pdf

Health, Quality and Safety Commission, New Zealand. "No place for bullying in New Zealand's health system". 15 September 2015. Accessed 27 February 2017.
    http://www.hqsc.govt.nz/our-programmes/safe-surgery-nz/news-and-events/news/2307/

Hernandez, P.N. "Reading Homer in the 21st Century." *College Literature* 34 (2007): 29-54.

Hesiod. *Theogony and Works and Days.* Translated by West, M.L. Oxford: Oxford University Press, 2008.

Hillman, J. *The Dream and the Underworld*, New York: Harper Perennial, 1979.

—. *Re-Visioning Psychology.* New York: HarperPerennial, (Reissue), 1992.

—. *A Terrible Love of War.* Harmondsworth: Penguin Books, 2004.

Hillman, J., Roscher, W.H. *Pan and the Nightmare.* Dallas, TX: Spring Books, 2000.

Hirschberg, P. *MY INTESTINES! Yes, watch in horror as my bowels are cut open!* YouTube. 2009. Accessed December 15, 2016.
    https://www.youtube.com/watch?v=w89s28pkhrw

Hodges, B. "The Many and Conflicting Histories of Medical Education in Canada and the USA: An Introduction to the Paradigm Wars." *Medical Education* 39 (2005): 613–21.

Hodgkin, P. "Medicine is War: And Other Medical Metaphors." *British Medical Journal Clinical Research Edition* 291 (1985): 1820-1.

Hogan, H., Healey, F., Neale, G., Thomson, R., Vincent, C., and Black, N. "Preventable Deaths Due to Problems in Care in English Acute Hospitals: A Retrospective Case Record Review Study." *BMJ Quality and Safety,* 21 (2012): 737-45.

Hojat, M., Gonnella, J.S., Nasca, T.J., Mangione, S., Vergare, M., and Magee, M. "Physician Empathy: Definition, Components, Measurement, and Relationship to Gender and Specialty." *American Journal of Psychiatry* 159 (2002a): 1563-9.

Hojat, M., Gonnella, J.S., Mangione, S., Nasca, T.J., Veloski, J.J., Erdmann, J.B., Callahan, C.A., and Magee, M. "Empathy in Medical Students as Related to Academic Performance, Clinical Competence and Gender." *Medical Education* 36 (2002b): 522-7.

Hojat, M., Mangione, S., Nasca, T.J., Rattner, S., Erdmann, J.B., Gonnella, J.S., and Magee, M. "An Empirical Study of Decline in Empathy in Medical School." *Medical Education* 38 (2004): 934-41.

Hole, S.R. *A Little Tour in Ireland.* New York. W S Gottberger and Co., 1891.

Homer. *The Iliad,* Books 1-12. Ed. by Monro, D.B., Allen, T.W. Oxford: Oxford University Press, 3rd ed., 1920.

—. *The Iliad,* Books 13-24. Ed. By Monro, D.B., Allen, T.W. Oxford: Oxford University Press, 3rd ed., 1920.

—. *The Odyssey,* Books 1-12. Ed. by Allen, T.W. Oxford: Oxford University Press, 2nd ed., 1917.

—. *The Odyssey,* Books 13-24. Ed. by Allen, T.W. Oxford: Oxford University Press, 2nd ed., 1919.

Hooker, C., and Noonan, E. "Medical Humanities as Expressive of Western Culture." *Medical Humanities* 37 (2011): 79-84.

House of Commons Health Committee. 2009. *Patient Safety: Sixth Report of Session, 2008–09.*

Howe, A., Smajdor, A., and Stöckl, A. "Towards an Understanding of Resilience and its Relevance to Medical Training." *Medical Education* 46 (2012): 349–56.

Huffington, A. *The Sleep Revolution: Transforming Your Life, One Night at a Time.* New York, NY: Penguin Random House, 2016.

Hughes-Hallett L. *Heroes. Saviours, Traitors and Supermen.* London: Fourth Estate, 2004.

Hull, F.M. "Death, Dying and the Medical Student." *Medical Education* 25 (1991): 491-6.

Hunter, A.J., and Chandler, G.E. "Adolescent Resilience." *Image--The Journal of Nursing Scholarship* 31 (1999): 243-7.

Hunter, K.M. *Doctors' Stories. The Narrative Structure of Medical Knowledge.* Princeton, NJ: Princeton University Press, 1991.

Ikegami, E. *Bonds of Civility: Aesthetic Networks and the Political Origins of Japanese Culture.* Cambridge: Cambridge University Press, 2005.

Illich, I. *Tools for Conviviality.* London: Marion Boyars, 1973.

Institute for Safe Medication Practices. "Survey Shows Workplace Intimidation Adversely Affects Patient Safety." 2004. Accessed January 7, 2017.
www.ismp.org/pressroom/pr20040331

Jackson, M. *Asthma, the Biography.* Oxford: OUP, 2009.

Jackson, D., Firtko, A., and Edenborough, M. "Personal Resilience as a Strategy for Surviving and Thriving in the Face of Workplace Adversity: A Literature Review." *Journal of Advanced Nursing* 60 (2007): 1–9.

Jaques, H. "Whistleblowing Helpline Takes More Than 350 Calls in First Four Months." *British Medical Journal* 346 (2013a): f2774.

Jaques, H. "White doctors are almost three times more likely to land hospital jobs than ethnic minority doctors." *BMJ Careers*, 26 Sep 2013b. Accessed May 20, 2017.
www.http://careers.bmj.com/careers/advice/White_doctors_are_almost_th ree_times_more_likely_to_land_hospital_jobs_than_ethnic_minority_ doctors

Jones, C.P. *New Heroes in Antiquity: From Achilles to Antinoos.* Cambridge, MA: Harvard University Press, 2010.

Jones, P. *Homer's Odyssey. A Commentary Based on the Translation of Richard Lattimore.* London; Bristol Classical Press, 2002.

Johnson, S. "Four in Five NHS Staff Thought About Leaving." *The Guardian.* Friday 12 February 2016. Accessed February 14, 2017.
https://www.theguardian.com/society/2016/feb/12/four-in-five-nhs-staff-consider-quitting-job-stress-guardian-poll

Joseph, S. "Growth Following Adversity: Positive Psychological Perspectives on Posttraumatic Stress." *Psychological Topics, 18* (2009): 335-44.

Judkins, S., Arris, L., and Keener, E. "Program Evaluation in Graduate Nursing Education: Hardiness as a Predictor of Success Among Nursing Administration Students." *Journal of Professional Nursing* 21 (2005): 314-21.

Kalanithi, P. *When Breath Becomes Air*. London: Random House, 2016.

Kaldjian, L.C., Jones, E.W., Wu, B.J., Forman-Hoffman, V.L., Levi, B.H., and Rosenthal, G.E. "Disclosing Medical Errors to Patients: Attitudes and Practices of Physicians and Trainees." *Journal of General Internal Medicine* 22 (2007): 988–96.

Kane, F.J. "Faculty Views of Medical Student Abuse." *Academic Medicine* 70 (1995): 563-4.

Karthikesan, D. "Dear doctors, be kind to each other". 9th May, 2015. Accessed January 15, 2016.
http://dharmarajkarthikesan.com/2015/05/09/dear-doctors-be-kind-to-each-other/

Keane, J. *The Life and Death of Democracy*. London: Simon & Schuster, 2009.

Kelly, E., and Nisker, J. "Medical Students' First Clinical Experiences of Death." *Medical Education* 44 (2010): 421-28.

Kels, B.D., and Grant-Kels, J.M. "The Spectrum of Medical Errors: When Patients Sue." *International Journal of General Medicine* 5 (2012): 613-9.

Kérenyi, C. *The Gods of the Greeks*. London, Thames & Hudson, 1974.

Kirk, G.S. "Homer and Modern Oral Poetry; Some Confusions." *Classical Quarterly* 10 (1960): 271-81.

—. *The Iliad – A Commentary, Vol I*. Cambridge: Cambridge University Press, 2001.

Klamen, D., and Williams, R. "Using Standardized Clinical Encounters to Assess Physician Communication." In *Measuring Medical Professionalism*, edited by D.T. Stern, 53-74. Oxford: Oxford University Press, 2006.

Klein, A.S., and Forni, P.M. "Barbers of Civility." *Archives of Surgery* 146 (2011): 774-77.

Kleinman, A. *The Illness Narratives. Suffering, Healing and the Human Condition*. New York NY: Basic Books, 1988.

Kohn, L.T., Corrigan, J.M., and Donaldson, M.S., eds. *To Err is Human: Building a Safer Health System*. Washington (DC): National Academy Press, 2000.

Kurtz, S., Silverman, J., and Draper, J. *Teaching and Learning Communication Skills in Medicine*. Oxford: Radcliffe Medical Press Ltd., 1998.

LaCombe, M.A. "Letters of Intent." In *Empathy and the Practice of Medicine*: *Beyond Pills and the Scalpel*, edited by Spiro, H.M., McCrea Curnen, M.G. Peschel, E., St James, D. New Haven, CT: Yale University Press, 1993.

Laing, R.D. *Knots*. Harmondsworth: Penguin Books, 2nd ed., 1972.

Lakoff, G., Johnson, M. *Metaphors We Live By*. Chicago: University of Chicago Press, 1981.

Lane, H.P., McLachlan, S., Philip, J. "The War against Dementia: Are We Battle Weary Yet?" *Age and Ageing* 42 (2013): 281-3.

Latour, B. *Reassembling the Social: An Introduction to Actor-Network-Theory*. Oxford: Oxford University Press, 2007.

Laurance, J. 2011. "Doctors' basic errors are killing 1,000 patients a month." Accessed 16 December 2016. http://www.independent.co.uk/life-style/health-and-families/health-news/doctors-basic-errors-are-killing-1000-patients-a-month-7939674.html

Leape, L.L., Brennan, T.A., Laird, N., Lawthers, A.G., Localio, A.R., Barnes, B.A., Hebert, L., Newhouse, J.P., Paul C. Weiler, P.C., and Hiatt, H. The Nature of Adverse Events in Hospitalized Patients: Results of the Harvard Medical Practice Study II. *New England Journal of Medicine* 324 (1991): 377-84.

Lempp, H., and Seale, C. "The Hidden Curriculum in Undergraduate Medical Education: Qualitative Study of Medical Students' Perceptions of Teaching". *British Medical Journal* 329 (2004): 770-3.

Lennane, K.J. "Whistleblowing: A Health Issue." *British Medical Journal* 307 (1993): 667–70.

Levine, D., Bleakley, A. "Maximising Medicine Through Aphorisms." *Medical Education* 46 (2012): 153–62.

Lewis, N.J., Rees, C.E., Hudson, J.N., and Bleakley, A. "Emotional Intelligence in Medical Education: Measuring the Unmeasurable." *Advanced Health Science Education Theory Practice Journal* 10 (2005): 339-55.

Liddell, H.G., and Scott, R. *A Greek-English Lexicon*. Oxford, Oxford University Press, 1940.

Lindstrom, U.F., Hamberg, K., and Johansson, E.E. "Medical Students' Experiences of Shame in Professional Enculturation." *Medical Education* 45 (2011): 1016–024.

Lingard, L., Garwood, K., Schryer, C.F., and Spafford, M.M. "'Talking the Talk': School and Workplace Genre Tension in Clerkship Case Presentations." *Medical Education* 37 (2003): 612-20.

Lingard, L., Hodges, B., MacRae, H., and Freeman, R. "Expert and Trainee Determinations of Rhetorical Relevance in Referral and Consultation Letters." *Medical Education* 38 (2004): 168–76.

Logue, C. *Kings*. London: Faber and Faber, 1992.

—. *All Day Permanent Red*. London: Faber and Faber, 2003.

Loraux, N. *Born of the Earth: Myth and Politics in Athens.* Translated by Selina Stewart. Cornell University Press, 2000.

Lord, A.B. *The Singer of Tales.* Cambridge, Mass: Harvard University Press, 2003.

Lubarsky, S., Dory, V., Audétat, M-C., Custers, E., and Charlin, B. "Using Script Theory to Cultivate Illness Script Formation and Clinical Reasoning in Health Professions Education." *Canadian Medical Education Journal* 6 (2015): e61–e70.

Luthar, S.S., Cicchetti, D., and Becker, B. "The Construct of Resilience: A Critical Evaluation and Guidelines for Future Work." *Child Development* 71 (2000): 543–62.

Lynn-George, K. "Structures of Care in the *Iliad.*" *The Classical Quarterly* 46 (1996): 1-26.

McCann, C.M., Beddoe, E., McCormick, K., Huggard, P., Kedge, S., Adamson, C., and Huggard, J. "Resilience in the Medical Professions: A Review of Recent Literature." *International Journal of Wellbeing* 3 (2013): 60-81.

MacDonald, N., and Attaran, A. "Medical Errors, Apologies and Apology Laws." *Canadian Medical Association Journal* 180 (2009): 11.

MacDonald O. *Disruptive Physician Behavior.* Waltham, MA: QuantiaMD, 2011.

McGushin, E.F. *Foucault's Askesis: An Introduction to the Philosophical Life.* Evanston, Ill.: Northwestern University Press, 2007.

MacIntyre, A. *After Virtue.* London: Duckworth, 1985.

McIntyre, N. *How British Women Became Doctors: The Story of the Royal Free Hospital and its Medical School.* London, Wenrowave Press, 2014.

McKenzie, D. "South Africa cricket finds a new hero in Temba Bavuma." January 15 2016. Accessed December 16, 2016.
http://www.news18.com/cricketnext/videos/south-africa-cricket-finds-a-new-hero-in-temba-bavuma-1190432.html

Macleod, C.W., ed. *Homer: Iliad, Book 24.* Cambridge: Cambridge University Press, 1985.

McMains, V. "Johns Hopkins Study Suggests Medical Errors are Third-Leading Cause of Death in U.S." 2016. Accessed December 16, 2016.
https://hub.jhu.edu/2016/05/03/medical-errors-third-leading-cause-of-death/

MacNaughton, J. "The Dangerous Practice of Empathy." *The Lancet* 373 (2009): 1940-1.

Maguire, P., and Pitceathly, C. "Dealing with Strong Emotions and Difficult Personalities." In *Difficult conversations in medicine*, edited by Macdonald E. Oxford: Oxford University Press, 2004.

Makary, M., and Daniel, M. "Medical Error—The Third Leading Cause of Death in the US." *British Medical Journal* 353 (2016): i2139.

Mangus, R. S., Hawkings, C. E., and Miller, M. J. "Prevalence of Harassment and Discrimination Among 1996 Medical School Graduates." *Journal of the American Medical Association* 280 (1998): 851-3.

Mankaka, C.O., Waeber, G., and Gachoud, D. "Female Residents Experiencing Medical Errors in General Internal Medicine: A Qualitative Study. *BMC Medical Education* 14 (2014):140.

Manring, M.M., Hawk, A., Calhoun, J.H., and Andersen, R.C. "Treatment of War Wounds: A Historical Review." *Clinical Orthopaedics and Related Research* 467 (2009): 2168–91.

Mansbach, A. "Whistleblowing as Fearless Speech: The Radical Democratic Effects of Late Modern Parrhesia. In *Whistleblowing and Democratic Values*, edited by Lewis, D. and Vanderkerkove, W. E-book: International Whistleblowing Research Network, 2011.

Marsh, H. *Do No Harm: Stories of Life, Death and Brain Surgery.* London: Orion Publishing Group, 2014.

Marshall, R.J., and Bleakley, A. "Putting it Bluntly: Communication Skills in The Iliad." *Medical Humanities* 34 (2008): 30-4.

Marshall, R.J., and Bleakley, A. "The Death of Hector: Pity in Homer, Empathy in Medical Education." *Medical Humanities* 35 (2009): 7-12.

Marshall, R.J., and Bleakley, A. "Sing, Muse: Songs in Homer and in Hospital." *Medical Humanities* 37 (2011): 27-33.

Marshall, R.J., and Bleakley, A. "Lost in Translation. Homer in English; The Patient's Story in Medicine." *Medical Humanities* 39 (2013): 47-52.

Martin, A.J., and Marsh, H.W. "Academic Resilience and Academic Buoyancy: Multidimensional and Hierarchical Conceptual Framing of Causes, Correlates and Cognate Constructs." *Oxford Review of Education* 35 (2009): 353-70.

Martin, A.J., Ginns, P., Brackett, M.A., Malmberg, L-E., and Hall, J. "Academic Buoyancy and Psychological Risk: Exploring Reciprocal Relationships." *Learning and Individual Differences* 27 (2013): 128–33.

Martole, D.M. "Translation Practice Between Abusive Fidelity and Ethnocentric Reduction: *Vanity Fair* in Romanian." Undated. Accessed February 14, 2017.

http://oaji.net/articles/2016/2547-1452442166.pdf

Marzona, D., Grosenick, U. *Minimal Art.* Rome: Taschen, 2004.

Medew, J. 2015. Medical students under pressure amid reports of bullying in Australian hospitals. May 24 2015. *Sydney Morning Herald.* Accessed January 15, 2016. http://www.smh.com.au/national/medical-students-under-pressure-amid-reports-of-bullying-in-australian-hospitals-20150524-gh8jq5.html

Meier, C. *A Culture of Freedom: Ancient Greece & the Origins of Europe.* Oxford: Oxford University Press, 2011.

Mennin, S., Eoyang, G., and Nations, M. *Leadership in Medical Education: Future of the Health Professions Workforce.* Kindle Edition, 2016.

Meyer, J. *Minimalism: Art and Polemics in the Sixties.* New Haven, CT: Yale University Press, 2004.

Miller, L. "Doctor at War; Doctors Washing Feet." *Narrative Inquiry in Bioethics* 4 (2014): 202-4.

Mizrahi, T. "Managing Medical Mistakes: Ideology, Insularity and Accountability Among Internists-in-Training." *Social Science Medicine* 19 (1984): 135–46.

Mol, A. *The Body Multiple: Ontology in Medical Practice.* Durham NC: Duke University Press, 2002.

Monrouxe, L.V., Rees, C.E., Endacott, R., and Ternan, E. "'Even Now It Makes Me Angry': Health Care Students' Professionalism Dilemma Narratives." *Medical Education* 48 (2014): 502-17.

Montgomery, K. *How Doctors Think: Clinical Judgement and the Practice of Medicine.* Oxford: Oxford University Press, 2006.

Montgomery, S.L. "Illness and Image: On the Contents of Biomedical Discourse." In *The Scientific Voice* edited by Montgomery, S.L., 134-95. New York, NY: The Guilford Press, 1996.

Moscucci, O. "Gender and Cancer in Britain, 1860–1910. The Emergence of Cancer as a Public Health Concern." *Am J Public Health* 95 (2005): 1312–21.

Mulhern, J.J. "Parrhesia in Aristotle." In *Free Speech in Classical Antiquity*, edited by Sluite, I., Rosen, R.M. Leiden: Brill, 2004.

Myers, A. "Whistleblowing – Corruption Prevention and the Public Interest." Whistleblowing International Network, 2014. Accessed January 7, 2015. www.http://whistleblowingnetwork.org/what-win-wants/

Nader, R. *Breaking Through Power: It's Easier Than We Think.* San Francisco: City Lights Open Media, 2016.

Nagler, M.N. "Towards a Generative View of the Oral Formula." *Transactions and Proceedings of the American Philological Association* 98 (1967): 269-311.

Nagy, G. *The Ancient Greek Hero in 24 Hours.* Cambridge, Massachusetts, Harvard University Press, 2013.

Narang, A. 2014. "Cynicism in Medicine – Insights on Residency Training." April 28th 2014. Accessed January 15, 2016. http://blogs.jwatch.org/general-medicine/index.php/2014/04/cynicism-in-medicine/

National Institute for Occupational Safety and Health (NIOSH). "Violence Occupational Hazards in Hospitals." April, 2002. Accessed April 7, 2013. www.cdc.gov/niosh/docs/2002-101/

Needham, N. "Whistleblowing - A Dangerous Choice? Medical Students Have a Duty to Report on Substandard Care." *Student BMJ* 20(e7870) (2012): 14-16.

Nendaz, M.R., and Bordage, G. "Promoting Diagnostic Problem Representation." *Medical Education* 36 (2002): 760-66.

Neumann, M., Edelhöuser, F., Tauschel, D., Fischer, M.R., Wirtz, M., Woopen, C., Haramati, A., and Scheffer, C. "Empathy Decline and its Reasons: A Systematic Review of Studies with Medical Students and Residents." *Academic Medicine.* 86 (2011): 996-1009.

Nicolson, A. *The Mighty Dead. Why Homer Matters.* London: William Collins, 2015.

Nietzsche, F. "Preface to an Unwritten Book", 1872. Accessed February 3, 2017. https://archive.org/stream/cu31924021569151/cu31924021569151_djvu.txt

—. 2013. *On the Genealogy of Morals.* Harmondsworth: Penguin Classics, 2013.

North, A.C., Bland, V., and Ellis, N. 2005. "Distinguishing Heroes from Celebrities." *British Journal of Psychology* 96 (2005): 39-52.

Notopoulos, J.A. "Mnemosyne in Oral Literature." *Transactions and Proceedings of the American Philological Association* 69 (1938): 465-93.

Ong, W.J. *Orality and literacy; the technologizing of the word.* London: Methuen, 1982.

Onians, R.B. *The origins of European thought.* Cambridge: Cambridge University Press, 1988.

O'Reilly KB. "Call for civility aims to stop disruptive behavior in the OR." 1 August 2011. Accessed April 8, 2013.

www.pwrnewmedia.com/2011/joint_commission/big_news_august/do
wnload_jc/jc_Call_for_civility.pdf

Osler, W. *Aequanimitas. With Other Addresses to Medical Students, Nurses and Practitioners of Medicine.* London: H.K.Lewis and Co., 1946.

Oswald, A. *Memorial.* New York: W.W.Norton, 2012.

Oxtoby, K. "Do the Classic Specialty Stereotypes Still Hold True for Today's Doctors?" *British Medical Journal Careers* 17 Dec. 2013.

Padel, R. *In and out of the mind. Greek images of the tragic self.* Princeton, NJ: Princeton University Press, 1992.

—. *Whom gods destroy: elements of Greek and tragic madness.* Princeton, NJ: Princeton University Press, 1995.

Park, A. (Ed.) *Resemblance and Reality in Greek Thought: Essays in Honor of Peter M. Smith.* London: Routledge, 2016.

Parry, M. *The Making of Homeric Verse: The Collected Papers of Milman Parry,* edited by Adam Parry. Oxford: Clarendon Press, 1971.

Pauli, H.G., White, K.L., and McWhinney, I.R. "Medical Education, Research, and Scientific Thinking in the 21st Century." *Education for Health*, 13 (2000): 15-25, 165-172, 173-186.

Pedersen, R. "Empathy Development in Medical Education – A Critical Review. *Medical Teacher* 32 (2010): 593-600.

Pellegrino, E.D. "Some Things Ought Never Be Done: Moral Absolutes in Clinical Ethics." *Theoretical Medicine and Bioethics* 26 (2005): 469-86.

Pellegrino, E. "Toward an Expanded Medical Ethics: The Hippocratic Ethic Revisited." In *The Philosophy of Medicine Reborn: A Pellegrino Reader*. Edited by H. Engelhardt and F. Jotterand, 401. Notre Dame, Indiana: University of Notre Dame Press, 2008.

Pendleton, D., Schofield, T., Tate, P., and Havelock, P. *The Consultation: An Approach to Learning and Teaching.* Oxford: Oxford University Press, 1984.

Pendleton, D., Schofield, T., Tate, P., and Havelock, P. *The New Consultation. Developing Doctor-Patient Communication.* Oxford: Oxford University Press, 2004.

Penson, R.T., Svendsen, S.S., Chabner, B.A., Lynch, T.J., and Levinson, W. "Medical Mistakes: A Workshop on Personal Perspectives." *The Oncologist* 6 (2001): 92-9.

Peterkin, A., Bleakley, A. 2017. *Staying Human During the Foundation Programme: How to thrive after medical school.* Boca Raton, FLA: CRC Press.

Peterkin, A., and Brett-Maclean, P., eds. Keeping Reflection Fresh: A Practical Guide for Clinical Educators. Kent, OH: Kent State University Press, 2017.

Piemonte, N. "Last Laugh: Gallows Humor and Medical Education". *Journal of Medical Humanities* 36 (2015): 375-90.

Pinker, S. *The Better Angels of our Nature*. London: Penguin Books, 2012.

Plato. *Meno*. In *Protagoras and Meno*, translated by Guthrie, W.K.C. Harmondsworth: Penguin Books, 1956.

—. *Phaedrus*. London: Loeb Classical Library, William Heinemann Ltd., 1971.

Platt, F.W. "Clinical Hypocompetence: The Interview." *Annals of Internal Medicine* 91 (1979): 898-902.

Pliny the Elder. *The Natural History*, translated by Bostock, J. and Riley, H.T. London. Taylor and Francis, 1855. Accessed January 14, 2017. http://www.perseus.tufts.edu/hopper/text?doc=Perseus%3Atext%3A19 99.02.0137%3Abook%3D9%3Achapter%3D35

Pope, A. *The* Odyssey *of Homer*. London, 1725-6.

Popper K. *The Open Society and its Enemies*. London: Routledge, 1945.

Porter, M. "BMA View on Whistleblowing." *British Medical Journal* 339 (2009): b4405.

Postlethwaite, N. "Thersites in the *Iliad*." In *Homer. Greece and Rome Studies*, vol. 4, edited by McAuslan, I., Walcot, P., Oxford: Oxford University Press, 1998.

Rabin, C. "The linguistics of translation." In *Aspects of translation*, edited by A.D.Booth, 123-145. London: Secker and Warburg, 1958.

Ragland, D., and Brand, R. "Type A Behavior and Mortality from Coronary Heart Disease." *The New England Journal of Medicine* 318 (1988): 65–9.

Ramsay, M.A.E. "Conflict in the Health Care Workplace". *Proceedings (Baylor University. Medical Center)* 14 (2001): 138–9.

Ratanawongsa, N., Teherani, A., and Hauer, K.E. "Third-year Medical Students' Experiences with Dying Patients during the Internal Medicine Clerkship: A Qualitative Study of the Informal Curriculum." *Academic Medicine* 80 (2005): 641-7.

Ratzan, R.M. "Winged Words and Chief Complaints: Medical Case Histories and the Parry-Lord Oral-Formulaic Tradition." *Literature and Medicine* 11 (1992): 94-114.

Reason, J. "Stress and Cognitive Failure". In *Handbook of Life Stress and Cognition*, edited by Fisher, S and Reason, J., 405-21, Chichester, UK: John Wiley and Sons, 1988.

—. *Human Error*. Cambridge, Cambridge University Press, 1990.

—. "Human Error. Models and Management." *The Western Journal of Medicine* 172 (2000): 393–6.

—. *A Life in Error. From Little Slips to Big Disasters.* Farnham, UK: Ashgate, 2013.

Reason, J., and Mycielska, K. *Absent-Minded? The Psychology of Mental Lapses and Everyday Errors.* New Jersey, Prentice-Hall, 1982.

Redfield, J. *Nature and Culture in the* Iliad: *The Tragedy of Hector.* Durham, NC: Duke University Press, 1994.

Reece, S. *The Stranger's Welcome: Oral Theory and the Aesthetics of the Homeric Hospitality Scene. Michigan Monographs in Classical Antiquity.* Ann Arbor: University of Michigan, 1993.

Rees, C.E., Monrouxe, L.V., and McDonald, L.A. "Narrative, Emotion and Action: Analyzing 'Most Memorable' Professionalism Dilemmas. *Medical Education* 47 (2013): 80-96.

Reese, S. 2015. *Drug and Alcohol Abuse: Why Doctors Become Hooked.* Accessed December 25, 2016.
http://www.medscape.com/viewarticle/843758

Reisfield, G.M., and Wilson, G.R. "Use of Metaphor in the Discourse on Cancer." *Journal of Clinical Oncology* 22 (2004): 4024-7.

Riesman, D., Glazer, N., and Denney, R. *The Lonely Crowd.* New Haven, CT.: Yale University Press, 1950.

Rieu, D.C.H. Preface to *Homer. The Odyssey,* translated by E.V.Rieu, revised by D.C.H. Rieu and P.Jones. London: Penguin Books, 1991.

Rieu, E.V, trans. *The Iliad of Homer.* London: Penguin Books, 1950.

Robbennolt, J.K. "Apologies and Medical Error." *Clinical Orthopaedics and Related Research* 467 (2009): 376–82.

Robert, C., Wass, V., Jones, R., Sarangi, S., and Gillett, A. "A Discourse Analysis Study of 'Good' and 'Poor' Communication in an OSCE: A Proposed New Framework for Teaching Students." *Medical Education* 37 (2003): 192-201.

Robinson, D. *The translator's turn.* Baltimore, Maryland: The Johns Hopkins University Press, 1991.

Rodulson, V., Marshall, R.J., and Bleakley, A.D. "Whistleblowing in Medicine and in Homer's *Iliad*". *Medical Humanities* 41 (2015): 95-101.

Rogers, C. *Client-Centered Therapy: Its Current Practice, Implications and Theory.* London: Constable, 1951.

Rosenberg, D. A., and Silver. H. K. "Medical Student Abuse." *Journal of the American Medical Association* 251 (1984): 739-42.

Rosenstein, A.H., and O'Daniel, M. "Disruptive Behavior and Clinical Outcomes: Perceptions of Nurses and Physicians." *American Journal of Nursing* 105 (2005): 54-64.

Rosenthal, J.H. 2012. "Ethics and War in Homer's *Iliad*." 27 March 2012. Accessed January 15, 2016. http://www.carnegiecouncil.org/publications/articles_papers_reports/0 125.html.

Roter, D., and Hall, J. *Doctors Talking with Patients/Patients Talking with Doctors: Improving Communication in Medical Visits*. London: Praeger, 2006.

Sahakian, B.J. *Sex, Lies, and Brain Scans: How fMRI Reveals What Really Goes On In Our Brains*. Oxford: Oxford University Press, 2017.

Salinger, J.D. *Catcher in the Rye*. London, Penguin Books, 1994.

Sanders, L. *Diagnosis: Dispatches from the Frontlines of Medical Mysteries*. London: Icon Books, 2010.

Sanghavi, D. 2011. 'The phantom menace of sleep-deprived doctors', *New York Times Magazine*, 5 August. Accessed June 3, 2015. http://www.nytimes.com/2011/08/07/magazine/the-phantom-menace-of-sleep-deprived-doctors.html?_r=0,

Sartre, J-P. *Being and Nothingness: An Essay on Phenomenological Ontology*. London: Routledge, 2003.

Schein, S.L. *The Mortal Hero: An Introduction to Homer's Iliad*. Berkeley: University of California Press, 1984.

—. Introduction to *Reading the Odyssey*, edited by Schein, S.L. Princeton: Princeton University Press, 1996.

Scheinbaum, C. 2012. Scalpel-Throwing Surgeons Stun Anger Management Pioneer. Accessed April 9, 2013. http://www.bloomberg.com/news/2012-08-02/scalpel-throwing-surgeons-stun-anger-management-pioneer-health.html

Schmidt, M, ed. *The Harvill Book of Twentieth-Century Poetry in English*. London: The Harvill Press, 1999.

Schön, D. *Educating the Reflective Practitioner: Toward a New design for Teaching and Learning in the Professions*. London: Wiley, 1990 2nd ed. Schwappach, D.L., and Boluarte, T.A. "The Emotional Impact of Medical Error Involvement on Physicians: A Call for Leadership." *Swiss Medical Weekly* 138 (2008): 9-15.

Scodel, R. *Epic Facework. Self-presentation and Social Interaction in Homer*. Swansea: The Classical Press of Wales, 2008.

Scott, K. M., Caldwell, P. H. Y., Barnes, E. H., and Barrett, J. "'Teaching by Humiliation' and Mistreatment of Medical Students in Clinical

Rotations: A Pilot Study". *Medical Journal of Australia* 203 (2015): 185e1-6.

Seaford, R. *Reciprocity and Ritual: Homer and Tragedy in the Developing City-State.* Oxford: Oxford University Press, 1995.

Segal, J.Z. "Public Discourse and Public Policy: Some Ways That Metaphor Constrains Health (Care)." *Journal of Medical Humanities* 18 (1997): 217-31.

Selzer, R. *Letters to a Young Doctor.* San Diego: Harcourt Brace, 1996a.

—. *Mortal Lessons: Notes on the Art of Surgery.* San Diego: Harvest, 1996b.

Senga, M., Pringle, K., Ramsay, A., Brett-Major, D.M., Fowler, R.A., French, I., Vandi, M., Sellu, J., Pratt, C., Saidu, J., Shindo, N., and Bausch, D.G. "Factors Underlying Ebola Virus Infection Among Health Workers, Kenema, Sierra Leone, 2014-2015." *Clinical Infectious Diseases.* 2016. Accessed December 28, 2016. https://www.ncbi.nlm.nih.gov/pmc/articles/PMC4967603/

Sennett, R. *Together: The Rituals, Pleasures and Politics of Cooperation.* London: Penguin, 2013.

Seoane, L., Tompkins, L.M., De Conciliis, A., and Boysen, P.G. Virtues Education in Medical School: The Foundation for Professional Formation." *The Ochsner Journal* 16 (2016): 50-5.

Serpentine Gallery. Marina Abramović's durational performance '512 hours'. Accessed February 14 2014, 2016. http://www.serpentinegalleries.org/exhibitions-events/marina-abramovic-512-hours

Sexton, J.B., Thomas, E.J., and Helmreich, R.L "Error, Stress, and Teamwork in Medicine and Aviation: Cross Sectional Surveys." *British Medical Journal* 320 (2000): 745–9.

Shapiro, J. "Illness Narratives: Reliability, Authenticity and the Empathic Witness." *Medical Humanities* 37 (2011): 68-72.

Shay J. *Achilles in Vietnam: Combat Trauma and the Undoing of Character.* New York: Scribner, 1994.

—. *Odysseus in America. Combat Trauma and the Trials of Homecoming.* New York: Scribner, 2002.

Sheather, J., and Hawkins, V. "Medicine Under Fire." *British Medical Journal* 355 (2016): i6464.

Shen, W. "Is the Quest to Build a Kinder, Gentler Surgeon Misguided?" *Pacific Standard.* Jul 14 2014. Accessed February 14, 2017. https://psmag.com/is-the-quest-to-build-a-kinder-gentler-surgeon-misguided-3950dee829fa#.tebhsfolk

Shorter Edition of the Oxford English Dictionary. Oxford: OUP, 1971.

Shrira I. "The occupation with the highest suicide rate." *Psychology Today* blog. Accessed April 9 2013. www.psychologytoday.com/blog/the-narcissus-in-all-us/200908/the-occupation-the-highest-suicide-rate

Shulman, L. "Signature Pedagogies in the Professions." *Daedalus* 134 (2005): 52-9.

Shuttle, P., and Redgrove, P. *The Wise Wound*. London: Marion Boyars Publishers Ltd; Reprinted edition, 2005.

Silver, H.K., and Glicken, A.D. "Medical Student Abuse: Incidence, Severity, and Significance." *Journal of the American Medical Association* 263 (1990): 527-32.

Sinclair, S. *Making Doctors: An Institutional Apprenticeship*. Oxford: Berg 3PL, 1997.

'skeptical scalpel' weblog. August 19 2014. Accessed January 12, 2017. http://www.kevinmd.com/blog/2014/08/selecting-grittier-surgeons-harder-think.html

Skott, C. "Expressive Metaphors in Cancer Narratives. *Cancer Nursing* 25 (2002): 230-5.

Slobod, D., and Fuks, A. "Military Metaphors and Friendly Fire." *Canadian Medical Association Journal* 184 (2012): 144.

Sluiter, I., and Rosen,R. "General Introduction". In *Free Speech in Classical Antiquity,* edited by Sluite, I., Rosen, R.M. Leiden: Brill, 2004.

Smiles, S. 1859. *Self Help.* Accessed February 14, 2017. http://files.libertyfund.org/files/297/Smiles_0379.*pdf*

Smith, B.W., Dalen, J., Wiggins, K., Tooley, E., Christopher, P., and Bernard. J. "The Brief Resilience Scale: Assessing the Ability to Bounce Back." *International Journal of Behavioral Medicine* 15 (2008): 194–200.

Smith-Han, K., Martyn, H., Barrett, A., and Nicholson, H. "'That's Not What You Expect To Do as a Doctor, You Know, You Don't Expect Your Patients to Die.' Death as a Learning Experience for Undergraduate Medical Students." *BioMed Central Medical Education* 16 (2016):108.

Snell, B. *The Discovery of the Mind: The Greek Origins of European Thought*. Cambridge, Massachusetts: Harvard University Press, 1953.

Sontag, S. *Against Interpretation and Other Essays*. London: Penguin Classics, 2009.

—. *Illness as Metaphor and AIDS and its Metaphors*. Harmondsworth: Penguin Classics, 2009.

Sophocles. *Oedipus Tyrannus.* In Sophocles' Fabulae edited by Pearson, A.C. Oxford: Oxford University Press, 1971.

Southwick, S.M., and Charney, D.S. *Resilience. The Science of Mastering Life's Greatest Challenges.* Cambridge University Press, Cambridge, 2014.

Spiro, H.M., McCrea, M.G., Curnen, E.P., Peschel, E., and St James, D, eds. *Empathy and the Practice of Medicine: Beyond Pills and the Scalpel.* New Haven, CT: Yale University Press, 1993.

Spivak, G.C. *Outside in the Teaching Machine.* New York, NY: Routledge, 1993.

Sritharan, K., Thillai, M. *Royal Society of Medicine Career Handbook: ST3 Senior Doctor.* Boca Raton: FLA.: CRC Press, Taylor & Francis Group, 2012.

Stanford, W.B. *The Ulysses Theme.* Dallas, TX: Spring Publications, 1968/ 1992.

Stangierski, A., Warmuz-Stangierska, I., Ruchała, M., Zdanowska, J., Głowacka, M.D., Sowiński, J., and Ruchała, P. "Medical Errors – Not Only Patients' Problem" *Archives of Medical Science* 8 (2012): 569-74.

Starfield B. "Is US Health Really the Best in the World?" *Journal of the American Medical Association.* 284 (2000): 483-5.

Statman, D., ed. *Virtue Ethics: A Critical Reader.* Edinburgh: Edinburgh University Press, 1997.

Stern, D.T., ed. *Measuring Medical Professionalism.* Oxford: Oxford University Press, 2006.

Stockholm Resilience Centre. Accessed November 27, 2016. http://www.stockholmresilience.org/research/research-news/2015-02-19-what-is-resilience.html

Strawson, G. "Against Narrativity." *Ratio (new series)* 17 (2004): 428-52.

Stringsandfretboards. "Medicine and Culture and the Strange Way We Learn." May 26. 2015. Accessed January 15, 2016. https://stringsandfretboards.wordpress.com/2015/05/26/medicine-and-culture-and-the-strange-way-we-learn/

Sun Tzu. *The Art of War.* London: Hodder Paperbacks, 2004.

Sutcliffe, K.M. *Defining and Classifying Medical Error: Lessons for Learning. Quality and Safety in Health Care* 13 (2004): 8–9.

Swaminath, G., and Raguram, R. "Medical Errors II, The Aftermath: Mea Culpa!" *Indian Journal of Psychiatry* 53 (2011): 9–12.

Szczegielniak A, Skowronek A, Krysta K,and Krupka-Matuszczyk I. "Aggression in the Work Environment of Physiotherapists." *Psychiatria Danubiana* 24 Suppl 1 (2012): S147-52.

Taft, L. "Apology and Medical Mistake: Opportunity or Foil?" *Annals of Health Law* 14 (2005): 55–94.

Tatum, J. *The Mourner's Song: War and Remembrance from the Iliad to Vietnam.* Chicago: The University of Chicago Press, 2004.

Taylor, C. "Unreported Bullying Plaguing Junior Doctors." 27 May 2015. Accessed January 15, 2016. http://www.hcamag.com/hr-news/unreported-bullying-plaguing-junior-doctors-200952.aspx

Thomas, E.J., Studdert, D.M., Burstin, H.R., Orav, E.J., Zeena, T., Williams, E.J., Howard, K.M., Weiler, P.C., and Brennan, T.A. "Incidence and Types of Adverse Events and Negligent Care in Utah and Colorado." *Medical Care* 38 (2000): 261-71.

Thorson, J.A., and Powell, F.C. "Medical students' attitudes towards ageing and death: a cross-sequential study." *Medical Education* 25 (1991): 32-7.

Truog, R.D., Browning, D.M., Johnson, J.A., and Gallagher, T.H. *Talking with Patients and Families about Medical Error.* Baltimore, MD: The Johns Hopkins University Press, 2011.

Tusaie, K., Dyer, J. "Resilience: A Historical Review of the Construct." *Holistic Nursing Practice* 18 (2004): 3-10.

University of Dundee press release 1 July 2013. "Patient Care Suffering Because of Senior Practitioners' Professionalism Lapses." Accessed January 7, 2015. www.http://app.dundee.ac.uk/pressreleases/2013/july13/patientcare.htm

van Raalte, M. "Socratic Parrhesia and Its Afterlife in Plato's Laws." In *Free Speech in Classical Antiquity*, edited by Sluite, I., Rosen, R.M., 279-312. Leiden: Brill, 2004.

Veloski, J., and Hojat, M. "Measuring Specific Elements of Professionalism: Empathy, Teamwork, and Lifelong Learning." In *Measuring Medical Professionalism*, edited by D.T. Stern, 117-46. Oxford: Oxford University Press, 2006.

Venuti, L. "Translation as Cultural Politics: Regimes of Domestication in English." *Textual Practice* 7 (1993): 208-23.

—. *The translator's invisibility. A history of translation.* London: Routledge, 2002.

Verghese, A. *The Tennis Partner.* New York: HarperCollins, 1999.

—. "Culture Shock – Patient as Icon, Icon as Patient." *New England Journal of Medicine* 359 (2008): 26.

Vincent, C.A. "Risk, Safety, and the Dark Side of Quality." *British Medical Journal* 314 (1997): 1775-6.

Vincent, C. "Adverse Events in British Hospitals: Preliminary Retrospective Record Review." *British Medical Journal* 322 (2001): 1395.

Walsh, T.R. *Fighting Words and Feuding Words: Anger and the Homeric Poems*. Lanham, MD: Lexington Books, 2005.

Waterman, A.D., Garbutt, J., Hazel, E., Dunagan, W.C., Levinson, W., Fraser, V.J., and Gallagher, T.H. "The Emotional Impact of Medical Errors on Practicing Physicians in the United States and Canada." *Joint Commission Journal on Quality and Patient Safety* 33 (2007): 467–76.

Watling, C., Driessen, E., van der Vleuten, C. P. M., Vanstone, M. and Lingard, L. "Understanding Responses to Feedback: The Potential and Limitations of Regulatory Focus Theory." *Medical Education* 46 (2012): 593–603.

Wear, W., and Aultman, J.M. "The Limits of Narrative: Medical Student Resistance to Confronting Inequality and Oppression in Literature and Beyond." *Medical Education* 39 (2005):1056–65.

Wears, R.L., and Wu, A.W. "Dealing with Failure: The Aftermath of Errors and Adverse Events." *Annals of Emergency Medicine* 39 (2002): 344–6.

Weissbort, D., and Eysteinsson, A. *Translation – theory and practice. A historical reader*. Oxford: Oxford University Press, 2006.

Wellbery, C. "The Value of Medical Uncertainty?" *The Lancet* 375 (2010): 1686-7.

Wender, D. *The Last Scenes of the Odyssey*. Leiden, NL: EJ Brill, 1978.

Wendland, C.L. *A Heart for the Work: Journeys through an African Medical School*. Chicago, ILL.: University of Chicago Press, 2010.

West, C.P., Huschka, M.M., Novotny, P.J., Sloan, J.A., Kolars, J.C., Habermann, T.M., and Shanafelt, T.D. "Association of Perceived Medical Errors with Resident Distress and Empathy. A Prospective Longitudinal Study." *Journal of the American Medical Association* 296 (2006): 1071-8.

West, M.L., trans. *Hesiod's Theogony and Works and Days*. Oxford: Oxford University Press, 2008.

Westman, M., and Eden, D. Effects of a Respite from Work on Burnout: Vacation Relief and Fade-out. *Journal of Applied Psychology* 82 (1997): 516–27.

Westman, M., and Etzion, D. The Impact of Vacation and Job Stress on Burnout and Absenteeism. *Psychology and Health* 16 (2001): 595 – 606.

Wheatstone, R. "Hero striking junior doctor leaves picket line after man
    collapses in the street near protest." 12 January 2016. Accessed
    December 27, 2016.
    http://www.mirror.co.uk/news/uk-news/hero-striking-junior-doctor-
    leaves-7166661
Wheeler, H.B. "Healing and Heroism." *New England Journal of Medicine*
    322 (1990): 1540-8.
Whistleblowing Helpline. 2013. *Public Interest Disclosure Act.* Accessed
    February 14, 2017.
    www.http://wbhelpline.org.uk/resources/public-interest-disclosure-act/
White, C. "Was There Ever a Golden Age for Junior Doctors?" *British
    Medical Journal* 354 (2016): i3662
Whitehouse H. In their own words: students share their views on smart
    drugs. *The Guardian* Tues 1 Mar 2016. Accessed 25 May 2017.
    https://www.theguardian.com/education/2016/mar/01/in-their-own-
    words-students-share-their-views-on-smart-drugs
Whiting R. 2016. BMA News, 26 May.
Willis, S.C., Jones, A., and O'Neill, P.A. "Can Undergraduate Education
    Have an Effect on the Ways in which Pre-Registration House Officers
    Conceptualise Communication?" *Medical Education* 37 (2003): 603-8.
Wilmer, H.A. "The Doctor-Patient Relationship and Issues of Pity,
    Sympathy and Empathy." *British Journal of Medical Psychology* 41
    (1968): 243-8.
Windle, G., Bennett, K.M., and Noyes, J. "A Methodological Review of
    Resilience Measurement Scales." *Health and Quality of Life Outcome*s, 9
    (2011): 8.
Wiseman, R. *Night School: The Life-Changing Science of Sleep.*
    Basingstoke: Macmillan, 2014.
Wiskar, K. "Physician Health: A Review of Lifestyle Behaviors and
    Preventive Health." *British Columbia Medical Journal* 54 (2012): 419-
    23.
Wispé, L. *The psychology of sympathy.* Dordrecht, Netherlands: Kluwer/
    Plenum, 1991.
Wolf-Hartmut, F. *Wounding and Death in the Iliad: Homeric Techniques
    of Description.* Translated by Peter Jones and Gabriele Wright.
    London: Gerald Duckworth and Co. Ltd., 2003.
Wu, A.W. "Medical Error: The Second Victim. The Doctor Who Makes
    the Mistake Needs Help Too." *British Medical Journal* 320 (2000):
    726–7.

Wu, A.W., Folkman, S., McPhee, S.J., and Lo, B. "Do House Officers Learn from their Mistakes?" *Quality and Safety in Health Care* 12 (2003): 221–8.

Wu, A.W., Huang, I-C., Stokes, S., Pronovost, P.J. "Disclosing Medical Errors to Patients: It's Not What You Say, It's What They Hear." *Journal of General Internal Medicine* 24 (2009): 1012–7.

Xyrichis, A., Ream, E. "Teamwork: A Concept Analysis." *Journal of Advanced Nursing* 61 (2008): 232-41.

Yates, F.A. *The art of memory.* London: Pimlico, 2001.

Youngson, R., and Blennerhassett, M. "Humanising Healthcare." *British Medical Journal* 355 (2016): i6262.

Zautra, A.J., Hall, J.S., and Murray, K. "Community Development and Community Resilience: An Integrative Approach." *Community Development* 39 (2008):130–47.

Zetteler, J. "Hero Today, Gone Tomorrow?" *British Journal of General Practice* 55 (2005): 644-5

Zhang, J., Patel, V.L., Johnson, T.R., and Shortliffe, E.H. "Toward a Cognitive Taxonomy of Medical Errors." *Proceedings of the AMIA Symposium. American Medical Informatics Association* (2002): 934-8.

Zolli, A., and Healy, A.M. *Resilience.* Headline Publishing Group, London, 2013.

INDEX

A

Abramović, Marina, 217
abuse, 193–210
  in medicine, 146
  statistics in medicine, 195–98
Achaeans, 245
Achilles, 16, 70, 184, 254, 258, 261
  and courage, 19
  and death, 32
  and death of Hector, 212
  and early death, 19, 32
  and embassy, 49, 152
  and heroism, 15–47
  and home, 164
  and Patroclus, 30, 36, 44, 153
  and Priam, 117, 171
  and rage, 19, 39, 151
  foretelling of death, 19,57
  in the underworld, 19, 33, 35
  running berserk, 144
  speaking bluntly, 188
Achilles' tendon, 252
Achilles' heel, 238
acronyms, 69
Aegisthus, 236, 257
Aeneas, 42, 45, 251
Aeolia, 260
Agamemnon, 38, 40, 47, 70, 118,
  151, 166, 184, 191, 205, 245–54,
  257, 261
  and abuse, 200
  and apology, 172
  and error, 157
  and folly, 158, 167, 169, 172
  and the embassy scene, 52
aidos. See shame
Ajax, 16, 45, 52, 200, 249
Alcinous, 258, 259

Aleppo, 25
Alice Oswald, Alice, 16, 18, 25, 130
All Day Permanent Red, 17
ambiguity, 9, 14, 22, 45, 49, 54, 68,
  91, 93, 106, 109, 111, 112, 119,
  170, 187, 221
anatomy, 7, 12, 18, 28, 31
Andromache, 17, 239, 249, 253
  and Hector, 107
anger. See rage
Anticleia, 261
anti-heroes, 22, 31, 36, 45
Antilochus, 45
Antinous, 256, 263
Aphrodite, 23, 33, 249
Apollo, 31, 32, 221, 246
apology, 171
archetype, 18, 22, 28, 29, 45, 58,
  186, 257
Ares, 33, 213
Argives, 243
Aristotle, 188, 255
Armstrong, Lance, 21, 26
Asclepius, 30, 219, 222
Atē. See Folly
Athene, 40, 70, 151, 212, 245-254,
  254–66

B

Barnard, Christiaan, 17
Batmanghelidjh, Camila, 26
berserk behaviour, 32, 144, 151, 251
Biles, Simone, 21
black humour, 33, 125, 242
book 9
  and embassy scene, 49
Brecht, Bertolt, 46
Briseis, 52, 151, 247

Bristol heart scandal, 179, 181
British Medical Association, 179
British Medical Journal, 43
bullying, 3, 39, 40, 142-147, 174,
    185, 197, 206, 207
burnout, 216
Bush, George, 3

C

Calchas, 184-190, 247
Calypso, 23, 236, 255-257
Catcher in the Rye, 28
celebrity, 26
Chapman, George, 70
Charybdis, 262
Chesterton, GK, 12
Chryseis, 184, 246
Chryses, 184, 191, 246
Cicero, 60
Cicones, 259
Circe, 211, 260, 261
Clooney, George, 24
Clytemnestra, 257
collaboration, 22, 45, 100, 142, 162,
    180, 198, 203, 208, 241, 243
communication, 11, 48–62
    and Sophists, 59
    art of, 13
    as a skill, 48, 54, 104
    as instrumental skill, 50
    mechanistic, 48
compassion, 25, 104–21, 132, 153
consultants, 3, 55, 136, 196, 200,
    205, 210, 267
Crohn's disease, 122
Cyclopes, 259
cynicism, 33, 144, 146, 147, 194,
    199

D

Danaans, 245
Dante, 261
Deiphobus, 212, 252

democracy
    different types of, 190
Democritus, 116
Demodocus, 258
Demosthenes, 60
Derrida, Jacques, 76, 100
desecration, 17
Deucalion, 39, 144
Diomedes, 32, 42, 200, 205, 245–54
doctors
    and abuse, 193–210
    and alcohol abuse, 147
    and bravery, 34
    and burnout, 225
    and glory, 35
    and identity, 84
    and reputation, 174
    and shame, 174
    and suicide, 35, 147
    and vocation, 20
    as "dangerous", 47
    at war, 33
    needing resilience, 224–44
Dr Finlay, 38
Dr Kildare, 24, 37
drugs
    for wakefulness, 220
durational misperformance, 220

E

Ebola epidemic, 25, 34
einfühlung, 112
electronic patient record, 102
Elpenor, 261
emotion
    in the ancient world, 60
empathy, 104–21, 132
    and cynicism, 33
    and metaphor, 110
    and suffering, 33
empathy decline, 144
Epicaste, 42
Epictetus, 116
eroticism, 21, 23, 126, 158, 236

error, 155–76
    and error prone systems, 170
    and gender differences, 174
    and medical education, 160
    reactions to, 175
ethics, 6, 13, 33, 37, 60, 64, 77, 84,
    94, 157, 179-181, 244
    of translation, 76
    virtue ethics, 179
etymology of:
    compassion, 112
    confrontation, 153
    empathy, 112
    error, 159
    Odysseus, 147
    pity, 112
    resilience, 228
Eumaeus, 263
Euripides
    Bacchae, 189
European Working Time Directive,
    219
Eurycleia, 264, 265
Eurylochus, 262
exhaustion, 212–23

F

faithfulness, 16, 21, 72-74, 81
Fate, 251
feedback, 208
feminine care, 5
feminine values, 227
Flexner, Abraham,5, 29, 37, 270
folly, 53, 156, 158, 167
formula, 86, 89
Foucault, Michel, 77, 116, 149, 182,
    190-192, 208, 276, 285
Freud, Sigmund, 35, 112, 126, 129,
    144, 147, 276

G

Gates, Bill and Melinda, 26
General Medical Council, 105, 113,
    179

and whistleblowing, 186
general practitioners, 3
Glaucus, 32
gods, 158
Greeks, 245–54
grit, 201, 224-44
guilt culture, 173, 175, 202-207

H

Hades, 261, 265
Hawking, Stephen, 24, 26
Hector, 16, 153, 166, 245–54
    and Andromache, 235
    death of, 212
    dragged behind Achilles' chariot,
        3
    faces Achilles, 234
    recovery of his body, 171
Hecuba, 249, 253
Hegel, 28, 46
Helen, 10, 21, 23, 119, 245–54, 257
Hephaestus, 250
Hera, 169, 248, 250
Hermes, 253, 260
heroes, 47
    and anti-heroes, 189
    and charisma, 39
    and cults, 36
    and desecration of body, 17
    and error, 165
    and excess, 39
    and femininity, 29
    and individualism, 30
    and masculinity, 29
    and mortality, 30
    and teamwork, 30
    and their flaws, 23, 37
    are transgressive, 38
    as archetypes, 28
    as stereotypes, 37
heroines, 21
Hesiod, 12, 42, 152
hierarchy, 5, 11, 99, 140, 141, 167,
    171, 185, 186, 190, 197, 200-
    205, 212, 223, 243, 254

Hippocratic Oath, 180
Homer
    and abuse, 200
    and communication, 50, 85
    and error, 157
    and formula, 94
    and heroes, 42, 15–47
    and hospitality, 208
    and literacy, 102
    and orality, 84
    and rhetoric, 49
    and thinking otherwise, 12
    and whistleblowing, 183
    as a woman, 30
    present at Troy, 234
    hexameter metre, 71
    why read Homer, 10
    why read Homer?, 3
House MD, 38
humanism, 116
humiliation, 99, 205
Hypsenor, 45

I

iambics, 71
iatrogenic illness, 5, 131, 140
identity formation, 13 84, 99, 181,
    222
Idomeneus, 200
Iliad, 16
    and Alice Oswald's Memorial,
        25
    and masculinity, 30
    as text of war, 10
    performance, 85
    whistleblowing in, 184
Iliad and Odyssey
    composition, 85
    first written, 102
    two styles of hero, 44
Illich, Ivan 50
immortality, 16, 19, 35, 36, 97, 251
interprofessional teams, 5
Ithaca, 260, 263

J

Japanese society, 150, 202
jazz, 86, 87
Jex-Blake, Sophia, 29
junior doctors
    and hospitality, 152
    and performance, 99
    and politics, 5, 11
    strike, 11

K

Kalanithi, Paul, 23
Keats, 70
kleos, 11, 251
    and death, 32
    glory, 19

L

Laertes, 256, 265
Laocoon, 183
LGBT, 29
Logue, Christopher, 16, 71-80, 137,
    246, 265
London School of Medicine for
    Women, 29
Longinus, 254
Lord, Albert, 84
loss of face, 56, 173
Lotus Eaters, 259

M

Machaon, 250
Thatcher, Margaret, 213
Marsh, Henry, 23
martial metaphors, 8, 20
medical education, 3
    and critical reflexivity, 43
    and reflective practice, 43
medical error, 8, 78, 125-130, 148-
    163, 167, 172, 219, 227
medical humanities, 5

medical students, 185
    and abuse, 185, 195, 196, 198,
        206, 194–211
    and death, 31, 237
    and empathy decline, 128
    and performance, 86
    becoming de-sensitised, 119, 194
    learning resilience, 224–44
Medical students
    as high achievers, 19
medicine
    and anger, 136–54
    and democracy, 5, 76
    and error, 155–76
    and hierarchy, 5, 9
    and inequality, 186
    and lyricism, 122–34
    and oral tradition, 83–103
    and sexual identity, 29
    and the senses, 127
    and understaffing, 224
    and women, 11
    as art, 92
    as epic, 8, 125, 136
    as tragedy, 8, 125
    as vocation, 45
    as war, 10, 137–44, 208
    collaboration in, 5
    error statistics, 159
    shaped by metaphor, 208
    whistleblowing in, 178–92
Meleager, 53
Memorial, 16, 25
Menelaus, 245–54, 257
menis/menin. See rage
Mentor, 257
metaphor, 124, 137–44, 208
    and error, 156
    body as machine, 208
    medicine as war, 208
    of heroism, 21
mindfulness, 226
minimalism, 74, 84, 89, 90
misdiagnosis, 64
Mnemosyne, 96
moral relativism, 43

mortality, 15-18, 23, 30-35
Muse, 19, 87, 245, 256
Myrmidons, 39, 250

N

narrative
    humility, 64
National Health Service, 55, 128,
    163, 172, 199, 217, 226
Nausicaa, 258
Nestor, 42, 247, 249, 256
Nietzsche, 22, 43, 202, 208, 243,
    288
nostos, 11, 254
Nott, David, 34
nurses, 148
nursing care, 148

O

Odysseus, 6, 16, 238, 245–54, 254–
    66
    and Calypso, 236
    and Circe, 211
    and cunning, 19, 55
    and eloquence, 55
    and embassy scene, 52
    and error, 157, 162
    and exhaustion, 211–23
    and heroism, 15–47
    and his death, 33
    and homecoming, 19
    and rage, 41
    and resilience, 234
    and Thersites, 188, 201
    as trickster, 19
    as wanderer, 10
    concealing his identity, 238
    in Sophocles' Philoctetes, 59
    in the underworld, 33, 237
    meets his mother in Hades, 237
    much enduring, 236
    polymetis, 6
    slaying of the suitors, 41, 199,
        240

Odyssey
    and collaboration, 46
    and homecoming, 12
oral narrative, 85
OSCE (Objective Structured
    Clinical Examination), 109
Osler, William, 19, 35, 64, 232

P

Pandarus, 45
Paris, 10, 245–54
parrhesia, 179, 182-192
Parry, Milman, 84
paternalism, 11, 21, 22, 109, 180,
    272
pathology, 167
patient-centredness, 11, 46, 84, 98,
    115, 123, 147, 180, 181
patients
    and anger, 55
    and their history, 63, 101
Patroclus, 17, 166, 245–55
Peleus, 18, 117, 253
Pendleton's rules, 208
Penelope, 16, 21,199, 214, 239,
    254–66
perfectionism, 19, 34, 35
Pericles, 182
Phaeacians, 258, 262
Phoenix, 52, 249
phrenes, 215
pimping, 194
pity, 121, 153
Plato, 188
    Meno, 113
    Ion, 36
    Republic, 212
Pliny the Elder, 228
poetry, 194
Polyphemus, 237, 257, 259
Poseidon, 32, 183, 237, 254–66
post truth, 180, 192
postgraduates, 3, 49, 109, 236
Priam, 117, 153, 216, 245–55

professionalism, 6, 11, 13, 31, 38,
    44, 104-106, 113-116, 121, 128,
    146, 165, 178, 181, 191, 197,
    235
protocols, 38, 95, 136, 141, 157,
    160-162, 170, 176, 222
psychiatrists, 69
psychiatry
    bullying in, 185
psychologists, 69
    and resilience, 226

Q

quarrel, 205

R

radiology, 93
rage, 39, 40, 51, 246
rape, 61
reflection, 151
reflexivity, 6, 151
resilience, 224–44
    and the military, 233, 241 243
    definitions, 234ff
    education for, 236
    metaphors of, 229
    relation to grit, 224–44
return of the repressed, 8, 129, 144,
    147
rhapsodes, 85, 88
rhetoric
    and athletics, 114

S

Salinger, JD., 28
savagery
    in modern times, 120
    in the Iliad, 120
Savile, Jimmy, 25
saving face, 56
Scylla, 262
Shakespeare, 71
shamans, 16

shame, 158, 204
    differs from embarrassment, 205
shame culture, 173, 175, 202, 204,
    207, 210
Shay, Jonathan, 3, 238
simulation, 50, 109
Sirens, 262
Socrates, 192, 212
Sontag, Susan, 94
Sophocles
    Oedipus Rex, 189
stereotype, 24
stereotypes, 37, 201, 230
Sthenelus, 204
substance abuse, 21
suitors
    of Penelope, 19, 41, 169, 199,
        215, 237, 238, 239, 240, 255,
        256, 257, 258, 261, 263, 264,
        265, 266
Sun Tzu, 153
surgeons
    and rage, 41
    and the lyrical, 123
    orthopaedic surgeons and sex, 34
surgical safety checklist, 160, 162
Sydenham, Thomas 154
sympathy, 110

T

teamwork, 61
Teiresias, 237
Telemachus, 41, 199, 254–66
telomerase, 18
telomere, 18
Teucer, 45
the Aeneid, 183
The Art of War, 153
the wooden horse, 245
Thersites, 188, 189, 201, 248, 290
Thetis, 18, 245–54
thinking otherwise, 6, 11
three wise men system, 38, 55
thumos, 211, 214, 215, 235
timē

    as public honour, 203
Tiresias, 33, 261
tolerance of ambiguity, 6, 22
translation, 63–82, 101
    and contingency, 79
    and democracy, 79
    and faithfulness, 72
    and identity, 76
    and metaphor, 66
    and patient's history, 65
    and power, 78
    and practicality, 81
    of foreign languages, 65
Trojan War, 19, 23, 25, 30, 59, 164,
    199, 206, 234, 245, 246, 254,
    258
Trojans, 10, 17, 30, 36, 39, 40, 42,
    52, 57, 104, 144-158, 166, 169,
    183, 213, 245-252
Troy, 108
    sack of, 259
    the film, 120
Trump, Donald, 4, 213
Tydeus, 42

U

UK NHS
    and working hours, 43
undergraduates, 3, 195, 226
underworld, 19, 20, 33, 35, 218,
    221, 261

V

Vietnam War, 3, 150, 238
Virgil, 183, 261

W

wandering, 10, 159, 164, 165
whistleblowing, 178–92
WikiLeaks, 181
Williams, William Carlos, 91
women
    and loss of power, 47

and resilience, 239
and the heroic, 29
in medicine, 5, 11, 29, 37, 99,
        135, 174, 195, 214, 215, 239
World Trade Centre, 46, 241

X

xenia (hospitality), 119, 257, 262

Y

Yousafzai, Malala, 24

Z

Zeus, 40, 199, 245–54
    and folly, 169